Postgraduate Orthopaedics: Viva Guide for the FRCS (Tr & Orth) Examination

Postgraduate Orthopaedics: Viva Guide for the FRCS (Tr & Orth) Examination

Edited by

Paul A. Banaszkiewicz FRCS (Glas) FRCS (Ed) FRCS (Eng) FRCS (Tr & Orth) MClinEd FAcadMed

Consultant Orthopaedic Surgeon
Queen Elizabeth Hospital and North East NHS Surgical Centre (NENSC)
Gateshead, UK

Associate Editor

Deiary F. Kader MBChB FRCS (Ed) FRCS (Glas) FRCS (Tr & Orth) MFSEM (UK)

Visiting Professor in Sport and Exercise Sciences
Northumbria University, Newcastle upon Tyne
Consultant Orthopaedic Surgeon
Queen Elizabeth Hospital and North East NHS Surgical Centre (NENSC)
Gateshead, UK

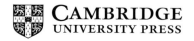
CAMBRIDGE
UNIVERSITY PRESS

CAMBRIDGE UNIVERSITY PRESS
Cambridge, New York, Melbourne, Madrid, Cape Town,
Singapore, São Paulo, Delhi, Mexico City

Cambridge University Press
The Edinburgh Building, Cambridge CB2 8RU, UK

Published in the United States of America
by Cambridge University Press, New York

www.cambridge.org
Information on this title: www.cambridge.org/9781107627369

© Cambridge University Press 2012

First published 2012

Printed and Bound in the United Kingdom by the MPG Books group

*A catalogue record for this publication is available from the British
Library*

ISBN 978-1-107-62736-9 Paperback

Contents

List of contributors   vi
Foreword   viii
Preface   ix

Section 1 – The FRCS (Tr & Orth) Oral Examination

1   General guidance for the FRCS (Tr & Orth)   1
Tom Symes and Paul A. Banaszkiewicz

Section 2 – Adult Elective Orthopaedics and Spine

2   Hip structured oral questions   13
Paul A. Banaszkiewicz and Rahul Kakkar

3   Knee structured oral questions   43
Michael Maru and Deiary F. Kader

4   Foot and ankle structured oral questions   55
N. Jane Madeley and Neil Forrest

5   Spine structured oral questions   69
Alexander D. L. Baker

6   Shoulder and elbow structured oral questions   86
Asir Aster

7   Orthopaedic oncology   100
Thomas B. Beckingsale

Section 3 – Trauma

8   Lower limb trauma   111
Mohammed Al-Maiyah and Ali S. Bajwa

9   Upper limb trauma   126
Gunasekaran Kumar

10   Pelvic and spinal trauma   135
Gunasekaran Kumar and Sherief Elsayed

Section 4 – Hand and Upper Limb/ Children's Orthopaedics

11   Hand and upper limb   149
John Harrison and Santosh Venkatachalam

12   Children's orthopaedics   159
Sattar Alshryda and Akinwande Adedapo

Section 5 – Applied Basic Science

13   Anatomy and surgical approaches   201
Tom Symes

14   Pathology   208
Sunit Patil

15   Biomaterials and biomechanics   223
Iain McNamara and Andrew P. Sprowson

16   Tissues of the musculoskeletal system   231
Andrew P. Sprowson and Iain McNamara

17   Evidence-based practice   241
Sattar Alshryda and James Mason

18   Imaging and investigative techniques   257
Rajesh Kakwani and Mike Newby

Section 6 – Diagrams for the FRCS (Tr & Orth)

19   Diagrams for the FRCS (Tr & Orth)   267
Asir Aster and Muthu Jeyam

Illustrations for Viva   277
Asir Aster and Muthu Jeyam

Index   281
The colour plate section is found between pages 150 and 151.

Contributors

Mr Akinwande Adedapo MBBS FRCS (Eng) FRCS (Glas)
James Cook University Hospital, Middlesborough, UK

Mr Mohammed Al-Maiyah MBChB FICMS FRCS Msc Orthop FRCS (Tr & Orth)
James Cook University Hospital, Middlesborough, UK

Mr Sattar Alshryda MRCS FRCS (Tr & Orth) MSc PhD
Freeman Hospital, Newcastle upon Tyne, UK

Mr Asir Aster MBBS FRCS (Surg) MSc (Ortho Eng) FRCS (Tr & Orth)
Hope Hospital, Salford Royal NHS Foundation Trust, UK

Mr Ali S. Bajwa MBBS MRCS (Ed) MSc Orth MPhil (Cantab) DSEM (UK) MFSEM UK FRCS (Tr & Orth)
James Cook University Hospital, Middlesbrough & Friarage Hospital Northallerton, UK

Mr Alexander D. L. Baker FRCS BSc MBChB MRCS MSc FRCS (Tr & Orth)
Lancashire Teaching Hospitals NHS Trust, Royal Preston Hospital, UK

Mr Paul A. Banaszkiewicz FRCS (Glas) FRCS (Ed) FRCS (Eng) FRCS (Tr & Orth) MClinEd FAcadMed
Queen Elizabeth Hospital, Gateshead, UK

Mr Thomas B. Beckingsale FRCS (Tr & Orth)
Freeman Hospital, Newcastle Upon Tyne, UK

Mr Sherief Elsayed MB BCh MRCS (Eng) FRCS (Tr & Orth)
Centre for Spinal Studies & Surgery, Queens Medical Centre, Nottingham, UK

Mr Neil Forrest MRCS FRCS (Tr & Orth)
Woodend Hospital, Aberdeen, UK

Mr John Harrison MSc FRCS (Ed) FRCS (Tr & Orth) MFSEM (UK)
Queen Elizabeth Hospital, Gateshead, UK

Mr Muthu Jeyam MBBS FRCS M.Phil FRCS (Tr & Orth)
Hope Hospital, Salford, UK

Mr Deiary F. Kader MBChB FRCS (Ed) FRCSGlas FRCS (Tr & Orth) MFSEM (UK)
Queen Elizabeth Hospital, Gateshead, UK

Mr Rahul Kakkar MBBS MRCS MS (Orth) FRCS (Tr & Orth)
Queen Elizabeth Hospital, Gateshead, UK

Mr Rajesh Kakwani MS (Orth) MRCS MCh (Orth) Dip SEM FRCS (Orth)
Queen Elizabeth Hospital, Gateshead, UK

Mr Gunasekaran Kumar FRCS (Tr & Orth)
Royal Liverpool University Hospital, Liverpool, UK

Mr Iain McNamara MA (Cantab) BM BCh (Oxon) MRCP FRCS (Tr & Orth) MD
Orthopaedic Research Unit, University of Cambridge, Cambridge, UK

Miss N. Jane Madeley FRCS (Tr & Orth)
Glasgow Royal Infirmary, Glasgow, UK

Mr Michael Maru MBChB MRCS MSc FRCS (Tr & Orth)
Golden Jubilee National Hospital, Glasgow, UK

Professor James Mason DPhil MSc BSc (Hons)
Director of Research, School of Medicine and Health Durham University, UK

Mr Mike Newby FRCR
Queen Elizabeth Hospital, Gateshead, UK

Mr Sunit Patil MSc FRCS (Tr & Orth)
Specialist Registrar, Northern Deanery, Newcastle
Upon Tyne, UK

Mr Andrew P. Sprowson MD FRCS (Tr & Orth)
Clinical Sciences Research Institute, Coventry, UK

Mr Tom Symes MBChB MSc FRCS (Tr & Orth)
Hull and East Yorkshire Hospitals NHS Trust, UK

**Mr Santosh Venkatachalam MBBS MS (Orth)
DNB (Orth) MRCS (Ed) FRCS (Tr & Orth)**
Queen Elizabeth Hospital, Gateshead, UK

Foreword

Exam success depends as much upon technique as it does upon knowledge. In this respect *Postgraduate Orthopaedics: Viva Guide for the FRCS (Tr & Orth) Examination* is a logical and, no doubt will become, a most welcome addition to the highly successful text, *Postgraduate Orthopaedics*. Its strength relies on the first-hand experience of surgeons who have recently sat and successfully passed the FRCS (Tr & Orth) examination. Each chapter has a totally different feel, in part due to the topics covered, but more importantly to the style with which each of the viva scenarios has been written. This eclectic approach keeps the text refreshing and also reflects the personal experiences of candidates undergoing the stress of this examination; sentiments that a heavily edited text would have lost.

I also like the first chapter that attempts to remove much of the mystique from the viva process and helps candidates to benchmark just what is expected of them to pass this examination.

I only wish that texts like this had been available in my day since so many of us struggled to come to terms with what the exam was all about and made the mistake of thinking that pure knowledge of orthopaedics was the key to success: if only!

Professor Alan J. Johnstone
Orthopaedic Trauma Unit
Aberdeen Royal Infirmary
Aberdeen, UK

Preface

This book has been written specifically to guide candidates better through the FRCS (Trauma and Orthopaedic) viva exam or structured oral examination, as the Intercollegiate Specialty Board (ISB) prefers to call it.

The oral exam is regarded by many as a poor relative of the clinicals; the intermediate and short cases being the most difficult part of the exam to pass and the section most candidates tend to fail.

Despite this the oral part of the exam should not be underestimated. The often-heard mutterings that the orals are fairly straightforward to pass can lull candidates into a false sense of security.

Candidates with good core knowledge may still end up failing one or more oral sections if technique is poor.

The book takes the form of the major four oral sections of the examination, namely adult elective orthopaedics, trauma, hand and upper limb/children's orthopaedics and applied basic science. There is an introduction section on general guidance and a chapter dealing with common diagrams that you may be asked to draw out in the examinations.

We have tried to pitch the oral dialogue at the standard of a good to outstanding pass believing that more is better than less. By way of comparison we occasionally include a poor substandard answer from a candidate. More often you learn more from the viva answers that go wrong than from questions that don't challenge you.

Each chapter has a slightly different style reflecting differing authors' focus and opinions regarding the keys for success in the examination. We think this makes the book more interesting and believe this approach is more challenging as it forces you to think a bit more for yourself and will help you to define and refine your viva tactics.

For better or worse we have continued to use examiner/candidates discussion in the oral sections. Even more so with the viva, it is the back-and–forth dialogue between examiner and candidate that candidates need to focus on.

Finally we wish you well in the examination and hope that this book will provide you with invaluable tactics and tips for success in the oral section of the FRCS (Tr & Orth) exam.

General guidance for the FRCS (Tr & Orth)

Tom Symes and Paul A. Banaszkiewicz

The FRCS (Tr & Orth) exam sets out to provide an assessment of the knowledge and skills and the ability to use these to the required standards of a consultant orthopaedic surgeon working in the National Health Service in the UK. It is a significant career hurdle to pass and involves an intensive 6–12-month period of study during which time everyday life and activities increasingly assume secondary importance to passing 'the exam'.

The viva exam or 'structured oral examination' as the Intercollegiate Specialty Board (ISB) prefers to call it is an important component of this exam. Whilst most candidates are more fearful of the clinical component, the oral section is never as clear-cut or straightforward as some examiners (or consultant non-examiners) would have us believe.

This general introduction provides an overview of how to improve your score and pass the oral exam with flying colours.

Careful tactical planning is required beforehand as on the days of the exam it is usually too late to alter your game plan and poorly thought-out tactics may lead to your downfall.

We have avoided the temptation of solely focusing on what successful candidates believe are the important tips and tricks that will get you through the oral exams. We have additionally looked at the exam process itself and what it sets out to test. The logic is that if you understand how and why the exam acts as an assessment tool you will increase your chances of success.

At most revision exam courses current or past examiners and recently successful candidates give a 5–10-minute talk on the key features needed to pass the exam. Most advice is fairly reasonable but opinions and views may occasionally be counterproductive and best ignored.

Remember that advice is always a personal issue for each individual candidate and what works best for you may not necessarily work well for the candidate sitting next to you.

Be a bit sceptical and question in your own mind the value of any guidance that you might receive. It could be completely wrong or include tactics and plans you have tried before which just don't work for you. Work out in detail your own individual viva tactics, before exam day, and stick to this strategy. During the exam only change your game plan if it is absolutely crystal clear you have adopted the wrong exam approach but this shouldn't be the case if you have done your homework correctly!

The FRCS (Tr & Orth) examination is the final hurdle at the end of higher surgical training. It usually enables the successful candidate to apply for his or her Certificate of Completion of Training and therefore a consultant post. In turn it leads to largely unsupervised surgical practice.

The FRCS is split into two sections, with part 1 comprising the written exam and part 2 the clinicals. Part 2 in turn is divided into clinical cases and the structured oral interviews or vivas. Half of the marks for the part 2 section are allocated in the clinical cases and half in the vivas.

The examiners are not looking for a narrow inflexible candidate but rather a safe surgeon with broad knowledge and sound basic principles that they would trust as a consultant colleague. It is with this standard in mind that the viva should be approached.

The viva examination is a test not only of knowledge but of the ability to convey the required information to the examiners in a confident and coherent way that persuades them you are a safe orthopaedic surgeon.

Postgraduate Orthopaedics: Viva Guide for the FRCS (Tr & Orth) Examination, ed. Paul A. Banaszkiewicz and Deiary F. Kader. Published by Cambridge University Press. © Cambridge University Press 2012.

All the basic knowledge required for the orals should have been acquired in preparation for the Part 1 exam. This does not mean, however, that you can relax and assume that you can give a good verbal answer based on this knowledge. We have all been in trauma meetings when, put on the spot by a consultant, we have seen colleagues clam up and deliver a rushed, illogical answer when the trainee knows the answer but cannot present his or her thoughts clearly.

The focus for preparation should therefore be on practising technique and formulating logical answers to any possible questions. Quite a task!

How to improve your viva technique
Before the exam
1.   Know your stuff

In general your knowledge needs to be broad and basic rather than narrow and very detailed so that you can talk about anything on the curriculum.

Having said this, drawing up a list of important topics in each section of the viva is a good idea so you can focus your viva practice. It is relatively easy to predict what topics will come up in the viva (but be prepared for the odd surprise!). For example, in the paediatric viva you are likely to be asked about developmental dysplasia of the hip (DDH), slipped upper femoral epiphysis (SUFE), clubfoot, septic arthritis of hip and Legg–Calvé–Perthes disease (LCPD). For the trauma viva you must know hip fractures, ankle fractures and wrist fractures very well but basic principles of fracture management will also be tested. In the basic science viva surgical approaches are often asked and knowledge of the structure of cartilage, bone, meniscus and tendon is essential.

There are a number of drawings and diagrams that you can be asked to reproduce. You may be asked to draw the brachial plexus or a stress–strain curve and label it – if practised these are easy, but they are also easy to make mistakes with if you are not familiar with them.

There are a number of websites with example viva questions. Don't try to answer them all. It is better to try to answer a few from each section well to practise the technique of constructing a logical structured answer.

http://www.bota.org.uk/cms.php?id=137
http://frcsorthexam.co.uk/viva_topics.html

2.   Practise with colleagues

Rehearsing your viva technique with colleagues who are also taking the exam is an excellent way of building confidence. Try to simulate the exam scenario by sticking to one topic and making the questions get harder and harder. Revising with colleagues of a similar ability is great but be careful one 'hotshot' doesn't try to dominate the group and render the exercise futile by answering all the questions. It is less about knowing all the answers, rather more being able to think on your feet, applying basic principles to questions and constructing logical and if possible evidence-based answers. Remember it's an exam about common sense and making sensible decisions. If you come out with something outrageous and can't back it up, you will fail.

3.   Practise with an examiner

If there is an examiner in your region who is happy to conduct a practise viva then jump at the chance. He or she knows the structure and standard of the exam and this will give you an idea of the level you have to achieve.

4.   Practise with your trainer

You spend a lot of time with your trainer, so ask him or her to grill you in theatre, in trauma meetings and in clinic, and use opportunities running up to the exam to get used to answering questions on a wide range of topics. Consultants are busy and don't always seem to have time for formal teaching but there are usually a few minutes between cases in theatre for a short session.

5.   Practise with your partner, dog, mirror. Practise, practise, practise!

You don't always have colleagues taking the exam at the same time or an understanding boss but you can give your partner some prompts and then practise talking orthopaedics. The dog may have more patience than your long-suffering other half! Joking aside, the more time you spend verbalising your answers the better you will get at giving a good answer. Practice highlights mannerisms that you can try to avoid in the exam and provides an experience that you can draw on when it comes to the real thing.

6. Go on a course

There are an increasing number of exam/viva preparation courses and these can give excellent viva practice. Many of the courses are very expensive and really not worth the money, but some provide you with a real insight into the exam – ask your colleagues for recommendations.

7. Know what to expect

Having knowledge about how the exam works and how the vivas are divided up helps you prepare and you will feel more confident when it comes to the real thing. Ask colleagues who have recently taken the exam what they were asked, the standard of questioning, whether they were asked to reference studies etc.

On the day
Before the exam

The viva part of the exam takes place one or two days after the clinical cases. Half the candidates will be examined on one day and half on the second. The time in between is stressful and difficult to spend productively as you mull over your performance in the clinical cases. Try not to convince yourself you have failed, as you probably haven't and need a confident performance in the vivas.

Often several different surgical specialties hold exams on the same day so there will be lots of trainees milling around. Listen for when you are to enter the examination hall.

Before each viva you line up in groups of eight and are then led into the hall where you sit at lines of tables.

The viva is in four sections:

Adult elective orthopaedics and spine

Trauma

Paediatric orthopaedics and hand surgery

Applied basic sciences related to orthopaedics

You have 30 minutes for each oral. Some candidates will have all four in close succession; others will have long gaps between them.

In the examination hall

There are two examiners per desk and sometimes a third who is mainly assessing the examiners. One of the examiners will ask questions for 15 minutes and then they swap over. The oral interviews are conducted by non-specialists, that is, a hand surgeon may ask you questions about adult elective orthopaedics and a hip surgeon may examine you on paediatric orthopaedics. This is in an attempt to standardize the difficulty of the questions so that specialists do not focus on the minutiae of their topic and lose the big picture.

Marking

The scoring system is out of 8. A score of 6 is a pass, 7 is very good and 8 is excellent but difficult to achieve. A 5 is a close fail and 4 a poor fail. If you score 5 on one table you can make it up on the others. The marking system is described in detail later in this chapter.

Question format

The examiners often use objects in their questions. They may have a laptop with a photo of an implant, a histology slide or even an anatomical dissection. There may be laminated photos of X-rays or CT scans. There may be orthopaedic hardware on the table to look at, such as a trauma implant. You must be able to explain how plates, screws and nails work.

The structure of the viva has changed from spot diagnoses of pictures, X-rays and quick-fire questions to a fairly predictable set of three or four main topics from each examiner. This means the questions start (relatively) simple and become progressively more difficult until you will probably not be able to answer. If you cannot answer the first question, you are in trouble and the examiners can ask you a reserve question but this will probably result in you scoring a 4. If you answer 10 questions on the topic very well and only get stuck on question number 11 you are doing well and probably heading for a 7. The examiners will push you if you are doing well, usually until the point where you either say you don't know or guess. Examiners can usually detect guesswork so it is generally better to admit defeat at this point and move on to a new topic.

Listen to the question

Listen closely to the wording of the question.

If you are asked about management of a patient, start with history, examination, investigation and treatment. If the question is 'What implant would you use?' don't talk about all the different options, state what you would do and back it up with reasons and evidence. If you are asked 'What would you do?' don't say 'My boss did this', you must give an opinion and justify it. When answering the question don't try to make up an answer if you really don't know. The examiners will see through this and will know immediately. Be honest, if you don't know just admit it and they will move on so you have a better chance. If you try and blag it you may become unstuck!

You may not understand the question and in this scenario you are perfectly justified to ask the examiner to repeat it.

Answering the question

Before you answer the question take a few seconds to compose yourself, mentally construct a checklist of the main points you want to make and then start calmly with your answer. This avoids blurting out the first thing that comes into your head and gives the examiners the impression you are giving a considered response. If you do come out with something nonsensical, just admit that you said the wrong thing and correct it.

If you are confident on a topic keep talking, keep to the question that was asked and show off! Avoid going off on a tangent since you don't score points for this. If you can direct the answer onto a topic you know well, try to do this. Once you have finished your answer stop and keep quiet. Try to avoid the temptation to add extras on the end of your answer, this sounds like you are waffling and can annoy the examiners. It can also bring you into an area you really didn't want to talk about, which is bad. The examiners may cut you off; it can happen whether you are doing well or not so don't let this put you off. Just concentrate on the next question.

Remember that the examiners are looking to pass the candidate that sounds like a safe, new consultant. This means that you need to give sensible answers but not be a world expert on anything in particular. You should approach the answer as if it is your first week as a consultant.

Quoting references

We suggest trying to remember the main author, journal title and year of a few important papers, for example long-term results of the joint replacement you use and joint registry survival data for your implant of choice. If you have time to read the last few editions of JBJS then this may come in useful but concentrate on the high-quality studies.

Recently there has been a focus in the orthopaedic literature on national joint registries, and knowing the basics of how these are organized and the results (at least of the England and Wales registry) is a good idea.

Viva voce and the new structured oral examination

The ISB makes a clear distinction between the traditional viva voce and the new structured oral examination.

The viva voce was the traditional form of oral exam, where one or more examiners fired random questions at a candidate in a face-to-face interview or discussion. Each candidate might receive a different exam with regard to the assessment content, item difficulty and examiner leniency. The occasional examiner could be quite unpleasant and demoralizing to candidates who were struggling with their performance. One or two senior examiners seemed to take a perverse pleasure in asking impossible basic science questions and failing as many candidates as possible.

This has all changed with the introduction of blueprinting, structure and careful standard setting. The current exam is a fair, consistent, valid and reliable method of assessment.

The importance of probing the higher cognitive processes of candidates has been emphasized by the ICB and sampling of the curriculum is more robust.

An assessment blueprint confirms that the exam tests a representative sample of all the appropriate curriculum outcomes and a representative sample of all the curriculum content.

The complex nature of assessment in high-stakes exit exams, and the need for high validity and reliability, make the assessment blueprint an essential tool for examination planning and ensure content validity of the exam.

The latest education evidence is applied to assessment methods and continually updated to ensure best educational practice.

Political correctness is better observed these days. The examiners have to remind the candidate which oral they are sitting in order to give them time to settle and must be polite at all times. They are not allowed to give much candidate feedback at all such as 'well done' or 'excellent' and certainly no harassment of candidates is ever allowed and will be stopped by the co-examiner.

A good robust discussion is a grey area; it may quickly turn into a robust argument and is probably best avoided.

Examiners are not testing a candidate's ability to stand up to rapid quick-fire questions and excessive probing. This was the norm in the late 1990s and could bring out the best in a candidate – has political correctness gone too far these days?

In truth these methods were old fashioned and more often terrified and stressed candidates into performing poorly.

Practicalities of the oral exam

The viva or structured oral examination consists of four 30-minute orals: trauma, adult elective orthopaedics, children's orthopaedics/hand and upper limb and applied basic sciences. Each viva section lasts 30 minutes during which time you will be asked six questions.

Examiners are encouraged to keep their own discussion to a minimum to allow candidates the maximum opportunity to speak and score marks.

Questions are set at the level of a newly appointed consultant at day one in a District General Hospital. The questions consist of a default question, competency question and advanced question.

The FRCS (Tr & Orth) is a structured blueprinted exam. The material on which candidates are to be tested is made available to examiners on each morning of the exams.

Each oral exam is divided into two halves lasting 15 minutes each. One examiner asks three questions of approximately 5 minutes 'to read minutes' duration whilst the other examiner makes notes. At the first bell (15 minutes) the examiners reverse roles and a further three questions are asked.

Each pair of examiners will decide between themselves which half of the oral exam (and three questions) they are going to take with the exception of the children's orthopaedics/hand and upper limb section in which an examiner is already allocated to each specialty well in advance of the exams.[1]

The examiner who is not asking questions will be writing detailed notes, which inform the marking process. This is used for feedback purposes for unsuccessful candidates. Notes need to be objective, fair, balanced and informative and deal with what was actually said by candidates, rather than a vague subjective statement that may be difficult to defend if a failed candidate challenges the decision. Comments need to be factually correct, phrased in a professional manner and no comment should be made that the examiner would not be prepared to make to the candidate in person.

The examiners independently assess the performance in each of the six questions. The two examiners do not confer and as such any accusations that one examiner may exert undue pressure on the other during the marking process is avoided.

It is important not to be too discouraged or downhearted should an oral exam question go particularly badly. You must leave it behind you, remain focused and hope that you can redeem the situation by answering the other oral exam questions well. The same sentiments apply if, say, the trauma or adult general orthopaedics oral goes poorly. Again, stay focused and put things behind you as sometimes you can lose all sense of perspective in gauging how well or otherwise you are performing. There are classic stories of candidates thinking that they have badly failed an oral only to gain a good pass but then failing the subsequent oral as they were too distracted with worries that followed them into the next oral exam. Today there is really no excuse for carrying forward negative sentiments from one oral into another. At the very worst, examiners are only allowed to give you neutral feedback even if you have performed extremely badly. At the beginning of the millennium examiners frequently made very discouraging and negative comments during an oral exam if you were performing poorly. Candidates were left in little doubt that they were going to be failed in that section of the exam.

Marking system

A closed marking system is used from 4 to 8 and this equates to the following:

- 4 – Poor fail.
- 5 – Fail.
- 6 – Pass.
- 7 – Good pass.
- 8 – Exceptional pass.

Examiners assess nine trainee characteristics during the standardized oral examination.

1. Personal qualities.
2. Communication skills.
3. Professionalism.
4. Surgical experience.
5. Organizational and logical, step-wise sequencing of thought processes, ability to focus on the answers quickly.
6. Clinical reasoning and decision making.
7. Ability to handle stress.
8. Ability to deal with grey areas in practice and complex issues.
9. Ability to justify an answer with evidence from the literature.

This list has been simplified into three domains.

Overall professional capability/patient care

- Personal qualities, professionalism and ethics, surgical experience, ability to deal with grey areas.

Knowledge and judgement

- Knowledge, ability to justify, clinical reasoning.

Quality of response

- Communication skills, organization and logical thought process. Assess questions, answers and prompting (QAP).

Marking in detail

4 – Unsafe and potentially dangerous. A very poor answer. Gross basic mistakes and poor knowledge. Should not be sitting the exam. The examiners have severe reservations about the candidate's performance and are essentially flagging this up. Too ignorant of the fundamentals of orthopaedic practice to pass. Difficult to salvage even if other marks are 7 or 8, which is probably unlikely if the candidate is scoring a 4 in the first instance.

Did not get beyond the default questions, fails in all/most competencies. Poor basic knowledge/judgement/understanding to a level of concern.

5 – Some hesitancy and indecisiveness. The answer is really not good enough with too many deficiencies. Too many basic errors and not getting to the nub of the issue. Wandering off at tangents and not staying focused on the question. Misinterpreting the question, wrong examination advice for tactics.

The same ATLS and/or radiograph talk with each oral viva question.

Difficulty in prioritising, large gaps in knowledge, poor deductive skills, patchy performance, struggled to apply knowledge and judgement. Confused or disorganized answer. Poor higher-order thinking.

6 – Satisfactory performance. Covered the basics well, safe and would be a sound consultant. No concerns. Performance acceptable but not anything special or outstanding.

Good knowledge and judgement of common problems. Important points mentioned, no major errors and requires only minor prompting.

7 – Good performance. Would make a good consultant. Articulate and to the point. Able to quote papers, knows various guidelines and publications.

Coped well with difficult topics/problems. Goes beyond the competency questions. Logical answers. Strong interpretation/judgement but wasn't able to quote or use the literature effectively. Good supporting reasons for answers.

No prompting needed for answers but prompting required for the literature.

8 – Potential gold medal or prize-winning performance. Smooth, articulate and polished. Able to succinctly discuss controversial orthopaedic issues in a sensible way. Excellent command of the literature. Switched on and makes the examiners feel very reassured. Looks and talks the part.

Stretches the examiners, no prompting necessary. Confident, clear, logical and focused answers.

The marking system should allow exceptional candidates to be identified and should in theory allow feedback to be given to unsuccessful candidates.

The two examiners give separate independent marks without conferring with each other.

The marking system may be reviewed in the future and one suggestion is to reduce the choice to poor fail, fail and pass in an attempt to reduce potential bias and variability. Any change to the marking system will throw up a number of conflicting issues and opinions and may not necessarily improve on the current method.

Within a 2-hour period (120 minutes) eight examiners can independently assess each trainee on a total of 24 topics. This generates 48 test scores, which should provide a reliable and valid measure of a candidate's ability in terms of the educational domains being assessed, namely professionalism/patient care, knowledge and judgement and quality of response.

Viva tactics

It very rapidly becomes apparent to the examiners how well a candidate has prepared for the structured oral examination. Usually within the first two minutes or so a score is formulated and tends to stay constant. It is unusual for a candidate to significantly change their performance throughout the remainder of the oral viva.

The viva should start easy and progress depending on how a candidate performs. The questions are never asked to trick a candidate. An examiner's performance is constantly scrutinized and any erratic or unduly harsh or lenient marking is flagged up and fed back to the examiners.

Unless a candidate is doing exceptionally well they will not be asked difficult or obscure questions. A candidate who is performing poorly is never put through this ordeal.

- If you don't know an answer to a question say so and the examiners can move on to a different question. Easier said than done if the question is at the beginning of a topic and is straightforward. Not knowing the answer is going to go down like a lead balloon with the examiners. With only three topics per examiner in the oral you can't afford to stall at the first hurdle with a topic and have nothing to say. If this scenario could occur it is perhaps wiser to delay sitting the exam to the next scheduled set of exams.
- If you wish to clarify a question then do so. Don't however keep clarifying every single question with the examiners, as this will annoy them immensely.
- If you are challenged about an answer take the hint you may be wrong even if you think you are right. That said, some examiners suggest standing your ground if you are convinced you are correct. The decision depends very much on the context of the question and how well you are doing and what sort of rapport you have developed with the examiners. If you are the 'irritating I know everything candidate type' then perhaps better not to argue.
- Try to quote papers if you are able to as this will impress the examiners and boost your marks.

Appearance and affect

Does it matter if you dress unconventionally, in poor taste or even unkempt and scruffily? It shouldn't matter and most examiners would deny it would influence their marking. However, conventional wisdom suggests it may convey the subliminal impression that you are unprofessional and may affect your overall mark.

You should wear something conventional, smart and comfortable that you have worn before. Dressing formally focuses the mind for the task ahead. If you are neat and tidy in appearance, perhaps your thoughts will be well ordered too. Forget loud or novelty ties. In the end you are not in the exam to score fashion points or use it to make a visible statement on your value system – you just want to pass the exam.

Examiners are also aware that the stress of the examination may make candidates do strange things. The examiners will make every effort to put you at ease and relax you. The occasional grimace or bizarre facial expression will be pardoned. However we remain unconvinced that you would pass the exam if you repeatedly behave in an odd or weird manner.

Winding up the examiners

Forget it as it is not worth the effort and you are at a significant disadvantage in terms of outcome.

- Don't ask me that question.
- I'll probably know the answer when you tell me it.
- Do not say 'in my experience'. It is highly likely that your experience is minimal.
- What I think you are trying to ask me is . . .
- Can I interest you in the complications of elbow replacements?
- Just get on with it.
- No thank you, stop interrupting me, I wish to finish my answer.
- I am having a bad day I don't like oral exams.
- I think you have got a bit mixed up with the answer.
- That's not right, you are wrong.
- I don't think we are on the same wavelength.
- I think we have a problem with communication.

Examiners are advised not to respond to inappropriate behaviour by the candidate. However they can only be tolerant and open minded up to a point and the overall impression you are creating will not be reassuring.

Examiner conduct

Each examiner is encouraged to be polite and put candidates at ease. They are not allowed to examine a candidate that they know on a personal basis or if the candidate has worked for them in the recent past. Examiners are reminded that excessive stress is unpleasant and damages a potentially good candidate's performance. All candidates are treated the same and the mark is based on performance only and not behaviour.

Oral exam questions

On average you will spend 5 minutes on each oral viva topic. Should a question have a somewhat limited scope or your knowledge is poor you will spend a little less time on it, but consistency demands that the examiners divide the time more or less equally. The oral vivas are structured so that the examiners have no choice of questions. In the past the oral viva consisted of as many questions as the examiner wanted to ask the candidate. The oral viva could include upwards of 15 topics with a spot diagnosis and very brief discussion of management of the condition shown.

Previously examiners in the hands oral were all hand surgeons and likewise in the children's oral all examiners were paediatric orthopaedic surgeons. It is now highly unlikely an examiner is able to examine you in their chosen subspecialty. The aim is to avoid them asking you excessive depth in an area of special interest or area of expertise. The aim of the exam is to test your knowledge to the level of a day one orthopaedic consultant in a District General Hospital and not to the chosen expert subspecialty level of the examiner. Thus a hip surgeon may have to ask you about hand topics or a shoulder surgeon about paediatric orthopaedic topics. The examiners may not necessarily be ignorant on these subjects but it is fair to say your own clinical experience may well be more recent and well informed than theirs. This should give you some confidence to speak with experience but don't overdo it and rub up the examiners the wrong way.

It has been suggested that the structured nature of the exam reduces the likelihood of an examiner being able to question you in excessive depth about a subject. This is especially so as the examiner is only likely to have general rather than subspecialty interest in the subject. We would counter this with saying that it is surprising how much ground one can cover in 5 minutes. In addition it is surprising how much an examiner will know outside their area of interest. The vast majority of examiners are conscientious and keep themselves up to date with orthopaedics. Also,

examiners would definitely want to avoid the potential embarrassment of a candidate being more informed on a topic than they are.

It is better not to argue with the examiners but if your answer reflects current thinking on a subject and is at odds with the examiner explain the evidence and up-to-date thinking. You may get the sense that the examiner is unhappy with your answer mainly because it does not match with what is written on the sheet so have the confidence to explain the new thinking. Offer your considered reasoning of the issue without being patronizing or causing embarrassment to the examiner.

The other concern with the format of the structured oral is that it may lack fluency and spontaneity. Some examiners may simply introduce the question before initiating a discussion with only occasional reference to the answer sheet. This is usually because they are experienced, are familiar with the material and have the self-assurance to allow the oral to run a more spontaneous course. They are confident enough in their own ability to access the answers. An examiner who is less certain of an answer, less comfortable with the topic and who is less certain of the criteria against which the answers are to be judged is likely to spend more time referring to the answer sheet. Then again the examiner may be particularly pedantic in their interpretation of how a structured viva should be conducted or be paranoid that the examiner assessor will pull them in and reprimand them for straying too far from the structured oral examining process. You may be able to detect clues as to what type of examiner you have by how he/she phrases the question. If the examiner looks down onto a sheet and reads the question from it without looking up at you and making eye contact they are in the second category. These examiners want facts, and ideally the facts that are listed on the answer paper.

You can refine your answering technique to improve your performance and the overall impression that you create. Some candidates may need a lot of prompting whilst others can get into a rhythm and quickly impress examiners with their knowledge. Examiners like a candidate who can take control and make life easy for them.

Most candidates usually require a bit of help from the examiner. If you have a reasonable knowledge of a subject then with oral examination practice you can train yourself to deliver the information with more facility and polish.

Do not worry about the pace of the oral exam. It is the responsibility of the examiners to ensure that the requisite points are covered, and the guided answer sheets from which they are working contain more information than all but the most talented candidates will cover. That said, do not stall the oral exam hoping the examiners will run out of time and only be able to ask you a few questions at the beginning rather than the more difficult ones at the end. This tactic is obvious to examiners and it annoys them immensely so that they will downgrade your mark.

The examiners' answer sheet also contains a list of prompts to guide the candidate back onto the subject if they stray too far and go off at a tangent from the question.

Every second an examiner talks provides less time for a candidate to show if he or she is competent. Therefore examiners are encouraged to allow candidates the maximum time to talk as much as possible. This process is helped by clear explicit questions. This contrasts to the old days when examiners would go off at tangents and tell you stories or anecdotes, although in all fairness you had usually passed the viva exam by that stage!

Examiners are now strongly encouraged to stop hammering on if a candidate can't answer a question, and just move on to another question. This is very different from the early millennium when many candidates frequently complained that some examiners would just keep at it in the vivas looking for the magical word to unlock the door.

Oral exam questions are prepared so as to be crystal clear and explicit with default questions if candidates are unable to answer. Tutorials are avoided, although again in the old days you had usually failed by the tutorial stage. It was not unheard of for examiners to stop formally examining candidates and give them an anatomy tutorial if they had messed up the anatomy section and failed outright.

Examiners may use props such as slides, radiographs, pictures and charts or surgical implants (e.g. screws, plates, femoral stem, worn polyethylene) but are advised to make sure they are clear and unambiguous to the candidates. Laminated photographs are generally preferred to laptops.

Topics for the structured oral exam

Ideally topics should be asked that cannot be assessed in a hands-on setting at the clinical exams, e.g. trauma emergencies, critical condition and acute illnesses. Some topics such as avascular necrosis (AVN) find their way into both parts of the exam so this distinction isn't particularly clear-cut at times. The clinical scenario should be realistic and be able to generate enough questions. The scenario should be neither too long with too much information nor too short with insufficient data.

Lines of questions should easily be developed for the 'introduction', 'competence' and 'advanced' question categories.

Examiners have identified appropriate acceptable and unacceptable answers to the questions.

Oral viva courses for the FRCS (Tr & Orth)

There are many viva teaching courses to choose from. Some are well established with excellent candidate feedback whilst others are less well known and illustrious. Oral practice courses are less difficult to organize than clinical courses and this explains the wider choice available.

The sensible option is to ask the advice of several local trainees who have recently passed the exam as to which one they would recommend. Another useful source is the regional training programme websites that usually have an area in which candidates are encouraged to provide feedback from the various courses they have attended. This should give you some idea of which courses are worth going to or avoiding. This material may be restricted unless you are a local trainee.

What is the evidence? Do I need to know papers?

Yes, you do. We are not convinced when we hear people say 'you do not need to quote the literature'. Looking good by quoting the latest journal articles is impressive but not to your examiner if you are quoting papers inappropriately within an answer.

You would need to know the seminal papers on different subject areas within the last few years. There is a subtle difference between quoting journal articles to support four different ways to manage a tibial plateau fracture or saying 'This is what I would do ...' If the examiners ask 'Why?' you can then quote the literature.

If you want to score an 8 the examiners would expect that not only should you have an excellent command of the literature but be able to use the literature to justify and support your management decisions.

To score a 7 a candidate needs to be familiar with the literature and be able to quote papers but perhaps is not quite as expert using it to support arguments or justify management decisions. The examiners may need to occasionally prompt and help out the candidate with the current literature.

Scoring 6 suggests a candidate would probably know the seminal papers but struggle to get further beyond this. With good knowledge and judgement and the important points mentioned a candidate may score a safe 6 without knowing any significant literature to back up the evidence.

A score of 5 suggests the literature doesn't really matter as you are struggling to keep your head above the water and are trying to get past the default questions onto the competency questions.

Scoring a 4 means you will have time to read the various key orthopaedic papers before you re-sit the examination.

Educational value of the structured, standardized oral exam

The oral examination questions are ideally sourced on patient care (i.e. clinical scenarios), designed to promote higher-order thinking (i.e. use of knowledge for decision making, interpretation, clinical judgement) and centred on a trainee's quality of answer (quality, focus, confidence displayed when answering and amount of prompting required).

Advantages of the oral exam include:

- It is a face-to-face exam. It can therefore be used to assess aspects of trainees that other exams may fail to assess such as quality of responses.
- It is a flexible exam. The examiner can choose from a pool of predetermined questions to ask an easier or more difficult question, depending on the candidate's response to the earlier question.
- Oral exams can be used to assess the candidate's cognitive abilities related to clinical practice, such as problem solving and decision making.
- Oral exams may capture certain important examinee traits which other exams may fail to assess; e.g. fitness-to-practise, worthiness for recognition as senior clinicians, professionalism.

Disadvantages of the oral exam include:

- Meticulous planning is required to ensure the exam is structured according to the examination blueprint.
- Oral exams require a large number of examiners to maintain reliability.
- The examiners should be pre-trained to apply the same standards to each candidate using pre-validated rating scale descriptors.
- The organization and administration of an oral exam is costly and time consuming.
- It has been shown that oral exams may bias against some candidates, e.g. certain ethnic groups.
- Oral exams tend to assess certain candidate attributes which are not intended to be assessed, e.g. examinee style of speaking.
- Oral exams can feel threatening and stressful to the candidate.

Although it is outside of the scope of the book to discuss in detail educational principles behind assessment several theories do warrant a brief mention.

Miller's pyramid of assessment stresses that four levels of assessment need to be tested to obtain a comprehensive understanding of a trainee's ability (Table 1.1).

Bloom's taxonomy categorizes knowledge into six levels:

1. Knowledge recall.
2. Comprehension or understanding.
3. Application.
4. Analysis.
5. Synthesis.
6. Evaluation.

This is a hierachical classification with the lowest cognitive level being 'knowledge recall' and the highest 'evaluation of knowledge' (Table 1.2). The lower levels can be attained with a superficial approach to learning with memorizing lists and rote learning of facts but the upper levels involve higher-order thinking and can only be attained by deep learning.

The assessment of recall and comprehension of knowledge is essential, but if only recall and comprehension are tested, lower-order thinking will be promoted. In contrast, higher-order thinking is encouraged by assessing the knowledge at application,

Table 1.1 Miller's pyramid of assessment.

Knows	Knowledge or information that the candidate has learned	SBAs
Knows how	Application of knowledge to medically relevant situations	EMIs
Shows how	Simulated demonstration of skills in an examination situation	Intermediate case, short case
Does	Behaviour in real-life situations	

Table 1.2 Bloom's taxonomy.

Level	Learner action	Question cues
Knowledge	Recall content in the exact form that it was presented. Memorization of definitions, formulas, or procedures gives examples of knowledge-level functioning	List, define, label, identify, name
Comprehension	Restate material in their own words, or can recognize previously unseen examples of a concept	Describe, associate, categorize, summarize
Application	Apply rules to a problem, without being given the rule or formula for solving the problem	Apply, calculate, illustrate, solve
Analysis	Break complex concepts or situations down into their component parts, and analyse how the parts are related to one another	Analyse, compare, separate, order, explain
Synthesis	Rearrange component parts to form a new whole	Combine, modify, rearrange, 'what-if'
Evaluation	Evaluate or make judgements on the worth of a concept, object, etc. for a purpose	Assess, decide, grade, recommend, explain, judge

analysis, synthesis and evaluation levels. Context-free questions, i.e. questions that are not based on practical/clinical scenarios, encourage the consideration of simple answers, e.g. yes/no.

The promotion and assessment of higher-order thinking can be achieved by introducing context-rich questions, i.e. questions based on patient, practical or clinical scenarios, for knowledge assessments.

The six levels have been telescoped to:

A. Recall–comprehension of knowledge; i.e. reproducing and understanding.
B. Application–analysis; i.e. making use of knowledge.
C. Synthesis–evaluation; i.e. doing different things with knowledge and making use of judgement.

The Van der Vleuten utility index formula is used to analyse the usefulness of different assessment methods. It is defined as the product

Unity $= R \times V \times E \times C \times A$

Where
R = Reliability

For high reliability guidelines need to be rigidly followed by the examiners.
V = Validity
Clinical scenarios should be drawn from the assessment blueprint and biased on higher-order thinking.
E = Educational impact
If pre-validated questions probing higher-order thinking skills are used, the oral exam can focus the trainees on sound clinical practice.
C = Cost moderate
Running an oral examination is expensive to organize, requiring examiner time and infrastructure, but is less expensive than clinical exams involving patients.
A = Acceptability
Examiners may dislike the loss of autonomy that results from the imposed structure in the oral exam. High stress levels have been reported amongst candidates.
Additionally, **P = Practicability**
Some difficulties but generally much easier to organize than the clinical exams.

Higher-order thinking involves the learning of complex judgemental skills such as critical thinking and problem solving and is more difficult to learn but is also more valuable because such skills are more likely to be useable in everyday clinical practice. The simplest thinking skills are learning facts and recall, while higher-order skills include critical thinking, analysis and problem solving.

With the increasingly complex nature of orthopaedic practice, it is becoming even more important that orthopaedic surgeons are capable of thinking divergently and creatively.

Endnote

1. We believe this to be the case but the only thing consistent about the exam regulations is that they change from year to year.

Chapter

2

Hip structured oral questions

Paul A. Banaszkiewicz and Rahul Kakkar

All viva questions outlined here are examples of actual questions asked in the FRCS (Tr & Orth) exam. Currently each viva question lasts 5 minutes and examiners are advised against switching to another topic earlier even if a candidate knows the subject well. Therefore to give a more realistic 5-minute viva question some topics have been combined from several smaller disjointed accounts from the old-style viva.

We have aimed the candidates' answers for a 7–8 score so they are significantly more detailed than what would be required for a bare pass. Aiming for the minimum to pass will generally be unsuccessful and is not recommended. On a few occasions we have answered questions in a less detailed manner so as to allow readers to gauge the differences in potential scores.

Structured oral examination question 1

EXAMINER: This is a radiograph of a 77-year-old woman who sustained a displaced intracapsular fractured neck of femur 3 years earlier managed with a hemiarthroplasty of the hip (see Figure 2.1). She was admitted onto the orthopaedic ward last night because of increasing left hip pain and difficulty mobilizing.

CANDIDATE: This is an anteroposterior (AP) radiograph of the pelvis taken on the 11/5/11 demonstrating a cemented Thompson's hemiarthroplasty of the left hip. The neck cut is straight down on to the lesser trochanter. The prosthesis seems to have sunk below the lesser trochanter and there are radiolucencies in Gruen zones 1, 4, 5 and 7. There appears to be a faint rim of calcification in the soft tissues, adjacent to the lateral cortex of the femur. The femoral head size would seem to match the acetabulum so it is not under or oversized and the femoral stem orientation appears neutral, neither excessively anteverted

nor retroverted. I would like to see immediate postoperative radiographs to confirm whether there has been a change in stem position from the time of the original surgery and would also like to see an up-to-date lateral radiograph of the hip.

EXAMINER: Here is a lateral radiograph of the left hip that was taken on admission. (Figure 2.2.)

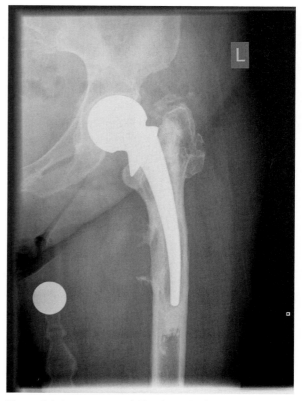

Figure 2.1 Anteroposterior (AP) radiograph of loose left cemented Thompson's hemiarthroplasty hip.

Postgraduate Orthopaedics: Viva Guide for the FRCS (Tr & Orth) Examination, ed. Paul A. Banaszkiewicz and Deiary F. Kader. Published by Cambridge University Press. © Cambridge University Press 2012.

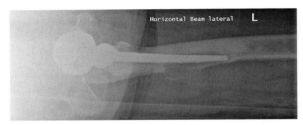

Figure 2.2 Lateral radiograph of loose left cemented Thompson's hemiarthroplasty hip.

CANDIDATE: The lateral radiograph demonstrates loosening of the Thompson's prosthesis with a large cortical lytic lesion surrounding the stem. There appears be reactive bone formation along the posteromedial diaphysis of the femur and a suggestion of a possible soft tissue mass. There is lateral cortical destruction at the tip of the stem.

EXAMINER: What do you think is going on?

CANDIDATE: The stem appears loose. The prosthesis has only been inserted for 3 years. I think the radiographs are highly suggestive of infection until proven otherwise.

EXAMINER: How would you investigate this patient?

CANDIDATE: I would perform routine blood tests including CRP and ESR to see if there are raised inflammatory markers.[1]

EXAMINER: How helpful are these?

CANDIDATE: They have relatively low sensitivity and low specificity as markers of prosthetic joint infection. Berbari *et al.* (Level II) published a systematic review in the JBJS American edition in 2010 on the use of inflammatory markers for diagnosis of prosthetic joint infection.[2] They concluded that IL-6 is a much more sensitive test for infection.

EXAMINER: What do you mean by sensitivity and specificity?[3]

CANDIDATE: Sensitivity is the ability of a test to pick up truly infected cases and specificity the ability of the test to exclude appropriately those cases which are not infected.

Or in more general terms sensitivity is the proportion of individuals with the disease (or condition) who are correctly identified by the test. Specificity is the proportion of individuals without the disease who are correctly identified by the test.

Positive predictive value is the probability that a patient with a positive result genuinely has infection and the negative predictive value is the probability that a patient with a negative result has genuinely avoided infection.[4]

EXAMINER. The paper actually reported that IL-6 was more accurate than CRP or ESR rather than sensitive. What do we mean by accuracy?

CANDIDATE: The accuracy of a test is defined as the proportion of tests that have given the correct result (true positives and true negatives).

EXAMINER: So how are you going to proceed with this patient?

CANDIDATE: I would want to take the patient to theatre and perform an aspiration of the hip to rule out infection.

EXAMINER: You are jumping in a bit fast. Is there anything else you might want find out beforehand?

CANDIDATE: I would want to take a full history from the patient. A number of patients who develop infection have early wound problems such as prolonged redness, induration, swelling or discharge. There may be a history of repeated courses of antibiotics. The wound may have become frankly infected requiring washout in theatre.

Onset of hip pain following a problem-free interval and an episode of sepsis is suggestive of haematogenous seeding of infective organisms from elsewhere. I would enquire if there was a history of bacteraemia from a UTI, chest infection or dental extraction.

Pain from an infected prosthesis is typically non-mechanical and unrelated to physical activity and not relieved by rest.

EXAMINER: The wound was oozy postoperatively but settled down. A large part of picking up periprosthetic infection is obtaining a good history and examination along with a high index of clinical suspicion.

How useful is a hip aspiration in diagnosing infection?

CANDIDATE: Spangehl *et al.* (level I) demonstrated a sensitivity of 0.86, a specificity of 0.94, a positive predictive value of 0.67 and a negative predictive value of 0.98 with initial image-guided aspiration in 180 patients undergoing revision hip arthroplasties.[5] They reported that aspiration alone is not sufficient for the diagnosis because of the risk of false-positive and false-negative results. They suggested in low-probability cases with a normal ESR and CRP that aspiration was not necessary. Aspiration would be indicated if pretest probability for infection was high (acute onset of pain, systemic illness, sinus formation) particularly if the CRP/ESR was normal or in all cases where the CRP or ESR was high.

EXAMINER: Joint aspiration was negative. How are you going to manage this patient?

CANDIDATE: I would need to get more history from the patient, most importantly what her symptomatic complaints are and also fully assess her fitness for anaesthesia and surgery.

EXAMINER: She has a 2-year history of intermittent progressively worsening hip pain worse with activities such as walking or rising from a chair. She is not the fittest patient for surgery; she developed pseudo-bowel obstruction and aspiration pneumonia postoperatively after the hemiarthroplasty requiring HDU admission.

CANDIDATE: I would need to sit down with the patient and fully discuss what her expectations from surgery were. We would need to reach an agreement on whether she would wish to proceed with revision hip surgery taking on board/ taking into account/accepting the potential risks and complications of the surgery weighed against the probable benefits of the procedure.[6]

EXAMINER: She can't live with her pain – she wants you to do something!

CANDIDATE: I would still be very suspicious that the hemiarthroplasty has a low-grade infection and perform a two-stage hip revision operation for her.

EXAMINER: Are there any other tests you might want to perform that could diagnose infection before going ahead with surgery?

CANDIDATE: The use of nuclear imaging (technetium-99 triple-phase bone scan, gallium imaging, labelled-leukocyte scans or FDG-PET imaging) for the detection of periprosthetic joint infection is worth considering but controversial. The recent AAOS clinical practice guidelines summary from 2010 reported a weak recommendation for their use.[7]

EXAMINER: How do you classify periprosthetic hip infection?

CANDIDATE: Tsukayama et al. proposed a 4-stage system consisting of early postoperative, late chronic and acute haematogenous infections, and positive intraoperative cultures of specimens obtained during revision of a presumed aseptically loose THA.[8,9]

Early postoperative infection presents less than 1 month after surgery with a febrile patient and a red swollen discharging wound. With late postoperative infection the patient is well, the wound has healed well, there is a worsening of hip pain and a never pain-free interval. Acute haematogenous infection can occur several years after surgery with a history of bacteraemia (UTI or other source of infection) and severe hip pain in a previously well-functioning hip. Positive intraoperative culture (at least three samples from different locations taken with clean instruments) occurs when a preoperative presumptive diagnosis of aseptic loosening was made.

McPherson et al. have also developed a staging system for periprosthetic hip infections that included three categories: infection type (acute versus chronic), the overall medical and immune health status of the patient, and the local extremity (wound) grade.[10]

EXAMINER: Why are you discounting a one-stage procedure?

CANDIDATE: Although there are advantages to performing a one-stage procedure such as low treatment cost and preservation of patient function it is a controversial option as the success rate is less than a two-stage procedure. The procedure involves removal of the prosthesis, thorough debridement and re-implantation at a single sitting.

EXAMINER: What are the prerequisites for a one-stage procedure?

CANDIDATE: There may be a case for performing a single-stage revision in a specialist centre with a large experience in dealing with infected hips.

EXAMINER: That's not quite the question I asked.

CANDIDATE: Prerequisites include a known organism sensitive to antibiotics, no pus present, elderly patients or patients with multiple medical problems. It is also indicated in healthy individuals devoid of re-infection risk who have adequate bone and soft tissue for reconstruction and a low virulence pathogen.

EXAMINER: What are the reported success rates for a single-stage revision?

CANDIDATE: Buchholz et al. who pioneered one-stage revisions at the Endo-Klinic in Hamburg reported a success rate of 77% in 583 revisions, but only after extensive bone and soft-tissue resection, which compromised long-term function.[11] These results were published in 1981 and can be viewed as somewhat historic now. Raut et al. from Wrightington reported a success rate of 86% in 57 cases at average follow-up of 7 years despite many discharging sinuses.[12,13] Hanssen and Rand summarized the results of single-stage exchange and found a cumulative success rate of 83% when antibiotic-loaded cement was used but only 60% when it was not.[14]

EXAMINER: What are the advantages to performing a two-stage procedure?

CANDIDATE: It is particularly important to perform a two-stage revision with more severe infections or virulent organisms, as the success rate of a single-stage procedure is much less in these situations.

EXAMINER: That's not what I asked.

CANDIDATE: It is more versatile for reconstruction allowing the use of either cemented or cementless components and bone allograft in patients with severe bone loss. It allows clinical assessment of the response to antibiotics prior to re-implantation.

EXAMINER: What are the disadvantages of a two-stage procedure?

CANDIDATE: It can be difficult to nurse patients between stages and the second-stage surgery can be difficult due to soft tissue scarring, limb shortening, disuse atrophy, loss of bone density and distortion of anatomy. If a PROSTALAC spacer is used it can dislocate or fracture and it is more costly to perform a two-stage procedure.

EXAMINER: So you perform the first-stage revision, how long will you keep the patient on antibiotics? (Figure 2.3.)

CANDIDATE: Duration of antibiotic treatment and timing between stages remains controversial. Current practice suggests delaying the second stage for at least 6 weeks pending good clinical progress with antibiotics and wound healing. A number of surgeons re-implant at 3 months treating the patient with 6 weeks of antibiotics and then further 6 weeks without antibiotics regularly monitoring the CRP/ESR for any signs of elevation and checking clinical progress for any signs of reoccurrence of infection such as sinus discharge or increasing hip pain. Some surgeons would routinely re-aspirate the hip to exclude any residue infection before going ahead with the second stage.

EXAMINER: Five of my last six THAs have become infected – what should I do?

CANDIDATE: Stop operating and investigate.

EXAMINER: Go on.

CANDIDATE: I would want to know if the same organism had been identified in the five cases particularly if the organism was *Staphylococcus aureus* as this may suggest a nasal carrier in theatre. Nasal swab cultures would need to be taken of relevant theatre staff and appropriate treatment started.

We would want to investigate for a breakdown in theatre sterility. I would involve microbiology and investigate the laminar flow system to see if it was working correctly.

There may be issues with the preparation of the instruments set such as packaging integrity and expiry date. A sterilization indicator should be present and the packaging must be dry.

There may be a breakdown in the precautions that must be taken by the scrub practitioner during the procedure such as

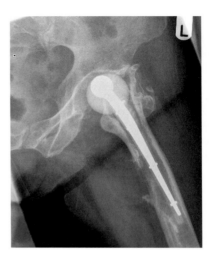

Figure 2.3
Anteroposterior (AP) radiograph of first stage PROSTALAC spacer.

the sterile field not being constantly observed and too much movement around the sterile field, including the opening and closing of doors and a wide space not being observed between scrubbed staff.

Taylor and Bannister showed that sets opened outside the confines of the laminar hood have significantly higher colony forming unit (CFU) counts during and after surgery.[15] Very few centres follow Sir John Charnley's technique of opening the instrument sets under the canopy at each stage of the operation.

Madhavan *et al.*'s paper from Bristol in the *Annals of the Royal College of Surgeons England* specifically looked at breakdown in theatre discipline during total joint replacement.[16] They noted a slackness had crept into theatre protocol such as corridor from changing room to theatre and theatre personnel attire.

EXAMINER: Do you know any papers that have looked at theatre sterility?

CANDIDATE: The classic paper on theatre sterility was published by Lidwell *et al.* in 1982.[17] This was an MRC randomized study which showed a decrease in infection rates following joint replacements carried out in ultra-clean theatres.

The deep infection rate was 3.4% in conventional theatres, 1.7% with ultraclean air and body exhaust and 0.2% when this was combined with prophylactic antibiotics.

EXAMINER: That's fine. Let's move on.

Alternative scenario

Differential diagnosis of the lesion would be granulomatous reaction to wear debris from Thompson's hemiarthroplasty. This is much more likely with a metal-on-polyethylene bearing THA interface. Other important differentials include metastatic disease and soft tissue sarcoma.

The examiner could lead you down the path of investigation of a possible tumour mass. A bone scan and MRI would need to be ordered for further investigation. A computed tomography-guided fine-needle aspiration of the mass could be performed. See references 18 and 19 for a similar type of scenario.

Endnotes

1. The candidate has got out of sync with the examiner and flow of the question. Not a disaster. The candidate should have answered how they would manage the patient with the standard default answer of history, examination and investigations etc.

2. Berbari E, Mabry T, Tsaras G *et al*. Inflammatory blood laboratory levels as markers of prosthetic joint infection: a systematic review and meta-analysis. *J Bone Joint Surg Am* 2010;**92-A**:2102–2109.

3. These are double-bullet questions fired at the candidate from a high-powered rifle and the candidate has to give a precise, correct answer back and then the oral continues on.

4. In the oral exam it is better to explain these terms to the examiners by drawing a table but in this particular question it doesn't quite fit together with the interactions to do this.

5. Spangehl MJ, Masri BA, O'Connell JX *et al*. Prospective analysis of preoperative and intraoperative investigations for the diagnosis of infection at the sites of two hundred and two revision total hip arthroplasties. *J Bone Joint Surg Am* 1999;**81-A**:672–682.

6. Waffly answer but can't be helped – it is what needs to be said by the candidate to the examiners. A standard, safe, nondescript response.

7. It may be enough just to mention the uncertainties with nuclear imaging or one may have to quantify your answer a bit more fully. It is a judgement decision but don't persist with your answer if the examiners want to move on. ^{99m}-Technetium bone scans are sensitive but not specific. Some investigators have found that a negative scan rules out infection while others have reported that a scan can occasionally be negative in the presence of infection if there is inadequate blood supply to the bone. A ^{99m}-technetium bone scan identifies areas of increased bone activity through preferential uptake of the diphosphonate by metabolically active bone. Increased uptake occurs with loosening, infection, heterotopic bone formation, Paget's disease, stress fractures, modulus mismatch of a large uncemented stem, neoplasm, reflex sympathetic dystrophy, and other metabolic conditions. In the uncomplicated THA, uptake around the lesser trichinae and shaft is usually insignificant by 6 months, but in 10% of cases, uptake may persist at the greater trochanter, prosthesis tip and acetabulum for more than 2 years. The pattern of uptake has not been found to consistently reflect the presence or absence of infection. Gallium imaging likewise has a poor sensitivity and accuracy. The use of leukocyte scans is generally preferred, having a higher sensitivity (88–92%) and specificity (73–100%), but their usefulness for the diagnosis of infection continues to be debated. FDG-PET is expensive, limited to a few institutions and although very sensitive does not allow differentiation between an inflamed aseptically loosened prosthesis and an infected one.

8. Tsukayama DT, Estrada R, Gustilo RB. Infection after total hip arthroplasty. A study of one hundred and six infections. *J Bone Joint Surg Am* 1996;**78-A**:512–523.

9. This is sometimes referred to as Gustilo's classification. With due respect to the first author Gustilo is easier to remember.

10. McPherson EJ, Woodson C, Holtom P *et al*. Periprosthetic total hip infection. Outcomes using a staging system. *Clin Orthop Relat Res* 2002;**403**:8–15.

11. Buchholz HW, Elson RA, Engelbrecht E *et al*. Management of deep infection of total hip replacement. *J Bone Joint Surg Br* 1981;**63-B**:342–353.

12. Raut VV, Siney PD, Wroblewski BM. One-stage revision of infected total hip replacements with discharging sinuses. *J Bone Joint Surg Br* 1994;**76-B**:721–724.

13. With due respect although Raut is the first author I think 'Wroblewski from Wrightington has shown' is easier to remember. There is enough to learn already without making things difficult for yourself!

14. Hanssen AD, Rand JA. Evaluation and treatment of infection at the site of a total hip or knee arthroplasty. *J Bone Joint Surg Am* 1998;**80-A**:910–922.

15. Taylor GJS, Bannister GC. Infection and interposition between ultraclean air source and wound. *J Bone Joint Surg Br* 1993;**75-B**:503–504.

16. Madhavan P, Blom A, Karagkevrakis B *et al*. Deterioration of theatre discipline during total joint replacement – have theatre protocols been abandoned? *Ann R Coll Surg Engl* 1999;**81**:262–265.

17. Lidwell OM, Lowbury EJ, Whyte W *et al*. Effect of ultraclean air in operating rooms on deep sepsis in the joint after total hip or knee replacement: a randomised study. *Br Med J* 1982;**285**:10–14.

18. Hanna MW, Thornhill TS. Thigh mass and lytic diaphyseal femoral lesion associated with polyethylene wear after hybrid total knee arthroplasty. A case report. *J Bone Joint Surg Am* 2006;**88-A**:2473–2478.

19. Patterson P, Grigoris P, Raby N *et al*. A thigh mass associated with a total hip replacement in a 69-year-old woman. *Clin Orthopaed Related Res* 2002;**404**:373–377.

Structured oral examination question 2

EXAMINER: This is an anteroposterior (AP) radiograph of a 52-year-old woman who presents to your clinic with non-specific right hip pain. She had a right metal-on-metal hip resurfacing procedure performed 3 years ago. (Figure 2.4.)

CANDIDATE: The anteroposterior (AP) radiograph demonstrates a higher abduction angle (lateral opening) than normal. The current recommendations are for an acetabular abduction angle of 40°. Several studies have demonstrated the importance of optimal cup positioning with regard to wear, metal ion levels and the revision rate. High cup angle has been consistently reported to lead to greater wear and higher serum metal ion levels. The head size appears small; the current recommendations are that unless a minimum 46 mm head size can be used the procedure should not be performed because of the risks of ALVAL and pseudotumours. There is no radiolucency about the metaphyseal stem, no obvious narrowing of the neck and no divot sign.

EXAMINER: What do you mean by a divot sign?[1]

CANDIDATE: A divot sign is a depression in the neck contour just below the junction with the femoral component often associated with a reactive exostosis. It is believe to be caused by repetitive bone-to-component abutment due to impingement.

EXAMINER: What is a pseudotumour and what is the difference between ALVAL and pseudotumour?

CANDIDATE: ALVAL (aseptic lymphocyte-dominated vasculitis-associated lesion) is caused by metal particulate debris. Patients present with localized hip pain and a localized osteolytic reaction. A more severe inflammatory reaction is termed a pseudotumour.

Several studies have described an association between pseudotumours and increased wear of retrieved components. Influencing factors include implant size and implant design (clearance and cover [arc angle]). In addition acetabular component positioning and femoral head–neck offset influence the risk of impingement and edge loading usually associated with high wear rates.[2] Despite this Campbell *et al.* reported that in 32 THA revised due to pseudotumor several patients demonstrated minimum wear features suggesting a hypersensitivity cause.[3]

Therefore the origin of pseudotumours is probably multifactorial caused either by excessive wear, metal hypersensitivity, a combination of the two, or as yet an unknown cause. Pseudotumor-like reactions have also

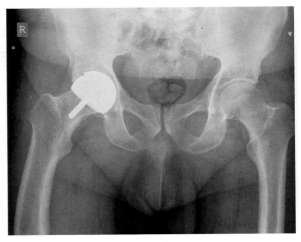

Figure 2.4 Anteroposterior (AP) radiograph right metal-on-metal hip resurfacing implant.

been reported in non-metal-on-metal bearings. In these cases, the histological findings showed accumulations of macrophages and giant cells, again suggesting an excessive wear origin.

EXAMINER: What are the risk factors for pseudotumours?

CANDIDATE: Significant risk factors for the development of pseudotumor include female sex, age less than 40 years, small component size, hip dysplasia and specific implant designs (ASR).

EXAMINER: How are you going to investigate this patient?

CANDIDATE: A careful history and examination of the patient is required. It is crucial to determine if the pain is arising from intrinsic (indicating hip pathology) or extrinsic sources (referred pain).

Extrinsic sources would include referred pain from the spine or pelvis, peripheral vascular disease, stress fracture, tendinitis or bursitis about the hip.

Intrinsic causes include aseptic loosening, avascular necrosis, infection [Long pause].

EXAMINER: What does the British Hip Society recommend [Prompt]?

CANDIDATE: Blood cobalt and chromium ions should be measured, as these are indicators of surface wear. If levels are raised the patient will require close observation. If levels are rising and the hip is painful it may be sensible to consider revising the implant.

I would also order an MRI scan with metal artifact reduction sequences (MARS). This is operator dependent but

(a)

(b)

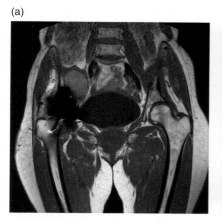
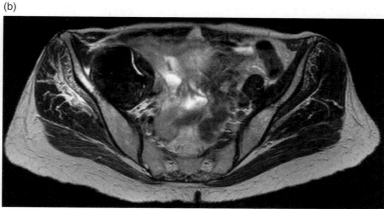

Figures 2.5a and 2.5b MRI of right MOM hip resurfacing implant demonstrating ALVAL mass.

can give clear images of fluid collections or solid lesions (pseudotumours) around the hip.

EXAMINER: This is the MRI scan obtained. What does it show? (Figure 2.5.)

CANDIDATE: The MRI is a T2-weighted image coronal view, which demonstrates an intra-pelvic mass.

EXAMINER: This was a pseudotumour. In fact the mass could be felt clinically when examining the abdomen.

EXAMINER: What are you going to do?

CANDIDATE: This patient requires urgent revision surgery to the hip.

EXAMINER: She is very scared of surgery and would prefer to avoid it.

CANDIDATE: I would stress the important of early revision surgery as the longer the MOM resurfacing implant is left in place the more extensive the soft tissue destruction will most likely be.

EXAMINER: What are the principles of surgery for pseudotumours?

CANDIDATE: The pseudotumour needs to be managed with aggressive debridement of all involved soft tissue. It is important to do a thorough debridement of the abnormal tissue similar to the treatment of infection. The surgery should be preformed by an experienced hip surgeon.

Although she is still relatively young I would use a metal-on-polyethylene bearing surface. A ceramic bearing surface has the potential for catastrophic fracture. We are already revising for a rare complication and we don't want anything to go wrong again. However I would use an uncemented implant. I would keep the option of using a constrained cup open as the

soft tissues may be so poorly compromised that the hip is unstable but obviously would prefer to avoid this, as components will loosen early in this situation.

It would be sensible to get a second opinion from an experienced hip surgeon as per British Hip Society guidelines to confirm and support the appropriateness of the management plan.

EXAMINER: Why bother with MOM hip resurfacing procedures? The old Charnley cemented hip replacement with trochanteric osteotomy works equally well with excellent long-term results reported from the surgeons at Wrightington.

CANDIDATE: Advantages of MOM hip resurfacings include better restoration of hip biomechanics, improved proprioceptive feedback, improved wear characteristics with no PE-induced osteolysis, increased levels of postsurgical activity, greater range of movement, reduced risk of dislocation, improved femoral bone stock mass because the neck and most of the head are retained and ease of conversion to a THA if the implant should fail.

EXAMINER: What are the contraindications for resurfacing?

CANDIDATE: These include severe osteoporosis, insufficient bone stock in the femoral head, large cysts at the femoral neck or head, a narrow femoral neck, notching of the femoral neck and severe obesity (BMI > 35 kg/m²).

Other contraindications include a history of chronic renal disease, metal hypersensitivity, those with anatomical abnormalities in the acetabulum or proximal femur and certainly caution in women of childbearing age.

EXAMINER: Is resurfacing contraindicated in women of childbearing age?

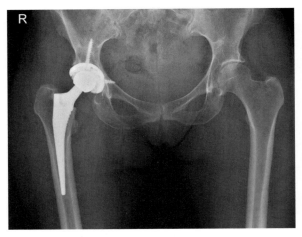

Figure 2.6 Anteroposterior (AP) radiograph of revised hip demonstrating uncemented THA with screw fixation into acetabulum.

CANDIDATE: No, although a recent annotation by De Smert in the JBJS British Edition reported that two-thirds of surgeons would exclude patients of childbearing age. Most surgeons (89%) believed that women should not be excluded.[4]

EXAMINER: I think most hip surgeons would now avoid a resurfacing procedure in a female regardless of whether they were of childbearing age or not.[5]

These are her postoperative radiographs. We kept her non-weightbearing for 6 weeks as there was quite an extensive anterior wall defect in the acetabulum but she has done very well. The hip pain has settled and the abdominal mass resolved. We were very lucky as the extensive soft tissue destruction that sometimes can be seem with this condition was absent. (Figure 2.6.)

EXAMINER: What are the outcomes of hip resurfacing compared with conventional THA?

CANDIDATE: Several recent studies report identical Harris hip scores but a greater percentage of patients with resurfacing involved in high demand activities. There is a higher revision rate in hip resurfacing compared with conventional THA.[6]

EXAMINER: What factors are associated with higher revision rates for hip resurfacing procedures?

CANDIDATE: These would include AVN, hip dysplasia, female sex, inflammatory arthritis, increased age, a small femoral implant and specific implant designs.

Endnotes

1. Occasionally if an examiner doesn't know what a candidate is discussing they will enquire further. Equally the examiner may let it pass so as not to reveal their own knowledge gap. Skilful, wily candidates may be able to bait and tempt the examiner into asking for clarification so as to then appear very studious and knowledgeable. Be careful however as there is a very real danger you may irritate the examiners by coming across as a 'know it all'.

2. An indirect way of letting the examiners know that you have read the various guidelines.

3. Campbell P, Ebramzadeh E, Nelson S et al. Histological features of pseudotumor-like tissues from metal-on-metal hips. Clin Orthop Relat Res 2010;**468**:2321–2327.

4. De Smet K, Campbell PA, Gill HS. Metal-on-metal hip resurfacing: a consensus from the Advanced Hip Resurfacing Course, Ghent, June 2009. J Bone Joint Surg Br 2010;**92**:335–336.

5. MOM hip resurfacing implants are being used much less now than previously. Whether this is an over-reaction to the ASR or not time will tell. However, from the exams perspective be very careful with what you are going to say or recommend to the examiners. Know the current guidelines and literature! Large MOM Jumbo hip replacements are now contraindicated as a primary procedure due to metal wear and corrosion at the trunnion.

6. Huo MH, Stockton KG, Mont MA et al. What's new in total hip arthroplasty? J Bone Joint Surg Am 2010;**92-A**:2959–2972.

Structured oral examination question 3

EXAMINER: This is an anteroposterior (AP) radiograph of a 78-year-old man presenting with increasing right hip pain. He had a THA performed 17 years ago.

CANDIDATE: The AP radiograph demonstrates severe osteolysis of both femoral and acetabular components. There are radiolucent lines at the bone–cement interface located circumferentially around all seven DeLee and Charnley zones in the acetabulum. The femoral component has separated from the femoral cement with lucencies in all seven Gruen zones.

The femoral implant is a Stanmore prosthesis and no cement plug has been used in the femur, so-called first generation cementing techniques.

EXAMINER: What do you mean by first-generation cementing techniques?

CANDIDATE: First-generation cementing techniques involved hand mixing of cement and finger packing of bone cement in the doughy phase into an unplugged, unwashed femoral canal. Clinical results with first-generation cementing have been variable and in general have produced some disappointing results due to the inability to produce a consistent cement mantle.

Second-generation techniques involved plugging the medullary canal, cleaning the canal with pulsed lavage and inserting cement in a retrograde manner using a cement gun. This reduced the incidence of gross voids and filling defects in the mantle.

Third-generation techniques involved porosity reduction via vacuum mixing or centrifugation and cement pressurization.

Fourth-generation cementing techniques include stem centralization both proximally and distally to ensure an adequate and symmetrical cement mantle. This is important as uneven and excessively thin cement mantles are associated with early failure and revision.

EXAMINER: How is cementing technique graded?

CANDIDATE: The quality of the cement mantle has been described by Harris and Barrack using a scale of A to D.[1]

Complete filling of the medullary cavity by cement, a so-called 'white-out' at the cement–bone interface is graded 'A'. Slight radiolucency of the cement–bone interface is defined as 'B'. Radiolucency involving 50% to 99% of the cement–bone interface or a defective or incomplete cement mantle is graded 'C'. Grade 'C2' is given to a defect where the tip of the stem abuts the cortex with no intervening cement. Radiolucency at the cement–bone interface of 100% in any projection, or a failure to fill the canal with cement such that the tip of the stem is not covered, is classified 'D'.

EXAMINER: What are you going to do?

CANDIDATE: I would want to take a full history from the patient. I would enquire about pain.

I would also want to exclude the possibility of infection (septic loosening) and would ask about problems with the hip postoperatively such as a wound infection requiring washout or a prolonged course of antibiotics. A history of fever, chills or a sinus tract suggests infection. Night pain, rest pain or constant pain would also suggest infection.

With aseptic loosening typically the pain is aggravated by weightbearing. Pain is significant with the first few steps of walking (start-up pain) which improves slightly with further walking only to worsen again with more walking. The pain is always improved with rest and rarely constant.

With aseptic loosening of a THA examination may reveal a shortening of the affected limb, antalgic gait and positive Trendelenberg sign. Pain at the extremes of movement suggests loosening.

It is important to exclude other causes of intrinsic hip pain such as trochanteric bursitis, tendinitis or impingement. Extrinsic sources of hip pain should also be excluded, particularly the lumbar spine especially if the pain has neurogenic features such as radiation below the knee, numbness, paraesthesia or dysaesthesias. Pulses and skin temperature should be checked to rule out a vascular cause for pain.

EXAMINER: Assume there is no infection in the hip and referred causes of pain have been ruled out. What are you going to do?

CANDIDATE: I would assess the patient. Find out how bad the pain is and whether the hip should be revised or whether symptoms are manageable and the patient can be reviewed regularly at the orthopaedic follow-up clinic.

EXAMINER: The patient can only walk about 200 yards before severe pain.

CANDIDATE: I would offer him revision hip surgery provided co-morbidity issues have been optimized and the risks of surgery had been discussed and understood. Both components would need to be revised.

EXAMINER: What are the complications that you would need to mention to the patient when consenting for surgery?

CANDIDATE: I would mention

- Infection.
- Dislocation. Usually component malpositioning or laxity of soft tissues around the hip.
- Fracture/perforation of femoral shaft.
- Nerve palsy (peroneal, sciatic, femoral) 2–7%.
- Vascular injury (femoral, iliac, obturator).
- Leg-length discrepancy.
- Heterotopic ossification.
- Death (cardiac/pulmonary).
- DVT/PE.

In addition the patient is going to require an extended trochanteric osteotomy (ETO) to remove the cement distally and this will increase operating time and blood loss. There is always the concern that the osteotomy site will go on to either malunion or non-union. Osteotomy migration or fracture can also occur.

EXAMINER: What about the bone loss? How do you plan for this?

CANDIDATE: Bone loss can be classified on the femoral side by using either the AAOS (Table 2.1) or the Paprosky classification system (Table 2.2).

The Paprosky classification evaluates the femoral diaphysis for its ability to support an uncemented, fully porous coated prosthesis. It is less detailed than the AAOS classification but is more useful in decision making if an uncemented revision is to be performed.

Table 2.1 AAOS classification system for femoral defects.

I Segmental defect
Proximal (partial or complete)
Intercalary
Greater trochanter

II Cavitary defect
Cancellous
Cortical
Ectasia (dilatation)

III Combined segmental and cavity defect

IV Malalignment
Rotational
Angular

V Femoral stenosis

VI Femoral discontinuity

Table 2.2 Paprosky classification system for femoral defects.

I Minimal metaphyseal cancellous bone loss/normal intact diaphysis

Type I defects are seen after removal of uncemented component without biological ingrowth on surface. Usually seen with Austin Moore type prosthesis or resurfacing procedures. The diaphysis and metaphysis are intact and there is partial loss of the calcar and anteroposterior (AP) bone stock

II Extensive metaphyseal cancellous bone loss/ normal intact diaphysis

Often seen after removal of cemented prosthesis. Calcar deficiency and major AP bone loss

IIIA Metaphysis severely damaged/ > 4 cm diaphyseal bone for distal fixation

Grossly loose femoral component
First-generation cementing techniques

IIIB Metaphysis severely damaged/ < 4 cm diaphyseal bone for distal fixation

Type IIIB defects extend slightly further than type IIIA, however reliable fixation can be achieved just past the isthmus of the femur
Cemented with cement restrictor
Uncemented with substantial distal osteolysis

IV Extensive metaphyseal and diaphyseal bone loss/isthmus non-supportive

Extensive defect with severe metaphyseal and diaphyseal bone loss and a widened canal that cannot provide adequate fixation for a long stem

Table 2.3 AAOS classification system for acetabular defects.

Type I Segmental defects

Peripheral – superior/anterior/posterior

Central – medial wall absent

Type II Cavitary defects

Peripheral – superior/anterior/posterior

Central – medial wall intact

Type III Combined segmental and cavitary bone loss

Type IV Pelvic discontinuity

Separation of anterior and posterior columns

Type V Arthrodesis

Table 2.4 Gross and associates classification system for acetabular bone defects.

Type	Description
I	No substantial loss of bone stock
II	Contained loss of bone stock (columns and/or rim intact)
III	Uncontained loss of bone stock (< 50% acetabulum)
IV	Uncontained loss of bone stock (> 50% acetabulum)
V	Contained loss of bone stock with pelvic discontinuity

Acetabular bone loss

Acetabular defect classification systems are used to predict the extent of intraoperative bone loss and guide reconstructive options.

Several classification systems exist; the three most commonly used are the American Academy of Orthopaedic Surgeons (AAOS) system (Table 2.3), the Gross and associates system (Table 2.4) and the Paprosky classification system (Table 2.5).

Gross and associates classification system (Table 2.4)

This classification is based on the nature of the bone graft needed for reconstruction on standard preoperative AP and lateral radiographs. A bone defect is considered uncontained if morselized bone graft cannot be used to fill the defect.

Table 2.5 Paprosky classification of acetabular bone defects.

Type	Radiographic finding	Intraoperative finding	Trial stability
I	No cup migration	Intact rim and no distortion. No major osteolysis. Bone loss minimal	Full
	No substantial bone loss	Small focal areas contained bone loss	
		Columns intact	
IIA	Superior (or superomedial) migration of < 3 cm	Superomedial bone loss	Full
	No substantial ischial lysis	Columns supportive and rim intact	
	No substantial teardrop lysis	Migration into defect under thin superior rim	
		Host-bone contact of > 50%	
IIB	Superior (or superolateral) migration of < 3 cm	Uncontained superior rim defect < 1/3	Full
		Columns supportive	
		Host-bone contact of > 50%	
IIC	Medial wall defect	Uncontained medial wall defect	Full
	Cup medial to Kohler line	Rim intact and rim columns supportive	
IIIA	Superolateral cup migration	Unsupportive dome	Partial
	Moderate ischial lysis	Columns intact	
	Partial teardrop destruction	Host-bone contact of 40–60%	
	Kohler line intact		
IIIB	Superomedial migration	Risk of pelvic discontinuity	None
	Severe ischial destruction	Bone contact of < 40%	
	Teardrop loss	Rim defect of > 50%	
	Migration medial to Kohler line		

Paprosky acetabular bone loss classification

This classification is based on information that can be obtained from AP radiographs. Four radiographic criteria are assessed:

1. **Superior migration of the hip centre**
   - Indicates damage to anterior and posterior columns.
   - Superomedial indicates greater damage to anterior column.
   - Superolateral indicates greater damage to posterior column.
2. **Ischial osteolysis**
   - Bone loss inferior posterior column and posterior column.
3. **Teardrop osteolysis**
   - Inferior anterior column and medial wall.
4. **Position of the implant relative to Kohler's line**
   - Deficiency of anterior column and/or medial wall deficiency.

A trial component with full inherent stability does not change position when the surgeon pushes its rim or performs a trial reduction. A trial component with partial inherent stability does not change position with removal of the inserter, but does not withstand the force of pushing on the rim or performance of a trial reduction. A trial component with no inherent stability changes position with the simple act of removing the inserter.

The Paprosky classification (Table 2.5) is often used clinically in preference to the AAOS classification as it not only predicts bone loss encountered intraoperatively but also assists in determining reconstructive options.

EXAMINER: How would you plan for surgery?

CANDIDATE:

- I would get an anaesthetic review to make sure the patient was fit enough for surgery and risks acceptable and also so they could order any special tests such as echocardiogram or pulmonary function tests etc.
- I would cross match for four units and make sure the cell saver was available.
- I would order one femoral head frozen allograft and have freeze dried allograft available if required.
- Implant removal kit which would include curved and straight osteotomes for the cemented cup and femur, ultrasonic tools, high speed burrs.
- Accurately template the revision implants required taking into account the level of the ETO.
- I would use uncemented components as generally they are preferred if previously cement was used. Cement would be relatively contraindicated if using an ETO as it may get into the osteotomy site and prevent healing.
- A long stem femoral implant, multihole revision (tantulum) acetabular shell and a metal-on-polyethylene bearing surface. I would attempt to use at least 32 mm head but preferably a 36 mm head as this significantly reduces the risk of postoperative dislocation.
- I would need Dall–Miles cables grip system to rewire the ETO back into place.
- I would need a flexible light source for visualizing the medullary canal of the femur.
- I would generally prefer a posterior approach with ETO unless the risk of dislocation was deemed high in which case I would use an anterolateral approach with ETO.

EXAMINER: How do you remove the cemented femoral component?

CANDIDATE: It is important to clear the shoulder of the prosthesis removing any cement or bone overhanging the proximal aspect of the greater trochanter as either stem removal will be obstructed or a greater trochanter fracture will occur with stem removal.

Flexible osteotomes and a small burr can then be used to further disrupt the cement/implant interface.

The ETO will greatly simplify implant and cement removal. I would use cement splitters to remove

cement along with ultrasonic tools. Cement is split radially and then removed.

EXAMINER: What about the acetabular component?

CANDIDATE: The safest way is to disrupt the PE cup from the cement using curved gouges. This prevents inadvertent damage to the bone of the acetabulum bed. After removal of the cup the cement is removed piecemeal. Sometimes a threaded extractor through a drill hole in the PE can be used. High-speed burrs are sometimes needed to debulk cement within acetabular anchoring holes.

Endnote

1. Barrack RL, Mulroy RD Jr, Harris WH. Improved cementing techniques and femoral component loosening in young patients with hip arthroplasty: a 12 year radiographic review. *J Bone Joint Surg Br* 1992;74:385–389.

This is a classic hip paper. You should know the key message, relevance and why it is important.

Structured oral examination question 4

EXAMINER: These are the radiographs of a 78-year-old lady who has been referred to the orthopaedic clinic by her GP because of increasing pain in her right hip. Would you care to comment on the radiographs? (Figure 2.7.)

CANDIDATE: This is an AP radiograph, demonstrating lower lumbar vertebrae, both hips and proximal femur. The most obvious features in the right hip are loss of joint space, osteophytes, sclerosis and bone cysts. The radiographic features are highly suggestive of osteoarthritis (OA) of the hip.

EXAMINER: How is osteoarthritis classified?

CANDIDATE: OA is classified into primary OA when obvious cause can be identified and secondary OA caused by such conditions as avascular necrosis, DDH, post traumatic, Paget's disease, slipped capital femoral epiphysis, protrusio acetabuli, Perthes' disease.

EXAMINER: What are the percentages of each type of OA?

CANDIDATE: Various studies have suggested that almost 90% of cases of OA are secondary.

EXAMINER: How are you going to manage this patient?

CANDIDATE: I would take a full history and examination from the patient, specifically I would want to know the location of pain, exclude referred pain from the spine. Hip pain is

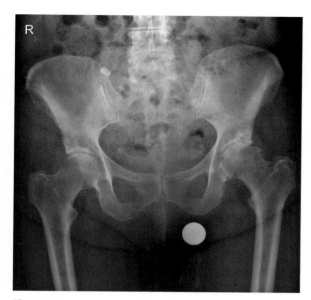

Figure 2.7 Anteroposterior (AP) radiograph demonstrating severe osteoarthritis of the left hip.

classically located in the buttock or groin radiating to the knee. Pain radiating below the knee to the foot is strongly suggestive of radicular type pain from the spine. I would inquire whether the patient had difficulty putting shoes and socks on, tying shoe laces, bending to pick up an object from the floor, getting in and out of a car [Examiner interrupts]

EXAMINER: The patient struggles to walk a quarter of a mile. She has typical symptoms of advanced OA. What are you going to do?

CANDIDATE: Assuming that all conservative options had been tried and have been unsuccessful I would offer her THA.

EXAMINER: What type of hip arthroplasty would you perform?

CANDIDATE: I would perform a cemented Exeter THA.

EXAMINER: Why this particular implant?

CANDIDATE: The Exeter THA has excellent peer-reviewed long-term data. It has a 10A ODEP rating for clinical use. It is an implant that I am very comfortable using, I have been trained to use this implant by my consultants, the instrumentation is straightforward and simple to use, the neck cut is not critical and the introducer allows for even pressure when inserting the implant.

EXAMINER: What are the design principles of the Exeter Stem?

CANDIDATE: The Exeter implant is a loaded taper model and becomes lodged as a wedge in the cement mantle during axial loading, reducing peak stresses in the proximal and distal

cement mantle. The stem is allowed to subside initially until radial compressive forces are created in the adjacent cement and transferred to the bone as hoop stresses.

EXAMINER: What approach would you use to the hip?

CANDIDATE: I am happy to use either the Hardinge or posterior approach to the hip.

EXAMINER: Make up your mind. Which one are you going to do?

CANDIDATE: For the majority of cases I would prefer to use the posterior approach to the hip. In rare instances I would use a Hardinge anterolateral approach if the risk of dislocation was high such as neurological or muscular weakness around the hip (Parkinson's disease/CVA), early dementia or substance abuse.

The posterior approach is considered easier to perform and is generally a quicker procedure, limiting operative complications such as blood loss and anaesthetic issues.

The abductor muscles are not disturbed significantly so there is generally no gait abnormality but the acetabulum is more difficult to see and can make prosthesis positioning difficult, possibly causing an increased dislocation rate due to component malpositioning. The sciatic nerve is at slightly more risk of being injured as well.

EXAMINER: There is approximately double the risk of sciatic nerve injury using the posterior approach. Most surgeons would say that there is no significant difference in surgical time between the two approaches; the posterior approach can take just as long as the anterolateral approach. The posterior approach is marginally technically easier than the anterolateral approach but this also depends on surgeon training, experience with using either approach and personal preference. I would argue about the acetabulum being less easy to visualize posteriorly as most surgeons believe the posterior approach provides better acetabular visualization especially for revision cases. The pelvis tends to tilt more and so the degree of cup anteversion is usually underestimated leading to an increased risk of dislocation. Where I think the posterior approach does make a difference is a reduced incidence of Trendelenberg gait postoperatively and improved Harris hip scores compared with the anterolateral approach. Whilst results have been a bit contradictory the risk of posterior dislocation is slightly higher posteriorly even with a careful repair of the soft tissues. Larger head sizes are being used now so this is becoming less of an issue.

EXAMINER: Talk me through the posterior approach to the hip.

CANDIDATE: Assuming full informed consent has been obtained, all relevant case notes and radiographs have been obtained, the leg has been marked and she has been suitably anaesthetized I would position the patient laterally, affected leg uppermost, with hip supports. I would then prepare and drip the patient and make an incision centred over the greater trochanter, approximately 15 cm in length.

I would cut through the skin, subcutaneous tissue, and open up the fascia lata, splitting the gluteus maximus along the line of muscle fibres, and then release the short external rotators from the greater trochanter. Finally, I would perform a capsulectomy and then dislocate the hip.

I would protect the sciatic nerve being aware of its position and avoid dissecting too near to it.

EXAMINER: What are the pathological processes involved in the development of osteoarthritis of the hip?

CANDIDATE: Disruption of the integrity of the collagen network occurs early in OA allowing hyperhydration. The increased water content of cartilage causes softening, decreases Young's modulus of elasticity and reduces its ability to bear load.

Initial changes in OA involve damage to the tangential zone immediately below the articular surface, with disorganization of the collagen network, loss of proteoglycans and swelling. This leads to a hypertrophic repair response with increased synthesis and accumulation of proteoglycan. However the repair process fails with loss of surface integrity, and fibrillation parallel to the surface. In regions of severe damage, there is a loss of cellularity and sporadic formation of cell clusters or clones.

Normal cartilage metabolism is a highly regulated balance between synthesis and degradation of the various matrix components. With OA the equilibrium between anabolism and catabolism is weighted in favour of degradation.

Cartilage catabolism results in release of breakdown products into synovial fluid, which then initiates an inflammatory response by synoviocytes.

These breakdown products include: chondroitin sulphate, keratan sulphate, PG fragments, type II collagen peptides and chondrocyte membranes.

Activated synovial macrophages then recruit PMNs establishing a synovitis. They also release cytokines, proteinases and oxygen free radicals (superoxide and nitric oxide) into adjacent synovial fluid. These mediators act on chondrocytes and synoviocytes modifying synthesis of PGs, collagen, and hyaluronan as well as promoting release of catabolic mediators.

Cartilage changes in osteoarthritis are characterized by increases in:

- Water content.
- Chondrocyte activity and proliferation.
- Stiffness of articular cartilage.
- Interleukin-1.
- Metalloproteinase levels.
- Cathepsins B and D levels.

and decreases in

- Quality of collagen.
- Proteoglycan quality and size.

Histology classically demonstrates:

- Loss of superficial chondrocytes.
- Replication and breakdown of the tidemark.
- Fibrillation.
- Cartilage destruction with eburnation (polished, shiny smooth with an appearance like ivory) of subchondral bone.

EXAMINER: Is OA simply an ageing process of cartilage?

CANDIDATE: Several differences between ageing cartilage and OA cartilage have been described suggesting a separate disease entity. For example OA and normal ageing cartilage differ in the amount of water content and in the ratio of chondroitin sulphate to keratin sulphate constituents.

EXAMINER: [Interrupting] That's fine that's okay.[1] What molecules are responsible for degrading the cartilage matrix?

CANDIDATE: The primary enzymes responsible for the degradation of cartilage are the matrix metalloproteinases (MMPs). These enzymes are secreted by both synovial cells and chondrocytes and are categorized into three general categories: (a) collagenases, (b) stromelysins and (c) gelatinases.

In OA, synthesis of MMPs is greatly enhanced and the available inhibitors are overwhelmed, resulting in net degradation. Interestingly, stromelysin can serve as an activator for its own proenzyme, as well as for procollagenase and prostromelysin, thus creating a positive feedback loop of pro-MMP activation in cartilage.

EXAMINER: What factors are responsible for inducing metalloprotease synthesis?

CANDIDATE: IL-1 is a potent pro-inflammatory cytokine that, in vitro, is capable of inducing chondrocytes and synovial cells to synthesize MMP. In addition IL-1 suppresses the synthesis of type II collagen and proteoglycans. Therefore in OA, IL-1 actively promotes cartilage degradation and may also suppress attempts at repair.

Endnote

1. Know the biochemical differences between ageing and osteo-arthritis in cartilage as your examiners may want you to continue answering the question.

Structured oral examination question 5

EXAMINER: This is the anteroposterior (AP) radiograph of a 48-year-old man who presents to your clinic with several weeks' history of progressively worsening bilateral hip pain. What do you think of the radiograph? (Figure 2.8.)

CANDIDATE 1: This is an anteroposterior (AP) view of the pelvis. The most obvious abnormality is patchy diffuse sclerosis with increased density in the superolateral aspect of the right femoral head (Ficat 2).

The left femoral head has a possibly minimal osteoporosis and/or blurring and poor definition of the bony trabeculae (Ficat 1). The radiograph is suspicious of bilateral AVN. I would like to obtain a frog-leg lateral radiograph of both hips. I would look for the crescent sign, indicating subchondral fracture, a feature of AVN that is more obvious on a frog-leg lateral than AP projection. This is because the anterior and posterior margins of the acetabulum on the AP projection are superimposed over the superior portion of the femoral head, the usual location of the sign. When AVN is bilateral, it usually occurs in each hip at different times, and the staging of disease in each hip is often different. [Candidate score 7–8]

CANDIDATE 2: This is an AP pelvic radiograph showing both hips. There is nothing very obvious staring at me. There are no features of osteoarthritis such as joint space narrowing, osteophytes or sclerosis.[1] [Candidate score 4]

EXAMINER: What do you mean by AVN?

CANDIDATE: Avascular necrosis occurs due to interruption of the blood supply to the femoral head leading to ischaemia and cellular death.

EXAMINER: What is the aetiology of AVN?

CANDIDATE: A number of conditions are associated with AVN. The most common cause is trauma secondary to fracture and/or dislocation of the femoral head. Other conditions include:

- Corticosteroid use.
- Alcohol abuse.

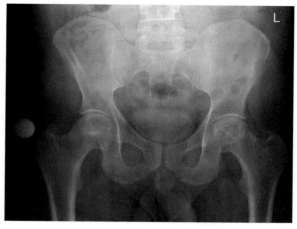

Figure 2.8 Anteroposterior (AP) radiograph of bilateral avascular necrosis.

- Smoking.
- Coagulopathies.
- Sickle cell anaemia.
- Caisson disease.
- Hypercholesterolaemia.
- Organ transplantation.
- Systemic lupus erythematosus.
- Gaucher's disease.
- Hypertriglyceridaemia.
- Intramedullary haemorrhages.
- Chronic pancreatitis.

AS IT GRIPS 3Cs (mnemonic)

Alcohol
Steroids
Idiopathic
Trauma
Gout, Gaucher's
Rheumatoid/radiation
Infection/increased lipids/inflammatory arteritis
Pancreatitis/pregnancy
SLE/sickle cell/smoking
CRF/chemotherapy/Caisson disease
In approximately 10–20% of cases no cause can be identified.

EXAMINER: What is the pathophysiology of AVN?

CANDIDATE: Aetiological factors in AVN are usually related to underlying pathological conditions that alter blood flow, leading to cellular necrosis and ultimately to collapse of the femoral head. This damage can occur in one of five vascular areas around the femoral head: arterial extraosseous, arterial intraosseous, venous intraosseous, extravascular intraosseous and extravascular extraosseous.

1. Extraosseous arterial factors are the most important. The femoral head is at increased risk because the blood supply is an end-organ system with poor collateral development. Blood supply can be interrupted by trauma, vasculitis (Raynaud's disease), or vasospasm (decompression sickness).

2. Intraosseous arterial factors may block the microcirculation of the femoral head through circulating microemboli. These can occur in sickle cell disease (SCD), fat embolization or air embolization from dysbaric phenomena.

3. Intraosseous venous factors affect the femoral head by reducing venous blood flow and causing stasis. These factors may accompany conditions such as Caisson disease, SCD or enlargement of intramedullary fat cells.

4. Intraosseous extravascular factors affect the hip by increasing the pressure, resulting in a femoral head compartment syndrome. For example: fat cells hypertrophy after steroid administration or abnormal cells, such as Gaucher and inflammatory cells, can encroach on intraosseous capillaries, reducing intramedullary circulation and contributing to compartment syndrome.

5. Extraosseus extravascular (capsular) factors involve the tamponade of the lateral epiphyseal vessels located within the synovial membrane, through increased intracapsular pressure. This manifests as trauma, infection and arthritis, causing hip effusion that may affect the blood supply to the epiphysis.

EXAMINER: Specifically how do steroids cause AVN?[2]

CANDIDATE: The mechanism postulated for steroid-induced AVN is still unclear.

Johnson proposed that fat cell hypertrophy within the bone marrow increases femoral head pressure resulting in sinusoidal vascular collapse and necrosis of the femoral head.[3] The exact mechanism of fat cell hypertrophy remains obscure but a disorder in fat metabolism is implicated.

Jaffe et al. believe patients undergoing steroid treatment are in a hyperlipidaemic state, which can increase the fat content within the femoral head and raise intracortical pressure producing sinusoidal collapse and finally necrosis.[4] Other investigators have proposed that this hyperlipidaemic state leads to fat embolism occluding the femoral head microvasculature, which initiates the pathophysiological process.[5] A recent study in rabbits suggests that the use of steroids can also damage endothelial and smooth muscle cells within the vasculature. This may result in interruption of the venous drainage from the femoral head, leading to blood stasis, an increase in intraosseous pressure and AVN.[6] Other studies suggest primary osteocyte cell death without any other features. This is seen with steroid use, in transplant patients and those who consume significant amounts of alcohol.

EXAMINER: How common are steroids as a cause of AVN?

CANDIDATE: High-dose corticosteroids are the most common cause of non-traumatic AVN accounting for 10–30% of cases. However only 10% of patients exposed to corticosteroids may develop AVN. Dosage is typically steroids > 2 g of prednisone, or its equivalent, within a 2–3-month period.

The period from the start of corticosteroid treatment to the diagnosis of AVN ranges from 1–16 months (mean 5.3 months), and the majority of patients are diagnosed within 1 year.

EXAMINER: You mentioned the crescent line, what is its significance?

CANDIDATE: Therapeutic interventions are less likely to halt progression of the disease once this sign appears.

EXAMINER: How does AVN of the hip present?

CANDIDATE: Although AVN can be clinically silent typically a patient complains of pain, usually localized to the groin area but occasionally to the ipsilateral buttock and knee. It is usually a deep intermittent, throbbing pain, with an insidious onset that eventually occurs at rest and may be present or even worsen at night. Physical examination reveals pain with both active and passive range of motion, especially with passive internal rotation. Range of motion is important as this helps determine the extent of the disease. In general, more limited flexion and abduction indicate more extensive articular damage, whereas limited rotation alone may indicate less destruction. A careful examination of the contralateral hip should always be undertaken as AVN is bilateral in 40–80% of cases.

EXAMINER: How is AVN classified?

CANDIDATE: Several classification systems for AVN exist. Ficat and Arlet is the most commonly known and consisted of four stages.[7] Hungerford and Lennox later added a fifth stage (Stage 0) when MRI became available.[8]

Stage 0 (preclinical). Suspected disease in the contralateral hip when the index joint has definitive findings. No clinical symptoms. MRI non-diagnostic.

Stage I (pre-radiological). Normal findings on radiographs and positive findings on MRI or bone scan. The MRI shows a double-line sign, consistent with a necrotic process.

Stage II (pre-collapse). Osteopenia, demineralization, sclerosis or cysts. A late finding is the crescent sign, a linear subcortical lucency, situated immediately beneath the subcortical bone, representing a fracture line and impending femoral head collapse.

Stage III (collapse). The femoral head is flattened and collapsed with the presence of sequestration manifested by a break in the articular margin without acetabular involvement.

Stage IV (progressive degenerative disease). Severe collapse and destruction of the femoral head, acetabular osteophytes. Osteoarthritis superimposed on a deformed femoral head.

EXAMINER: Any other classification systems?

CANDIDATE: Steinberg (Table 2.6) expanded the staging system into seven stages and quantified the amount of involvement of the femoral head into mild (< 15%), moderate (15–30%) and severe (> 30%), based on radiographs.[9] It is considered more useful than Ficat because it grades the severity and extent of the involvement, both of which are thought to affect prognosis.

EXAMINER: Any others?

CANDIDATE: Other classification systems include the ARCO (Association Research Circulation Osseous) classification, University of Pennsylvania system and the Mitchell MRI classification.

EXAMINER: What is the Kerboull necrotic angle and its importance?

CANDIDATE: The Kerboull necrotic angle is used to calculate the size of the necrotic segment. It is the sum of the angle of the necrotic segment as measured on both the anteroposterior and frog-lateral radiographs. Patients with a Kerboull angle > 200° more commonly have poor results with certain bone-preserving procedures.

EXAMINER: How are you going to manage this patient?

CANDIDATE: I would perform bilateral core decompression. The AVN is still at an early stage where it may be successful (Ficat stage I and II AVN). The procedure has no role in the management of Ficat stage III or IV disease. Results have been satisfactory when core decompression is combined with either non-vascularized or vascularized fibular grafts in patients with Ficat stage II lesions.

EXAMINER: What are the prerequisites for performing a free vascularized fibular graft (VFG)?

Table 2.6 Staging system of Steinberg *et al.*

Stage	Radiographic feature
0	Normal X-ray findings; normal bone scan and MRI. Diagnosed on histology
I	Normal X-ray findings; abnormal bone scan and/or MR findings IA: Mild (< 15% of femoral head affected) IB: Moderate (15–30% of femoral head affected) IC: Severe (> 30% of femoral head affected)
II	Cystic and sclerotic changes in the femoral head IIA: Mild (< 15% of femoral head affected) IIB: Moderate (15–30% of femoral head affected) IIC: Severe (> 30% of femoral head affected)
III	Subchondral collapse (crescent sign) without flattening IIIA: Mild (< 15% of femoral head affected) IIIB: Moderate (15–30% of femoral head affected) IIIC: Severe (> 30% of femoral head affected)
IV	Flattening of femoral head IVA: Mild (< 15% of surface and < 2-mm depression) IVB: Moderate (15–30% of surface or 2- to 4-mm depression) IVC: Severe (30% of surface)
V	Joint narrowing and/or acetabular changes (this stage can be graded according to severity)
VI	Advanced degenerative changes

CANDIDATE: VFG for AVN is a major operative procedure with a long rehabilitation time and therefore patient selection to minimize the potential for an unsuccessful operation is critical.

McKee from Toronto suggests the operation should be limited to patients:[10]

1. With 2 mm or less of femoral head collapse as measured on plain radiographs.
2. Who are 45 years of age or younger (and have a reasonable life expectancy).
3. Have had withdrawal of an identified aetiological agent.
4. Have no contractures about the hip.
5. Have a supple joint.

These are obviously general guidelines that may be adjusted somewhat depending on the individual patient.

EXAMINER: What are the advantages of performing a free vascularized fibular graft (VFG)?

CANDIDATE: Advantages of vascularized fibular grafting include:

- Being able to perform a core decompression of the femoral head.
- The ability to perform curettage and removal of the osteonecrotic focus.
- Impaction of autogenous cancellous graft to fill the defect created by removal of the osteonecrotic bone.
- The structural support of the subchondral surface provided by the fibular graft.
- The addition of vascularized bone and blood supply to the area of osteonecrosis enhances the revascularization process.

EXAMINER: What complications can occur with a free vascularized fibular graft?

CANDIDATE: Gaskill et al. from a tertiary centre in North Carolina performing a large volume of VFG reported a 16.9% complications rate, 4.3% of complications require reoperation or chronic pain management.[11,12]

Donor site morbidity

- Great-toe flexion contracture (4.3%). Majority asymptomatic noticeable only on clinical examination with the ankle fully dorsiflexed. Occasionally requires z-lengthening of the FHL tendon at the level of the medial malleolus. Flexion contracture of the second and third toes may co-exist in a small number of patients.
- Persistent weakness in the operated extremity (0.6%) either long toe flexors or peroneal group.
- Mild persistent pain and tenderness at the ankle or distal osteotomy site (4.1%) usually after prolonged standing or moderate activity such as jogging.
- Sensory deficits (1.7%). The sensory deficit was not always consistent with peripheral nerve or dermatomal distributions.
- Superficial infection.

Graft site complications

- Symptomatic lateral pin migration (2.4%). A Kirschner wire was used routinely to secure the fibular graft in its final position after placement in the femoral head.
- Symptomatic heterotopic ossification (1.4%).
- Femoral fracture (0.7%). All occurred in the intertrochanteric and subtrochanteric region after a fall.
- Deep venous thrombosis (0.3%).
- Superficial infection (4%).
- Deep infection (4%).
- Haematoma (1%).
- Trochanteric bursitis (1%).

EXAMINER: What are the other techniques that can be used to manage AVN hip?

CANDIDATE: The trapdoor procedure is performed with an arthrotomy to dislocate the hip anteriorly, followed by curettage of the necrotic segment of the head and packing of the defect with iliac crest bone graft through a cartilage window in the femoral head. This can be used for Ficat stage III and early Ficat stage IV and reasonable results reported.

EXAMINER: You have to be more specific than that – what do you mean by reasonable results?[13]

CANDIDATE: Michael Mont reported on a series of 30 hips Ficat stage III/IV at 5 years with 73% having good to excellent results.[14]

EXAMINER: Any other options?

CANDIDATE: Osteotomy has been used to treat Ficat stage III and IV disease but results have been variable because it is difficult to rotate the necrotic segment out from the weightbearing area, especially when the lesion is large. Sugioka et al. reported good to excellent results at 3 to 16 years of follow-up in 78% of 229 hips treated with the transtrochanteric anterior rotational osteotomy.[15] Their results with this technically demanding procedure have not been reproduced by others.

A success rate of approximately 30% at 5 years is common, with the best results reported in patients whose lesions do not result from trauma and who have less than 30% of the head involved.

EXAMINER: Any new technique that has emerged in the last 2 or 3 years?

CANDIDATE: Stem cells have been used to manage AVN.

EXAMINER: Go on – do you know about the technique or results?

CANDIDATE: Sorry that's all I know.

EXAMINER: Two techniques are being promoted. One is a three-stage procedure and the other is a single-stage procedure. The first method is by stem cell culture in the lab to multiply the number of cells several million fold. These cultured stem cells are reinjected into a previous core decompression site.

In the second method, bone marrow obtained from the pelvis is centrifuged in the operating room to yield a bone marrow concentrate rich in stem cells. The patient is supine on a traction table with a C arm image intensifier. Percutaneous core decompression drilling with a Kirschner wire (diameter 2.7 mm) is performed to perforate the interface between the necrotic lesion and healthy bone. Following this concentrated autologous bone marrow aspirate is slowly transplanted into the necrotic area under fluoroscopic control. This is still an experimental procedure but early results seem promising for early disease.

EXAMINER: The patient had surgery on both hips. These are his postoperative radiographs.

CANDIDATE: The AP radiograph demonstrates a metal core rod in the right hip. (Figure 2.9.)

EXAMINER: What do we call this?

CANDIDATE: The patient has had a tantalum rod inserted into the femoral head. The implant achieves decompression, supports the subchondral plate of the necrotic areas and probably induces bone regeneration.

EXAMINER: Anything else?

CANDIDATE: The use of a trabecular metal 'AVN rod' has a number of attractive theoretical advantages, including no donor site morbidity, improved rehabilitation, structural support of the femoral head and the potential for 'osseointegration' of the biologically friendly material.

EXAMINER: The patient had core decompression performed on the left hip and a core decompression with tantalum rod inserted in the right hip. He initially got good pain relief from the procedures for about a year or so but he returns to the orthopaedic clinic complaining both hips are now painful. The left side is worse than the right. What do you think of the radiographs?

CANDIDATE: The AP radiograph suggests AVN has progressed.

EXAMINER: What will you do?

CANDIDATE: I would offer him bilateral hip arthroplasty, the left one being more symptomatic first.

EXAMINER: What type of hip replacement would you use?

CANDIDATE: In view of his relatively young age I would perform an uncemented THA with a ceramic bearing surface.

EXAMINER: What are the advantages of using a ceramic bearing surface?

CANDIDATE: The advantages of using a ceramic bearing surface include superior lubrication, friction, and wear properties compared with other bearing surfaces in clinical use. Specifically it is an extremely hard material, very resistant to wear, with a low coefficient of friction, excellent abrasive resistance and excellent wettability properties for

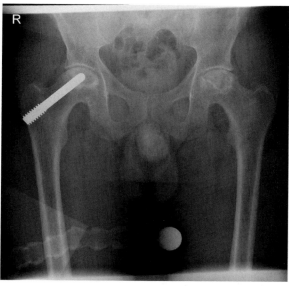

Figure 2.9 Anteroposterior (AP) radiograph pelvis with tantalum rod inserted into the right hip.

improved lubrication. It is presumed that the lower wear rates lead to a lower rate of aseptic loosening and the need for revision surgery.

Disadvantages include potential for catastrophic fracture, squeaking, chipping on insertion and reduced range of implant sizes.

EXAMINER: What is the incidence of squeaking?

CANDIDATE: The reported incidence of squeaking with alumina ceramic bearings varies widely from 0.45% in a series of 2716 ceramic implants to 7.0% in a series of 159 ceramic implants. Most reported series note that squeaking is rare and without clinical significance; however, on rare occasions, major squeaking has led to revision surgery.[16]

EXAMINER: Will there be any special issues removing the tantalum rod and performing THA?

CANDIDATE: I would contact the manufacturers of the implant as there is a special implant removal kit. Otherwise not using the removal kit makes the surgery much more difficult.
I would use a Gigli and reciprocating saw to section the head, implant removal corer to take out the tantalum rod and then perform a conventional uncemented THA.

EXAMINER: Are there any worries with tantalum material?

CANDIDATE: Studies suggest a trend towards an poorer outcome in patients following conversion of tantalum rod to THA.[17]

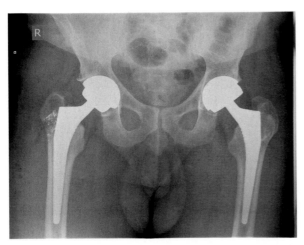

Figure 2.10 Anteroposterior (AP) radiograph left metal-on-metal (MOM) hip and right ceramic large jumbo hip arthroplasty.

There is also concern of tantalum residue within the joint space found in the majority of conversions. Although there is no catastrophic wear seen in studies there is the potential for accelerated joint damage in the medium to long term.

EXAMINER: These are his radiographs. He had a large jumbo head MOM performed on the left side and a large ceramic jumbo head THA performed on the right side. Do you have any worries? (Figure 2.10.)

CANDIDATE: The BOA released a statement after the annual conference at Torquay in 2011 reporting a higher than anticipated early failure rate for large jumbo head MOM hips. Concern was expressed regarding the trunnion at the 'Morse' taper where the large diameter metal head attaches to the stem. Various examples were shown of damage from either wear or corrosion or both resulting in either loosening of the acetabular component, loosening of the femoral component or a metal reaction with necrosis and soft tissue damage. As such its use should now be avoided. Excluding the ASR implant theses devices have a reported revision or impending revision rate of 12–15% at 5 years.

EXAMINER: What about follow-up?

CANDIDATE: This should be as per BHS guidelines for MOM bearing surfaces, yearly for the first 5 years and probably for life. Pain in this group of patients should be taken seriously and investigated appropriately with cobalt chromium levels and an MRI scan of the hip looking for any local reaction/tissue necrosis/presence of pseudotumour.

EXAMINER: What about the other ceramic hip?

CANDIDATE: There are some worries again regarding the trunnion, where the large ceramic head attaches to the stem which may be the source of excessive wear or corrosion, leading again to early failure, although the evidence is not as strong.

Endnotes

1. If you initially miss a subtle AVN spot diagnosis it is extremely difficult to recover the viva especially if the candidates before and after you spot it without prompting.

2. Take your pick. On the day steroids but you may be asked about alcohol, smoking, Caisson disease, sickle cell anaemia and transplant recipients etc. A few buzzwords may be sufficient to bluff your way through although it's more likely the examiner will want a more detailed explanation.

3. Johnson LC. *Histiogenesis of Avascular Necrosis.* Presented at the Conference on Aseptic Necrosis of the Femoral Head. St Louis, 1964.

4. Jaffe WL, Epstein M, Heyman N, Mankin HJ. The effect of cortisone on femoral and humeral heads in rabbits. An experimental study. *Clin Orthop Relat Res* 1972;**82**:221–228.

5. Jones JP Jr. Fat embolism, intravascular coagulation, and osteonecrosis. *Clin Orthop Relat Res* 1993; **292**:294–308.

6. Nishimura T, Matsumoto T, Nishino M, Tomita K. Histopathologic study of veins in steroid treated rabbits. *Clin Orthop Relat Res* 1997;**334**:37–42.

7. Ficat RP. Idiopathic bone necrosis of the femoral head. Early diagnosis and treatment. *J Bone Joint Surg Br* 1985;**67**(1):3–9.

8. Hungerford DS, Lennox DW. The importance of increased intraosseous pressure in the development of osteonecrosis of the femoral head: implications for treatment. *Orthop Clin North Am* 1985;**16**(4):635–654.

9. Steinberg ME, Hayken GD, Steinberg DR. A quantitative system for staging avascular necrosis. *J Bone Joint Surg Br* 1995;**77**:34–41. (Level 2/3 evidence).

10. McKee MD, Waddell JP, Kudo PA, Schemitsch EH, Richards RR. Osteonecrosis of the femoral head in men following short-course corticosteroid therapy: a report of 15 cases. *Can Med Assoc J* 2001;**164**:205–206.

11. Gaskill TR, Urbaniak JR, Aldridge JM 3rd. Free vascularized fibular transfer for femoral head osteonecrosis: donor and graft site morbidity. *J Bone Joint Surg Am* 2009;**91-A**:1861–1867.

12. Standard protocol is that Gaskill should be mentioned as the first author when quoting papers in the exam. Rules sometimes need to be bent and as Urbaniak is a recognized world expert in VFG the examiners may be more familiar with his research and therefore mentioning him as the lead author may be tactically more astute. There were 215 complications (a 16.9% rate) at the time of follow-up, at an average of 8.3 years, after the 1270 procedures. Quote papers and results but be sensible about it.

13. Sometimes you will get away with that type of general statement regarding results, other times the examiners may press you.

14. Mont MA, Einhorn TA, Sponseller PD, Hungerford DS. The trapdoor procedure using autogenous cortical and cancellous bone grafts for osteonecrosis of the femoral head. *J Bone Joint Surg Br* 1998;**80**:56–62.

15. Sugioka Y, Hotokebuchi T, Tsutsui H. Transtrochanteric anterior rotational osteotomy for idiopathic and steroid induced necrosis of the femoral head: indications and long-term results. Clin Orthop 1992;**277**:111–120.

16. Jarrett CA, Ranawat A, Bruzzone M *et al*. The squeaking hip: a phenomenon of ceramic-on-ceramic total hip arthroplasty. *J Bone Joint Surg Am* 2009;**91**-A:1344–1349.

17. Lewis P, Olsen M, McKee M, Waddell J, Schemitsch E. *Total Hip Arthroplasty Following Failure of Core Decompression and Tantalum Rod Insertion for Femoral Head Avascular Necrosis. 11th Congress Effort E poster content. 2–5 June 2010 Madrid, Spain.*

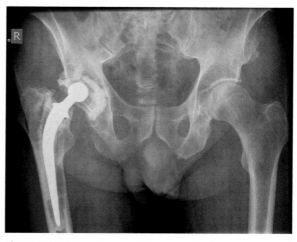

Figure 2.11 Anteroposterior (AP) radiograph of a loose cemented left THA.

Structured oral examination question 6

EXAMINER: This is an anteroposterior (AP) radiograph of a 72-year-old male who had a cemented THA performed 17 years ago. (Figure 2.11.)

CANDIDATE: The AP radiograph demonstrates a cemented THA suggestive of a Stanmore implant. The cup looks worn with the femoral head eccentric in the polyethylene socket. There are lucencies in all three DeLee and Charnley acetabular zones. There is a continuous radiolucency at the femoral cement–bone interface.

EXAMINER: What do we mean by the term wear?

CANDIDATE: Wear is defined as a progressive loss of bearing surface from a material as a result of chemical (corrosive) or mechanical action. Types of mechanical wear include adhesive, abrasive and fatigue.

EXAMINER: What exactly do you mean by abrasive and adhesive wear?

CANDIDATE: Abrasive wear occurs when two surfaces with microscopic irregularities or asperities slide past one another while in intimate contact. The interaction generates particles mainly from the softer material.

Adhesive wear occurs when two opposing materials bond under contact load. Actual transfer of material from one surface to the other may occur, forming transfer films. When motion resumes between the two surfaces, particles may be broken free from one or both surfaces. These new particles then further contribute to wear from third-body abrasive wear.

The wear of ultra-high-molecular-weight polyethylene (UHMWPE) in THA is mainly adhesive and abrasive.

EXAMINER: What is fretting wear?

CANDIDATE: Fretting occurs with small cyclic motions of one surface relative to another.

EXAMINER: What are the wear sources in joint replacement surgery?

CANDIDATE: Wear sources include the primary articulation surface, secondary articulation surfaces, cement/prosthesis micromotion, cement/bone or prosthesis/bone micromotion and third-body wear.

EXAMINER: What are the modes of wear in joint replacement surgery?

CANDIDATE: There are four modes of wear.

1. Mode 1 is the generation of wear debris that occurs with motion between the two bearing surfaces as intended by the designers.

2. Mode 2 refers to a primary bearing surface rubbing against a secondary surface in a manner not intended by the designers (for example, a femoral head articulating with an acetabular shell following wear-through of the polyethylene).

3. Mode 3 refers to two primary bearing surfaces with interposed third-body particles (such as bone, cement, metal and so on).

4. Mode 4 refers to two non-bearing surfaces rubbing together (such as back-sided wear of an acetabular liner, fretting of the Morse taper, stem–cement fretting).

While several modes of wear often occur simultaneously, mode 1 accounts for the majority of wear in well-functioning hip or knee replacements.

EXAMINER: What do we mean by effective joint space?

CANDIDATE: Schmalzreid *et al.* coined the term 'effective joint space' to refer to all periprosthetic regions to which joint fluid, and hence wear debris, can gain access.[1] In the acetabulum, wear debris can reach the interface through unfilled screw holes or via non-ingrown areas of the shell. On the femoral side, use of circumferential porous coating has reduced the incidence of diaphyseal osteolysis by blocking access of wear particles.

EXAMINER: What is osteolysis?

CANDIDATE: Osteolysis is a biological phenomenon that can result in the loosening of the implant principally caused by the UHMWPE wear particles. Metal or ceramic wear particles that are produced at the articulating surfaces of a hip prosthesis are also implicated but to a much lesser degree. Osteolysis is influenced by the size and morphology of the UHMWPE particles. Macrophages actively phagocytose (engulf) wear debris at the bone–implant interface. These cells release various enzymes and osteolytic mediators such as interleukin, tumour necrosis factor (TNF-α), and prostaglandin. These cytokines cause inflammation and trigger bone dissolution or resorption around the implanted region.

EXAMINER: What factors influence osteolysis (wear)?

CANDIDATE: Osteolysis (wear) is a multifactorial process dependent on surgical factors, implant design, patient factors and material composition.

Implant-specific factors that affect wear performance of THA (and TKA) are given in Table 2.7.[2,3]

Surgical factors (e.g. component position, soft tissue balancing) that affect joint loads and kinematics which influence wear performance of THA (and TKA) are given in Table 2.8.

Patient-specific factors that affect wear performance of THA (and TKA) are given in Table 2.9.

EXAMINER: What do you know about osteoblastic regulators?

CANDIDATE: Three osteoblastic regulators (RANK, RANKL and OPG) are involved in bone resorption. This is linked to TNF-α,

Table 2.7 Implant-specific factors affecting joint wear.

Implant design choices

- Modularity versus monoblock
- UHMWPE component thickness
- Bearing couple conformity
- Fixation (cemented versus ingrowth)
- Implant constraint
- Implant impingement

Material

- Metallic alloy (Co-Cr-Mo alloy versus titanium alloy)
- Ceramic (alumina, zirconia, oxidized zirconium alloy)
- UHMWPE (highly cross-linked versus conventional)

Bearing couple

- Metal-on-UHMWPE
- Ceramic-on-UHMWPE
- Metal-on-metal
- Ceramic-on-ceramic

Quality control

- Lot-to-lot variability
- Shelf life and packaging of UHMWPE components
- Sterilization process (radiation versus ethylene oxide)

a cytokine responsible for encouraging osteolysis through the facilitation and augmentation of osteoclast differentiation and activation of pre-existing osteoclasts.

Gold medal

Periprosthetic osteolysis is the loss of bone surrounding an artificial implant. The formation of a periprosthetic interfacial membrane between the bone and the implant is implicated in bone resorption. The interfacial membrane is composed primarily of two cell types, the macrophage and the fibroblast.

Aseptic osteolysis is thought to occur through a mechanism involving expression of bone resorptive cytokines such as interleukin-1β (IL-1β), interleukin-6 (IL-6), tumour necrosis factor-α (TNF-α), platelet-derived growth factor (PDGF) and receptor activator of nuclear factor-κ B ligand (RANKL).

Table 2.8 Surgical factors affecting joint wear.

- Surgical approach
- Component position
- Restoration of appropriate mechanical and rotational axes
- Initial stability and method of component fixation
- Soft-tissue balance (laxity versus overconstraint)
- Subluxation or dislocation
- Third-body wear
- Surgeon experience

Table 2.9 Patient-specific factors affecting joint wear.

- Activity level. Patients with active lifestyles often return to recreational activities that markedly increase joint-loading conditions (e.g. running, jumping, stair climbing)
- Body mass index and body weight. Increased body weight can be associated with increased magnitude of force and altered kinematics, although the detrimental effects of excessive weight can be counterbalanced by decreased activity levels and loading cycles that accompany a sedentary lifestyle
- Gait mechanics (level and stairs)
- Limb alignment
- Implant time in situ
- Preoperative diagnosis of post-traumatic arthritis and AVN have been associated with higher prosthesis failure rates as usually arthroplasty is performed in younger, more active patients
- Comorbidities. ACL and meniscal injuries predispose to osteoarthritis in a young age group
- Special cultural demands (e.g. kneeling in Middle Eastern and Asian populations). Deep flexion for kneeling loads implants beyond current design characteristics (TKA)
- Revision versus primary surgery

RANKL is a potent bone resorptive cytokine present on the membranes of bone marrow stromal cells, osteoblasts in bone, as well as on T-cells, and as a soluble molecule secreted into the bone microenvironment by these cells. Receptor activator of nuclear factor-κ B (RANK), a RANKL receptor, is expressed on the cell surface of preosteoclasts.

Macrophages express RANK and, when exposed to RANKL in the presence of macrophage colony-stimulating factor (M-CSF), have been shown to differentiate into mature osteoclasts capable of bone resorption. Osteoprotegerin (OPG) acts as a decoy receptor for RANKL by binding to RANKL and preventing the functional interaction of RANKL with RANK thereby blocking the osteoclast formation and the bone resorptive effects of RANKL. Osteoclast activation is thus blocked.

EXAMINER: What factors affect PE cup wear in THA?

CANDIDATE: Implant factors associated with an increased wear rate include non-cross linked PE, longer shelf-life for liners γ-irradiated in air, thickness of PE.

Patient factors include younger age due to higher activity levels, obesity due to increased joint loading.

Surgeon factors include position of the cup relative to Kohler's line, increase in cup abduction angle.

EXAMINER: What is the current thinking about UHMWPE?

CANDIDATE: Three approaches are currently being investigated in an attempt to modify highly cross-linked UHMWPE so that the increased wear resistance provided by cross-linking can be maintained without the reduced fracture resistance that accompanies cross-linking.[4]

1. Stabilization of free radicals through the impregnation of irradiated ultra-high molecular weight polyethylene with vitamin E. Vitamin E protects polyethylene against oxidation, which renders the melting step that normally follows cross-linking with radiation unnecessary. Vitamin E also quenches free radicals.

2. A second approach involves sequentially irradiating and annealing polyethylene. Irradiation is conducted in three steps with an interspersed annealing processes that together improve oxidative stability compared with that resulting from a single large dose of irradiation followed by annealing.

3. The third approach involves the photo-induced graft polymerization of 2-methacryloyloxyethyl phosphorylcholine (MPC) onto crosslinked polyethylene (CLPE). The concept is to create a hydrophilic layer with better wettability than a conventional polyethylene surface, thus increasing the chance for lubrication.

Endnotes

1. Schmalzreid TP, Jasty M, Harris WH. Periprosthetic bone loss in total hip arthroplasty: polyethylene wear debris and the concept of the effective joint space. *J Bone Joint Surg Am* 1992;**74-A**:849–863. This is a classic hip paper that you need

to know for the exam. With a classic paper ask yourself why the paper is important and how has it changed orthopaedic practice.

2. Tsao AK, Jones LC, Lewallen DG. What patient and surgical factors contribute to implant wear and osteolysis in total joint arthroplasty? *J Am Acad Orthop Surg* 2008;**16**:S7–S13.

3. For ease of learning and memorizing we have provided the information in table form. Be aware of the need to carefully apply this knowledge into an appropriate usable answer in the exam. If the radiograph demonstrates a malaligned THA (cup open or stem in varus etc.) tell this to the examiners as a probable cause of accelerated wear and then follow up with other surgeon-related factors. Be proactive and mention this sooner rather than later, especially if the topic is travelling down the wear rather than revision route. If the patient is young mention patient-related factors associated with wear such as activity or diagnosis (AVN).

4. Ramage SC, Urban NH, Jiranek WA, Maiti A, Beckman MJ. Expression of RANKL in osteolytic membranes: association with fibroblastic cell markers. *J Bone Joint Surg Am* 2007;**89-A**(4):841–848.

Structured oral examination question 7

EXAMINER: This is a radiograph of a 68-year-old woman who has been referred up to the orthopaedic clinic by the physiotherapist-led musculoskeletal clinic with an 18-month history of left hip pain and difficulty walking. (Figure 2.12.)

CANDIDATE: This is an anteroposterior (AP) radiograph of the pelvis demonstrating a coarsened trabecular pattern of the left hip, a thickened left cortex compared with the opposite hip, and increased density of the left hip compared with the right side. Both iliopectineal (Brim sign) and ilioischiatic lines are thickened. There is sclerosis involving the left pelvis (ileum, ischium and pubic rami), left femur and lower lumbar spine. The radiograph is highly suspicious of Paget's disease.

Differential diagnosis would include other causes of increased and disorganized bone turnover such as sclerotic bony metastasis (prostatic carcinoma), renal osteodystrophy, fibrous dysplasia, multiple myeloma, lymphoma, osteopetrosis and hyperparathyroidism.

EXAMINER: What is Paget's disease?

CANDIDATE: Paget's disease is a metabolic bone disorder of unknown aetiology characterized by a disorganized increase in osteoclastic bone resorption and compensatory osteoblastic new bone formation. There is accelerated but chaotic bone remodelling in which the bone is biomechanically weak and prone to deformity and fracture.

The disease can be divided into three major phases, lytic, mixed lytic/sclerotic and sclerotic, each of which is

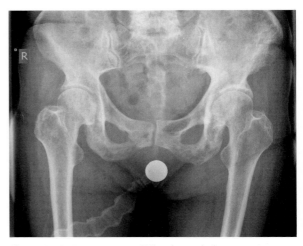

Figure 2.12 Anteroposterior (AP) radiograph demonstrating Paget's disease of the left hemipelvis.

associated with distinctive clinical, radiological and pathological features.

EXAMINER: What causes Paget's disease? What is the pathophysiology of Paget's disease?

CANDIDATE: The primary abnormality of Paget's disease is an intense focal resorption of normal bone by abnormal osteoclasts. These osteoclasts are abnormal in size, activity and quantity. The abnormal osteoclasts make large resorption cavities in the bone matrix. In response to the osteoclast resorption, osteoblasts are recruited, resulting in bone formation. The osteoblast activity is rapid such that the newly formed bone is not organized and remains irregular and woven in nature, less resistant and more elastic than typical lamellar bone; prone to deformity and fracture.

EXAMINER: What are the other radiographic features of Paget's disease?

CANDIDATE: Radiographic features of Paget's include:

- Advanced disease in the long bones is characterized by coarsened trabecula, bony sclerosis, bony enlargement and deformity. A 'candle flame' or 'blade of grass' sign represents a wedge- or V-shaped pattern of advancing lysis in the diaphysis of long bones. The femur develops a lateral curvature whilst the tibia develops an anterior curvature that may result in fracture. Fine cracks may appear (stress fractures) which resemble Looser zones but occur on the convex bone surface.

- Lateral radiographs of the lumbar spine demonstrate a 'picture-frame' vertebral body that is secondary to severe osteoporosis centrally and a thickened, sclerotic cortex.

- The skull is involved in 29–65% of cases. Inner and outer table involvement leads to diploic widening. Osteoporosis circumscripta is a well-defined lysis, most commonly involving the frontal bone, producing well-defined geographic lytic lesions in the skull. It is seen in the early or lytic phase, when osteoclastic resorption overwhelms bone production. At a later stage a 'cotton wool appearance' represents mixed lytic and blastic pattern of thickened calvarium.
- Protrusio deformity of the pelvis is a common occurrence with advanced Paget's disease.

EXAMINER: What are the current theories regarding the aetiology of Paget's disease?

CANDIDATE: The aetiology of Paget's disease is still unknown. Proposed theories include viral, genetic and environmental causes. Paramyxoviruses such as measles virus, respiratory syncytial virus, and canine distemper virus have been implicated. Electron microscopy has shown virus-like structures that resemble the paramyxovirus in osteoclast nuclei and cytoplasm of cells affected by Paget's disease. However, more recent studies have been unable to confirm the presence of specific viral antibodies in patients with Paget's disease. Environmental factors implicated include high levels of arsenic and an uncertain association with cats and dogs. Genetically 5–40% of patients have first-degree relatives with the disease.

EXAMINER: That's fine. I am however a bit sceptical about the cats and dogs theory. Moving on – what are the complications of Paget's disease?

CANDIDATE: Complications of Paget's disease include:

- Compression fractures of the vertebral body (commonest complication of spinal Paget's).
- Pagetic spinal stenosis, defined as compression of the spinal cord, cauda equina or spinal nerves by expanded pagetic bony tissue of the spine. Most common in the lumbar region and typically single level causing cord or nerve root compression.
- An enlarged and deformed skull can lead to increased intra-cranial pressure, hydrocephalus or cranial nerve deficits such as facial palsy (narrowing of neural foramina), hearing loss or blindness (pressure on optic nerve).
- High cardiac output secondary to increased bone vascularity (rare).
- Insufficiency fractures.
- Osteosarcoma, chondrosarcoma, malignant fibrous histiocytoma and giant cell tumours all have been reported with Paget's disease.

EXAMINER: What are the indications for THA in Paget's disease?

CANDIDATE: The indications are similar to non-Pagetoid disease. It is important to make sure that the pain is arising from the joint surface and not the bone. Bone pain with active Paget's is suggested by an increased alkaline phosphatase value. It is also important to exclude insufficiency fractures, neurological compression in the spine or Paget's sarcoma as a cause of pain.

EXAMINER: How do you assess disease activity?

CANDIDATE: Patients with active Paget's disease have a raised alkaline phosphatase (AlkPhos) and urine hydroxyproline values. The higher the level the more active the disease is. Patients with very high AlkPhos levels are thought to be at higher risk of bleeding and heterotrophic ossification formation.

EXAMINER: If the Paget's disease is active what will you do?

CANDIDATE: I would make a referral to one of my rheumatoid colleagues for a Pamidronate (Aredia) injection. This is a bisphosphonate, which is a potent inhibitor of osteoclastic activity, and hence bone resorption. This reduces bone vascularity and bleeding and possibly the incidence of heterotopic ossification.

EXAMINER: What are the technical issues of performing THA in Paget's disease?

CANDIDATE: There is tendency for excessive bleeding at surgery due to increased vascularity. Blood should ideally be cross-matched or at the least available from a group and save within 10 minutes. Bone can be very hard and sclerotic making it difficult to ream and broach. Burrs may be needed to enter the bone prior to reaming and/or broaching. Varus deformity of the proximal end of the femur predisposes to varus placement of the femoral component.

Protrusio as we have mentioned is a common finding and I would consider using bone graft medially to compensate. Some surgeons use lateral offset liners and antiprotrusio cages although this complicates surgery.

As Paget's bone is brittle there is a higher risk of both intra-operative and postoperative fracture.

There is some controversy as to whether there is an increased risk of heterotopic ossification occurring from the abnormalities of osteogenic differentiation in Paget's disease patients. Some surgeons routinely give prophylaxis to reduce the risk of HO. [Candidate score 6]

EXAMINER: There is a bit more than that when planning THA.

CANDIDATE: As bone pain is common in Paget's disease and does not necessarily improve with THA a diagnostic local anaesthetic injection to rule out concurrent bone pathology may be indicated. It is also important to exclude referred pain from spinal stenosis or radiculopathy and other causes of musculoskeletal pain.

Good quality, full-length radiographs to assess the degree of deformity and the extent of bone involvement. Radiographs should be scrutinized for the presence of a stress fracture that could account for hip pain. The fractures may be in the region of the femoral neck, intertrochanteric area or femoral shaft. They usually present as incomplete or fissure fractures on the tension side of the bone. Unrelenting hip pain and radiographic bone destruction suggest sarcomatous change.

Consider using cell salvage, hypotensive anaesthesia and predonation of autologous blood if intraoperative blood loss is anticipated to be high with active disease. Concurrent osteotomy may be needed if component alignment is difficult.

Marked protrusio can make hip dislocation very difficult.

EXAMINER: You mentioned osteotomy, how often do you perform osteotomy when you perform THA for Paget's disease?

CANDIDATE: In the majority of patients with Paget's THA can be performed without need for osteotomy. However, if deformity is severe, precluding implantation with a standard stem, then planning for reduction osteotomy to correct the deformity and/or the use of modular stems must be made preoperatively.

EXAMINER: What type of hip replacement would you use?

CANDIDATE: Although there has been a trend in recent years to use uncemented components in Paget's disease in this patient I would use a cemented THA. She is 68 and has Paget's disease and I think it is a reasonable option in this situation. If the patient is younger then the choice becomes more controversial. Although previous studies have recommended the use of cement in the last 20 years there has been a trend to use uncemented components. The worry that the altered morphology of pagetoid bone adversely influences ingrowth into cementless implants has not been borne out in practice. The biology of bone ingrowth for initial fixation of uncemented components depends, in part, on the ability of bone to proceed through the early phase of fracture healing.

Patients with Paget's disease are not known to have compromised ability for fracture healing and these patients progress through the biological process of fracture healing at normal speed.

Parvizi et al. reported on 21 cementless THA implanted against pagetoid bone; all were stable and demonstrated radiographic evidence of ingrowth at 7-year follow-up.[1] Lusty et al. from Sydney, Australia reported medium-term results of 23 uncemented THA at 6.7-year follow-up.[2] There were three revisions, one stem for aseptic loosening and two stems after periprosthetic fracture.

Some surgeons prefer cementless components especially when bone is very sclerotic or a concurrent osteotomy is done. Extremely sclerotic bleeding bone will make interdigitation of cement difficult and cement extravasation into the fracture gaps may occur after osteotomy. If using a cementless cup the use of adjuvant acetabular screws is recommended.

EXAMINER: Any special complications that can occur postoperatively?

CANDIDATE: There is a reported greater incidence of heterotopic ossification.

EXAMINER: Anything else?

CANDIDATE: Dislocation.

EXAMINER: No, I am not aware of an increased risk of dislocation. However, several studies have documented osteolysis following THA in patients with Paget's disease.[3] This is thought to be related to the increased metabolic turnover of the pathological bone. Other authors have reported that osteolysis is not a problem following THA in Paget's disease.[4]

Other complications include periprosthetic fracture around total hip implants, and the continuation of bone pain following arthroplasty, microfractures and malignant transformation to osteosarcoma.

Gold medal

EXAMINER: What causes have been identified for the increased number and activity of pagetic osteoclasts?

CANDIDATE: Causes identified include:

1. Osteoclastic precursors are hypersensitive to calcitriol (1,25 (OH) 2D3).
2. Osteoclasts are hyper-responsive to RANK ligand (RANKL), the osteoclast stimulatory factor that mediates the effects of most osteotropic factors on osteoclast formation.

3. Marrow stromal cells from pagetic lesions have increased RANKL expression.

4. Osteoclast precursor recruitment is increased by interleukin (IL) 6, which is increased in the blood of patients with active Paget's disease and is over-expressed in pagetic osteoclasts.

5. The antiapoptotic oncogene *Bcl-2* in pagetic bone is over expressed.

6. Expression of the proto-oncogene *c-fos*, which increases osteoclastic activity, is increased.

7. Numerous osteoblasts are recruited to active resorption sites and produce large amounts of new bone matrix. As a result, bone turnover is high and bone mass is normal or increased, not reduced.

Endnotes

1. Parvizi J, Schall DM, Lewallen DG, Sim FH. Outcome of uncemented hip arthroplasty components in patients with Paget's disease. *Clin Orthop Relat Res* 2002;**403**:127–134.

2. Lusty PJ, Walter WL, Walter WK, Zicat B. Cementless hip arthroplasty in Paget's disease at medium-term follow-up (average of 6.7 years). *J Arthroplasty* 2007;**22**(5):692–696.

3. Alexakis PG, Brown BA, Howl WM. Porous hip replacement in Paget's disease: an 8–2/3-year follow-up. *Clin Orthop Relat Res* 1998;**350**:138–142.

4. Ludkowski P, Wilson-MacDonald J. Total arthroplasty in Paget's disease of the hip: a clinical review and review of the literature. *Clin Orthop Relat Res* 1990;**255**:160–167.

Structured oral examination question 8

When reviewing various hip topics to include in this chapter DDH was the most common viva question that was regularly asked in the oral viva examination in the last 15 years. We would guess this is because it is a fairly common hip condition with a lot to talk about. The story can go in many different directions.

EXAMINER: These are the anteroposterior (AP) radiographs of a 66-year-old woman with bilateral hip pain. (Figure 2.13.) Would you like to pass comment on them?

CANDIDATE 1: The AP radiographs demonstrate a severely dysplastic hip on the right side with secondary OA changes. On the left side again there is dysplasia but to a lesser degree with again secondary OA changes present. [Candidate score 5]

CANDIDATE 2: This is an AP radiograph of the hips and pelvis of a 66-year-old woman taken on the 16/5/11, which demonstrates severe bilateral dysplasia.[1] There is a high

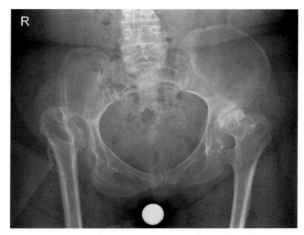

Figure 2.13 Anteroposterior (AP) radiograph of the pelvis of severe bilateral developmental dysplasia of the hip (DDH).

dislocation on the right side, Crowe IV or Hartofilakidis III hip. There is no contact between the true and false acetabulum. The femoral head appears poorly developed and probably absent with the femoral neck articulating against the iliac crest. The view of the proximal portion of the femoral canal on the right side suggests a very narrow medullary canal. On the left side there is a Crowe III hip or Hartofilakidis II hip. There is a low dislocation and secondary osteoarthritis.[2] [Candidate score 6–7]

EXAMINER: The left side is a Hartofilakidis I hip as the femoral head is still contained within the original acetabulum. With a low dislocation the femoral head is in contact, at least in part, with the true acetabulum and in this situation this is the most severe deformity. In high dislocation, the femoral head and acetabulum make no contact and the head has migrated superiorly and posteriorly. Often in this situation, the true acetabulum is reasonably well preserved although underdeveloped and osteoporotic.[3]

EXAMINER: What do you mean by dysplasia?

CANDIDATE: Dysplasia is lack of coverage of the femoral head, whether it is subluxed or dislocated.

EXAMINER: How do you classify dysplasia?

CANDIDATE: Crowe classified dysplasia radiographically into four categories based on the proximal migration of the femoral head. The migration is calculated on an AP radiograph by measuring the vertical distance between the inter-teardrop line and the junction between the femoral head and medial edge of the neck.

Crowe I is less than 50% subluxation, Crowe II hips have between 50% and 75% subluxation.

EXAMINER: [Interrupting] That's fine. That's okay. Any other classification systems that you know?

CANDIDATE: [Sharp intake of breath, shaking of head and then silence.] No.

EXAMINER: Have you heard of the Hartofilakidis classification?

CANDIDATE: I have but I can't remember the specifics.

EXAMINER: The Hartofilakidis classification system divides DDH in adults into three types: dysplasia, low dislocation and high dislocation. Many surgeons prefer this system, as it is more practical and simpler to use.

What are the anatomical issues associated with DDH?

CANDIDATE: The anatomical differences are divided into acetabular, femur and soft tissue issues. The acetabulum is shallow and anteverted; the femur has a small deformed head and short anteverted valgus neck.

EXAMINER: That's not all the differences. There are some you have missed. Do you know any more?

CANDIDATE: Muscles around the hip are usually shortened and er, er . . .

EXAMINER: The greater trochanter is small and posteriorly displaced, the femoral canal narrow, the acetabulum is usually small with poor bone quality, hip capsule elongated and redundant, psoas tendon hypertrophied and abductors orientated transversely as a result of the superior migration of the femoral head. The femoral and sciatic nerves may be shortened and therefore more vulnerable to injury during arthroplasty surgery.

EXAMINER: What is the role of a CT scan in planning an operation for DDH?[4]

CANDIDATE 1: CT scans can be used to determine the available acetabular coverage and to estimate the degree of femoral anteversion.

CANDIDATE 2: CT scans are useful in assessing available bone stock, and the morphology, dimensions and orientation of both the acetabulum and femur.

Any leg length discrepancy can be precisely evaluated and allow for design of custom femoral implants.

Various measurements include: femoral neck shaft angle, anteversion of the femoral neck, medial head offset, position of the isthmus and height can be measured.

The AP size of the acetabulum as measured by CT is often different from the supero-inferior size evaluated on plain radiographs.

Proximal femoral anteversion is calculated by measuring the angle between the posterior bicondylar axis and the mediolateral dimensions of the medullary canal 20 mm above the lesser trochanter.

EXAMINER: These measurements are useful to know but how are they actually going to help you to plan surgery?

CANDIDATE: In the acetabulum following the abnormal anatomy too closely might lead to anterior instability if the cup is overanteverted. It is important to recognize that a substantial amount of acetabular anteversion and deformity can be present with a relatively normal-looking AP pelvic radiograph.

In addition femoral anteversion may be difficult to recognize. Even in normal-looking AP radiographs a significant amount of anteversion may be present. Attempting to implant an uncemented stem in a deformed anteverted femur may result in a proximal femoral fracture.

EXAMINER: What are the technical difficulties in performing a THA in a DDH patient?

CANDIDATE: Crowe type II and III hips have a marked superolateral rim deficiency and anterior wall defect. Bulk autografting of the superolateral acetabulum with bone from the femoral head can be used to increase the cover and stability of the acetabular component. The graft and its bed need careful preparation, stable fixation and precise positioning. Graft resorption can occur leading to cup migration and loosening.

Although it is technically difficult for anatomical placement of the acetabular component the forces on the THA are significantly reduced. Linde et al. found a 42% rate of loosening of cemented Charnley components after a mean of 9 years if the component was positioned outside the true acetabulum compared with 13% if placed inside.[5,6]

EXAMINER: Any other options to deal with deficient superior coverage of the cup?

CANDIDATE: A small, uncemented cup can be placed in a high hip centre location. In this position the cup is completely covered with host bone and avoids the need for grafting. Disadvantages include decreased polyethylene thickness associated with a small acetabular component, difficulties with correction of leg length inequality and altered hip biomechanics. Hip instability is increased due to the use of a small femoral head component along with the risk of femoral–pelvic impingement either in flexion or extension.

EXAMINER: What do we mean by cotyloplasty?

CANDIDATE: Cotyloplasty involves a deliberate fracture of the medial wall of the acetabulum in order to place the acetabular component within the available iliac bone. The acetabulum is advanced medially by the creation of a controlled comminuted fracture of the medial acetabular wall. Mixed results have been reported but there is a worry that future revisions may be difficult because issues with restoration of bone stock have not been addressed.[7]

EXAMINER: How do you preoperatively plan for DDH surgery?

CANDIDATE: On the acetabulum side the position of the true acetabulum should be identified and a decision made whether to restore the acetabulum to its true position or not. The degree of anteversion of the acetabulum should be defined as well as the adequacy of bone stock for satisfactory cup fixation and coverage.

Preoperative planning would also include an estimation of the acetabular component size, the preferred method of fixation (cement/uncemented) and need for bone graft.

On the femoral side the size of the femoral canal and the need for special or custom implants should be assessed.

The need for femoral shortening should be made preoperatively. The method and amount of femoral shortening needs to be worked out beforehand.

Preoperative planning should also include the surgical approach to be used, solutions to deal with the hypoplastic acetabulum and femur, management of LLD and restoration of abductor function.

EXAMINER: What is the effect of anteversion of the femoral stem on THA?[8]

CANDIDATE: When there is more than 40° of anteversion, a corrective rotational osteotomy or a modular implant in which the version of the femoral neck can be varied may be necessary.

EXAMINER: That's not really the question I asked.

CANDIDATE: A large amount of femoral anteversion increases the risk of dislocation.

EXAMINER: That's correct but not the whole story. You have already partly answered the question earlier on.

CANDIDATE: I am sorry, I don't understand.[9]

EXAMINER: Attempting to implant an uncemented stem in a deformed femur may result in a proximal femoral fracture. In this situation you may want to use either a cemented or modular stem that allows control of anteversion. Also excessive anteversion of the femoral component can lead to internal rotational contracture of the hip.

EXAMINER: How do you correct length inequality in DDH?

CANDIDATE: With Crowe type III and IV hips if the cup is placed in the anatomical position femoral shortening is required. Without femoral shortening it is very difficult to reduce the prosthetic head into the acetabular component because of soft tissue contractures.

If one attempts to fully correct a significant leg length discrepancy a sciatic nerve palsy may occur. If permanent this can be a disabling complication from surgery and which patients are less willing to accept these days. The exact amount of lengthening that results in sciatic nerve palsy is not known. Acute limb lengthening of more than 2–4 cm during arthroplasty is associated with an increased risk of neural injury. Therefore as a general rule the hip should be lengthened the minimum amount required to re-establish reasonable function and hip stability. Any lengthening more than 4 cm becomes very risky for a sciatic nerve injury and is generally not advised.

Shortening is performed either by sequential resecting of the proximal femur or by performing a shortening subtrochanteric osteotomy.

Sequential proximal resection results in a small straight femoral tube with a small metaphyseal flare which is usually unsuitable for an uncemented femoral implant. Typically a small cemented DDH stem needs to be used with a straight proximal medial geometry and without a metaphyseal flare.

Advantages of a subtrochanteric shortening osteotomy include preservation of the metaphyseal femoral region (which provides most of the rotational stability of the implant) and allowing concomitant correction of angular and anteversion deformities. It is technically difficult and there is a risk of non-union.

EXAMINER: How do you reduce the risk of non-union?

CANDIDATE: Different subtrochanteric osteotomy geometries can be used. These include transverse, oblique, stepcut and double Chevron osteotomies. A transverse osteotomy is simplest and the resected bone can be used as an onlay graft.

Avoiding the use of a cemented stem prevents the risk of the cement interfering with healing of the osteotomy site. A press fit achieves distal fixation of the prosthesis. Strut allograft and circlage cables may also be needed for support.

EXAMINER: What are the principles of revision hip surgery with DDH?

CANDIDATE: Two major concerns are deficient acetabular bone stock and the position of the acetabular cup particularly if the centre of the hip has not been restored during the primary procedure.

Several surgeons have advocated the use of a high hip centre in order to take advantage of the remaining bone stock and to avoid the use of a structured graft.

However, a high hip centre does not correct leg length discrepancy, does not provide good bone stock for revision hip surgery and is associated with early acetabular loosening and a higher rate of dislocation because of ischial impingement.

The pattern of bone loss associated with DDH is a reduced AP diameter combined with poor superior support. This loss is further increased by surgical bone loss at the time of the index operation, migration of the cup and osteolysis.

Bone graft would need to be ordered along with special equipment such as universal screwdrivers, screw extractors, high speed burrs and metal cutters.

Endnotes

1. It is not unreasonable to mention the patient's age and when the radiograph was taken to the examiners with the first radiograph shown in the viva exam. Just like the trauma viva and the 'I would initially manage the patient with the ATLS protocol' if you keep repeating the catch phrase it will severely annoy the examiners. Once is reasonable to let the examiners know it is part of your standard practice. Any more is irritating and wastes time.

2. The score is 6–7, as the candidate didn't classify the left side correctly. If the candidate had correctly identified a Hartofilakidis I hip it would be more towards a 7–8 mark. The candidate would have correctly used two classification systems to grade the severity of the DDH. He or she has already pre-empted questions on DDH classification.

3. The examiners have the answers in front of them so it is easy for them to point out the differences between a Hartofilakidis I hip and Hartofilakidis II hip. Unless they had a hip interest the examiners probably wouldn't be familiar with this depth of knowledge in everyday clinical practice. Expanding on this it would then be fair to say this level of knowledge is probably not needed as the viva attempts to standardize answers to a newly qualified day one consultant in a DGH. These are guidelines but unfortunately in real life the exam is an artificial situation and never quite that straightforward.

4. This is probably one of the pre-agreed oral viva questions that the examiners need to ask. The examiners have a set standard answer with various bullet points provided so as to be able to mark candidates accordingly.

5. Linde F, Jensen J, Pilgaard S. Charnley arthroplasty in osteoarthritis secondary to congenital dislocation or subluxation of the hip. *Clin Orthop* 1988;**227**:164–171.

6. The candidate's answer isn't particularly well structured.

7. Candidates can either volunteer this extra information or perhaps wait for the examiners to ask it!

8. Technically the candidate hasn't really answered the question.

9. The candidate is not quite getting what the examiner wants and has just gone a bit blank in the stress of the moment.

Chapter

3

Knee structured oral questions

Michael Maru and Deiary F. Kader

Structured oral examination question 1: TKR in valgus knee

EXAMINER: This is a radiograph of a 72-year-old lady complaining of pain and gradual deformity of both knees. She has been referred to your clinic to be considered for total knee arthroplasty. What can you see? (Figure 3.1.)

CANDIDATE: These are weightbearing anteroposterior (AP) views of a 72-year-old lady demonstrating narrowing of joint spaces with bone-on-bone contact in the lateral compartments of both knees. There is early arthrosis affecting the medial compartments of both knees. There is moderate valgus deformity.

EXAMINER: What conditions are associated with this pattern of joint disease?

CANDIDATE: The valgus deformity of the knee with arthritis is commonly seen in women and in inflammatory joint conditions such as rheumatoid arthritis. It can also occur in primary osteoarthritis, overcorrection of high tibial osteotomy (HTO), post-traumatic arthritis following lateral meniscectomy and osteonecrosis.

EXAMINER: What are the perioperative considerations for total knee arthroplasty in valgus knee?

CANDIDATE: The preoperative assessment should include a thorough history and examination to establish if there are any predisposing factors such as rheumatoid arthritis and the success of non-surgical management. The competency of the knee collateral ligaments and degree of deformity correction should be assessed in order to plan on type of implants. I would use a medial parapatellar because this gives good access to the whole knee and better soft tissue cover. I am aware that a lateral approach can also be used.

EXAMINER: What is the theoretical advantage of a lateral approach?

CANDIDATE: It is a direct approach providing easier access and preserves the neurovascular supply to the extensor mechanism.

EXAMINER: Tell me more about the intraoperative considerations.

CANDIDATE: In valgus knees the lateral femoral condyle is deficient, therefore the femur is internally rotated and tibia is externally rotated. The medial structures are stretched while lateral and posterior structures are contracted. The vastus lateralis acts as a subluxing or dislocating force to the patella. In mild valgus deformity (7–10°) a distal femoral cut of 7° can improve patella tracking and avoid the need for lateral retinacular release. Due to the posterior femoral condyle deficiency, the standard 3° posterior condylar referencing can result in internal rotation of the component. In this situation,

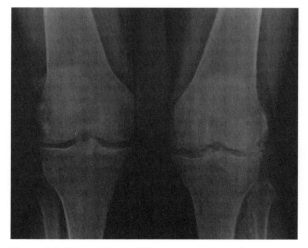

Figure 3.1 Anteroposterior (AP) radiograph bilateral knees.

Postgraduate Orthopaedics: Viva Guide for the FRCS (Tr & Orth) Examination, ed. Paul A. Banaszkiewicz and Deiary F. Kader. Published by Cambridge University Press. © Cambridge University Press 2012.

AP axis (Whiteside line) is used to prevent malrotation in the form of internal rotation. Patients with severe valgus deformity usually require lateral retinacular release to achieve proper patella tracking. With regards to flexion–extension gap, the release of lateral and posterior structures results in increased extension gap requiring a thicker insert which may elevate the joint line. Excessive PCL release usually requires cruciate sacrificing implants in order to balance the knee. With correction of significant valgus deformity, one has to watch for peroneal nerve palsy in the postoperative period.

Arima J, Whiteside LA, McCarthy D, White SE. Femoral rotational alignment based on the AP axis, in TKR in a valgus knee. *J Bone Joint Surg Am* 1995;77:1331–1334.

Structured oral examination question 2: Meniscus – basic science

EXAMINER: Tell me about the anatomy and function of the meniscus.

CANDIDATE: The menisci are crescentic cartilaginous structures interposed between the tibia and femoral condyles. They are triangular in cross-section. The peripheral borders are attached to the joint capsule. The medial meniscus is nearly semicircular with a wider posterior than anterior horn. This is attached anterior to the ACL insertion while the mid aspect is firmly attached to the deep MCL. The lateral meniscus is nearly circular with a larger surface than medial meniscus. The posterior horns of both menisci attach to the posterior intercondylar eminence. The attachment of the lateral meniscus to the capsule is interrupted by the popliteus tendon. Due to the loose attachment to the capsule, the lateral meniscus has twice the excursion of the medial meniscus. The anterior horns of both menisci are connected by intermeniscal ligaments.

Histologically, the menisci have an extracellular matrix composed mainly of water (70%) and primarily type 1 collagen fibres (60%), proteoglycans, elastin and glycoproteins. The main cellular component is the fibrochondrocytes that synthesize and maintain extracellular matrix. The blood supply to the meniscus comes from the lateral, middle and medial geniculate vessels with 20–30% of the peripheral portion being vascular. The main functions of the menisci are load transmission with estimated 50% in extension and 85% in flexion, joint conformity and articular congruity, distribution of synovial fluid aiding nutrition and joint lubrication. The menisci also have proprioceptive function,

act as shock absorbers and prevent soft tissue impingement during joint motion.

EXAMINER: What are the vascular zones of menisci?

CANDIDATE: The menisci are relatively avascular structures with peripheral blood supply from the premeniscal capillary plexus formed by branches from lateral and medial geniculate vessels. Studies have shown that the degree of peripheral vascular penetration is 10–30% of medial meniscal width and 10–25% of lateral meniscal width. This gives rise to the three zones of meniscal vasculature from peripheral to central, namely red–red, red–white and white–white. Therefore, peripheral tears are suitable for repair while central tears are not suitable due to lack of healing capacity.

Arnoczky SP, Warren RF. Microvasculature of the human meniscus. *Am J Sports Med* 1982;**10**:90–95.

EXAMINER: These are images belonging to a young professional footballer. What can you see? (Figure 3.2.)

CANDIDATE: This is a T2-weighted MRI of the knee showing sagittal and coronal images. There is absence of 'bow tie sign' of the medial meniscus and there is 'double PCL sign' suggestive of bucket-handle tear of medial meniscus.

EXAMINER: How would you manage this patient?

CANDIDATE: I would start by taking a detailed history and clinical examination . . . [Examiner interrupts]

EXAMINER: How would you treat this patient? [Examiner getting impatient]

CANDIDATE: I would offer this patient EUA, arthroscopy, repair or excision of bucket-handle tear.

EXAMINER: Good. Are you aware of any meniscal repair techniques?

CANDIDATE: The four main meniscal repair methods are open repair, inside out, outside in and all inside. The 'outside in' method is versatile and safe. [Examiner interrupts again]

EXAMINER: Let's move on . . .

Structured oral examination question 3: Infected total knee arthroplasty (TKA)

EXAMINER: A 78-year-old lady who underwent left TKA 2 years ago is referred to your Painful Arthroplasty Clinic because of increasing pain, stiffness and recurrent swelling of the left knee for 4 months. Prior to onset of symptoms, she was very active

(a)

(b)

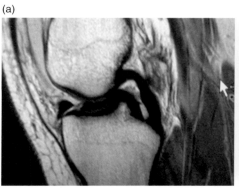
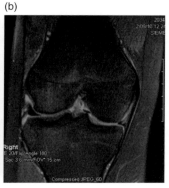

Figures 3.2a and 3.2b T2-weighted sagittal and coronal MRI scan images of knee.

(a)

(b)

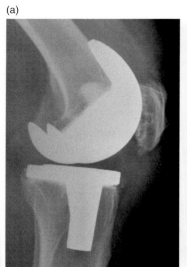
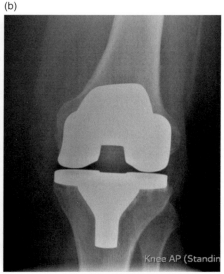

Figures 3.3a and 3.3b Anteroposterior (AP) and lateral radiographs of left TKA.

and enjoyed long-distance walking. She is systemically well. These are the plain radiographs. (Figure 3.3.)

CANDIDATE: This is an AP and lateral radiograph showing a cemented cruciate sacrificing total knee arthroplasty taken on 16/8/11. There is an area of subchondral radiolucency underneath the medial side of the tibial component. There is no obvious periosteal reaction. Both components appear to be well fixed. I would like to see the initial postoperative radiograph and compare it with the most recent radiograph.

EXAMINER: This is the most recent radiograph and there are no other postoperative radiographs available! What would you like to do for this patient?

CANDIDATE: I would start by taking a detailed history of the perioperative events, general health as well current problem. I would like to know the date of index operation,

if there was prolonged discharge from the wound, redness or persistent swelling in the immediate postoperative period. A pain-free interval after the operation followed by sudden deterioration may be suggestive of haematogenous spread precipitated by bacteraemia from UTI, URTI or dental procedure. I would also like to know the pattern of pain: mechanical or non-mechanical and whether it's relieved by rest. The clinical examination should be focused on identifying instability and localizing the problem.

EXAMINER: So you think this joint is infected?

CANDIDATE: My working diagnosis is infected TKA. My main differential diagnoses are aseptic loosening, inflammatory arthropathy in a prosthetic joint, instability and malalignment.

EXAMINER: How would you investigate this patient?

CANDIDATE: I would start with routine blood investigations including CRP and ESR.

EXAMINER: How sensitive and specific are these?

CANDIDATE: In a recent systematic review in the American JBJS by Berbari et al., the pooled sensitivities for ESR and CRP were 75% and 88% respectively while the pooled specificities were 70% and 74% respectively. The study also reported that interleukin 6 (IL-6) level assay was more sensitive and specific at 97% and 91% respectively. If the blood inflammatory markers are elevated, I would proceed with radioisotope bone scan and arrange for alignment check under image intensifier and joint aspiration in theatre.

EXAMINER: Are you aware of any guidelines regarding diagnosis of periprosthetic joint infections?

CANDIDATE: I am aware of the AAOS clinical guideline practice summary for diagnosis of periprosthetic joint infection of the knee. The working group strongly recommend:

- Testing ESR and CRP.
- Joint aspiration.
- The use of intraoperative frozen sections.
- Obtaining multiple intraoperative cultures.
- Against initiating antibiotic treatment until after cultures.
- Against the use of intraoperative Gram stain.

Nuclear imaging was weakly recommended as an option in patients in whom diagnosis of periprosthetic joint infection has not been established and who are not scheduled for re-operation.

Berbari E, Mabry T, Tsaras G et al. Inflammatory blood laboratory levels as markers of prosthetic joint infection: a systematic review and meta-analysis. J Bone Joint Surg Am 2010;92-A:2102–2109.

Della Valle C, Parvizi J, Bauer TW et al. Diagnosis of periprosthetic joint infections of the hip and knee. J Am Acad Orthopaed Surg 2010;18(12):760–770.

EXAMINER: Let's say the aspiration yields heavy growth of Staphylococcus aureus. How would you proceed from here?

CANDIDATE: With raised inflammatory markers and a positive bone scan and aspiration, I would offer this patient two-stage revision total knee replacement. I have opted for two-stage procedure because the investigations show severe infection caused by a virulent organism. The first stage would be extraction of the implants, debridement of joint and bone followed by application of antibiotic-loaded spacer. Antibiotic treatment depending on sensitivity is started after the first

stage usually for a period of 4–6 weeks with close monitoring of CRP and ESR as well as clinical progress. The timing of the second stage depends on achieving normal CRP and ESR, healing of wounds or sinus and general well-being of the patient. Recent studies have shown that two-stage revision has better infection eradication rate and no difference in clinical outcome (knee scores, range of motion) compared with single stage (Jämsen et al.). Some of the disadvantages of two-stage revision are soft tissue scarring, dislocation of spacers, disuse atrophy and loss of bone density which makes the second-stage procedure difficult. I am aware that some surgeons have reported encouraging results from single-stage revision such as Buechel et al. who reported infection eradication rate of 90.9% over an average follow-up of 10.2 years. This compared favourably with the results of two-stage revision surgery while remaining cost-effective. However, I believe that single-stage revision should be reserved for cases where the organism and its sensitivities are known and it is of low virulence; in the very elderly patients and those with multiple medical problems.

[Debrief: The examiner has allowed the candidate to talk about the topic without interrupting.]

Jämsen E, Stogiannidis I, Malmivaara A et al. Outcome of prosthesis exchange for infected knee arthroplasty: the effect of treatment approach. Acta Orthop 2009;80 (1):67–77.

Buechel FF, Femino FP, D'Alessio J. Primary exchange revision arthroplasty for infected total knee replacement: a long-term study. Am J Orthop (Belle Mead NJ) 2004;33 (4):190–198; discussion 198.

Structured oral examination question 4: Unicondylar knee arthroplasty (UKA) versus high tibial osteotomy (HTO)

EXAMINER: This is a radiograph of a 42-year-old man who is a bricklayer. He complains of pain over medial aspect of knee which has failed non-surgical management. He has come to your clinic for a consultation. What can you see? (Figure 3.4.)

CANDIDATE: This is a weightbearing AP radiograph of left knee demonstrating moderate medial compartment osteoarthritis. The lateral compartment appears normal. There is a varus deformity of less than 10°. I would like to take a history and examine the patient. The examination is focused mainly on localizing the tenderness, range of motion, if the varus deformity is correctable and stability of knee.

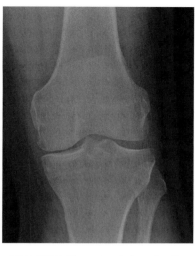

Figure 3.4
Anteroposterior (AP) radiograph left knee.

EXAMINER: The patient is fit and well, states that the pain is affecting his job and he would like to consider a surgical option. What would you offer him?

CANDIDATE: The options of surgical management once conservative measures have failed include HTO, unicondylar knee arthroplasty or total knee replacement. Since this patient has a high-demand physical job, I would offer him HTO.

EXAMINER: What are the prerequisites of HTO?

CANDIDATE: A physiological age of < 60 years, fixed varus deformity < 15° or valgus deformity < 12°, fixed flexion deformity of < 15°, > 90° flexion.

EXAMINER: Are you aware of any contraindication for HTO?

CANDIDATE: The main contraindications are inflammatory arthropathy such as rheumatoid arthritis and psoriatic arthropathy, incompetent medial collateral ligament or ACL, large varus thrust with coronal subluxation of > 1 cm, severe OA of medial compartment or lateral compartment/PFJ and more than 20° of correction. Obesity is also a contraindication because valgus knee is poorly tolerated due to medial thigh contact.

EXAMINER: The patient tells you that he has heard about partial knee replacement and is keen to consider the option. How do you proceed?

CANDIDATE: I would explain to the patient that UKA is an option; however, I would not recommend UKA for this particular patient because the highly physically demanding job could result in accelerated wear of UKA.

EXAMINER: So which patients would you offer UKA?

CANDIDATE: The indications and prerequisites for HTO and UKA are more or less the same. However women prefer the UKA because they do not tolerate the angular deformity created by HTO very well. In addition, patients who have low physical demand may benefit from UKA.

EXAMINER: Are you aware of any comparative studies of HTO versus UKA?

CANDIDATE: Yes. A recent review by Dettoni et al. reported that a few studies show slightly better results for UKA in terms of survivorship and functional outcome. Nevertheless, the differences are not remarkable, the study methods are not homogeneous and most of the papers report on closing wedge HTOs. They concluded that with the correct indications, both treatments produce durable and predictable outcomes in the treatment of medial unicompartmental arthrosis of the knee. There is no evidence of superior results of one treatment over the other.

Dettoni F, Bonasia DE, Castoldi F et al. High tibial osteotomy versus unicompartmental knee arthroplasty for medial compartment arthrosis of the knee: a review of the literature. Iowa Orthop J 2010;30:131–140.

EXAMINER: Let's say this patient has decided to go ahead with HTO. What type of HTO would you perform and why?

CANDIDATE: I am conversant with closing wedge osteotomy. This was considered the gold standard in the past and may entail proximal fibular osteotomy or disruption of tibial–fibular joint. It has the risk of peroneal nerve injury, there is also loss of bone stock making it technically difficult to perform TKA. Due to these reasons, the open wedge osteotomy has become popular recently even though it has the disadvantage of having to use bone graft and late collapse with loss of correction. No conclusions can be drawn on which techniques are to be preferred when comparing between closing wedge with opening wedge as none has shown significantly better outcome over the other.

Amendola A, Bonasia DE. Results of high tibial osteotomy: review of the literature. Int Orthop 2010;34(2):155–160.

EXAMINER: You mentioned difficulty with conversion of HTO to TKA. Tell me more about this.

CANDIDATE: Before the introduction of internal fixation and early motion in HTO, cast immobilization was part of the postoperative treatment and this resulted in patella baja following a lateral closing wedge osteotomy. This complication was probably due to contracture of the patellar tendon during

(a)

(b)

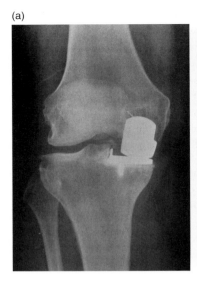

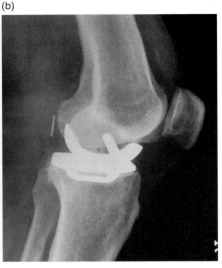

Figures 3.5a and 3.5b Anteroposterior (AP) and lateral radiographs UKA.

cast immobilization. More recent studies show that closing wedge osteotomy increases patellar height, whereas opening wedge osteotomy lowers patellar height and this can have implications following TKA. Van Raaij *et al.* performed a systematic review and reported prolonged surgical time, extra-operative procedures and less postoperative knee range of motion (ROM), but no increase in revision surgeries for patients receiving TKA after prior HTO compared with patients receiving primary TKA.

van Raaij TM, Reijman M, Furlan AD, Verhaar JAN. Total knee arthroplasty after high tibial osteotomy. A systematic review. *BMC Musculoskeletal Disord* 2009;**10**:88.

http://www.wheelessonline.com/image3/i1/knee6.jpg

Structured oral examination question 5: Unicondylar knee arthroplasty (UKA) versus total knee replacement (TKR)

EXAMINER: Have a look at these radiographs. What can you see? (Figure 3.5.)

CANDIDATE: Non-weightbearing AP and lateral radiographs of 54-year-old man showing a left medial UKA in situ. The components look well fixed and aligned. There are no obvious periprosthetic fractures. The lateral compartment and PFJ look relatively normal.

EXAMINER: What else can you see?

CANDIDATE: (A bit hesitant and moves closer to the computer screen. This is followed by period of silence before the examiner prompts.)

EXAMINER: The patient tells you that he fell while coming down the stairs sustaining injury to the left knee. He complains of global pain and swelling of the left knee and inability to flex it. What's going through your mind?

CANDIDATE: There is a faint radio-opaque line behind the femoral component. I would like to compare this with previous radiographs. The history and radiographs are suggestive of dislocation of mobile bearing spacer.

EXAMINER: Good. What are the advantages of UKA?

CANDIDATE: Some of the advantages of UKA are:

- Preservation of bone stock.
- Faster recovery and return to normal function.
- Prevention of PFJ overload.
- Retention of knee kinematics and increased flexion.
- Less blood loss, infection rate and reduced risk of thromboembolism.
- Easier revision to TKA than HTO.

EXAMINER: Does UKA perform as well as TKA?

CANDIDATE: Careful patient selection for UKA is critical if consistent and reliable results are to be obtained. In the early 1980s UKA became gradually unpopular mainly because of poor results due to poor patient selection, operative technique and polyethylene wear. With improvement in patient selection, operative technique and prosthesis design, the results of UKA became comparable to TKA. Latest reports show highly satisfactory survival rate and patient satisfaction for UKA particularly in activities requiring ROM such as going down stairs and kneeling. In a recent report from the Finnish

Arthroplasty Registry, Koskinen *et al.* published a 10-year survival rate of between 53% and 81% depending on prosthetic model implanted. The UK National Joint Registry (NJR) 8th Report showed an overall 5-year revision rate of TKA and UKA of 3% and 9.4% respectively.

Koskinen E, Paavolainen P, Eskelinen A, Pulkkinen P, Remes V. Unicondylar knee replacement for primary osteoarthritis. A prospective follow-up study of 1,819 patients from the Finnish Arthroplasty Register. *Acta Ortho Scand* 2007;**78**(1):128–135.

UK National Joint Registry (NJR) 8th Report. 2011; www.njrcentre.org.uk

Structured oral examination question 6: Anterior cruciate ligament (ACL) and posterior cruciate ligament (PCL) reconstruction

EXAMINER: These images belong to a 26-year-old rugby player. He gives a history of falling awkwardly on to his left knee after a heavy tackle. What can you see? (Figure 3.6.)

CANDIDATE: These are plain radiographs and MRI of the right knee. The most obvious abnormality is cortical disruption at the site of PCL insertion with displaced avulsed fragment. The lateral radiograph shows this is a large fragment which is displaced into the joint.

EXAMINER: How would you treat this patient?

CANDIDATE: I would offer this patient reattachment of the PCL avulsion through open procedure.

EXAMINER: What approach would you use?

CANDIDATE Posterior approach.

EXAMINER: Tell me about posterior approach to the knee.

CANDIDATE: The indications include removal of popliteal cysts and neoplasms, posterior synovectomy, open reduction and internal fixation of posterior tibial plateau shear fractures, fixation of bone avulsions associated with a posterior cruciate ligament (PCL) injury, repair of posterior vascular injuries, and more recently, posterior inlay PCL reconstructions. The patient is usually positioned prone with tourniquet high up in the thigh. The lazy S-shaped incision is made starting posterolaterally along the border of biceps femoris tendon crossing the popliteal fossa and ending posteromedially at the posterior border of semitendinosus tendon. The deep fascia is incised in the midline. The small saphenous nerve is identified

with accompanying sural nerve that must be preserved. The sural nerve is traced proximally where it pierces deep fascia from the tibial nerve trunk. At the apex of the fossa, the common peroneal nerve separates from tibial nerve. The tibial nerve lies posterior to the popliteal vein which in turn is superficial to popliteal artery. Popliteal vessels are displaced laterally and this usually requires ligation of middle geniculate and superior medial geniculate vessels. The medial head of gastrocnemius is identified, traced proximally and can be detached from its origin then retracted towards midline to expose the medial joint capsule. Similarly the lateral head of gastrocnemius can be detached to expose the posterolateral corner of the joint. The main structures at risk are the popliteal vessels, small saphenous vein and common peroneal nerve and tibial nerve.

EXAMINER: Have you been involved in any arthroscopic PCL reconstruction?

CANDIDATE: Yes (despite never having seen one!)

EXAMINER: What is the optimum tunnel placement?

CANDIDATE: The tunnel placement in PCL reconstruction depends on whether it is single-bundle or double-bundle reconstruction . . .

EXAMINER: Tell me about the one you have seen.

CANDIDATE: The optimum placement of PCL tunnel is controversial. The literature shows that the femoral tunnel for posterolateral bundle reconstruction should be placed at 1.30 o'clock . . .

EXAMINER: Are you sure? (Realizing that the candidate is bluffing.)

CANDIDATE: To be honest I have not seen many of these but I will check on it.

EXAMINER: Let's move on. Now tell me about the optimum tunnel placement for single bundle ACL reconstruction.

CANDIDATE: The principles of ACL reconstruction are placement of tunnel anatomically and isometrically, using biologically active grafts which are adequately tensioned to allow early rehabilitation. In single-bundle reconstruction, the aim is to place tunnel at the footprint of the posterolateral bundle of ACL. The anteromedial bundle is thought to be the most isometric but most surgeons feel that it's important to replace the posterolateral bundle. For the femoral tunnel the isometric point lies at about 10 to 10.30 o'clock for right knee and 1.30 to 2 for left knee. The most common mistake is to

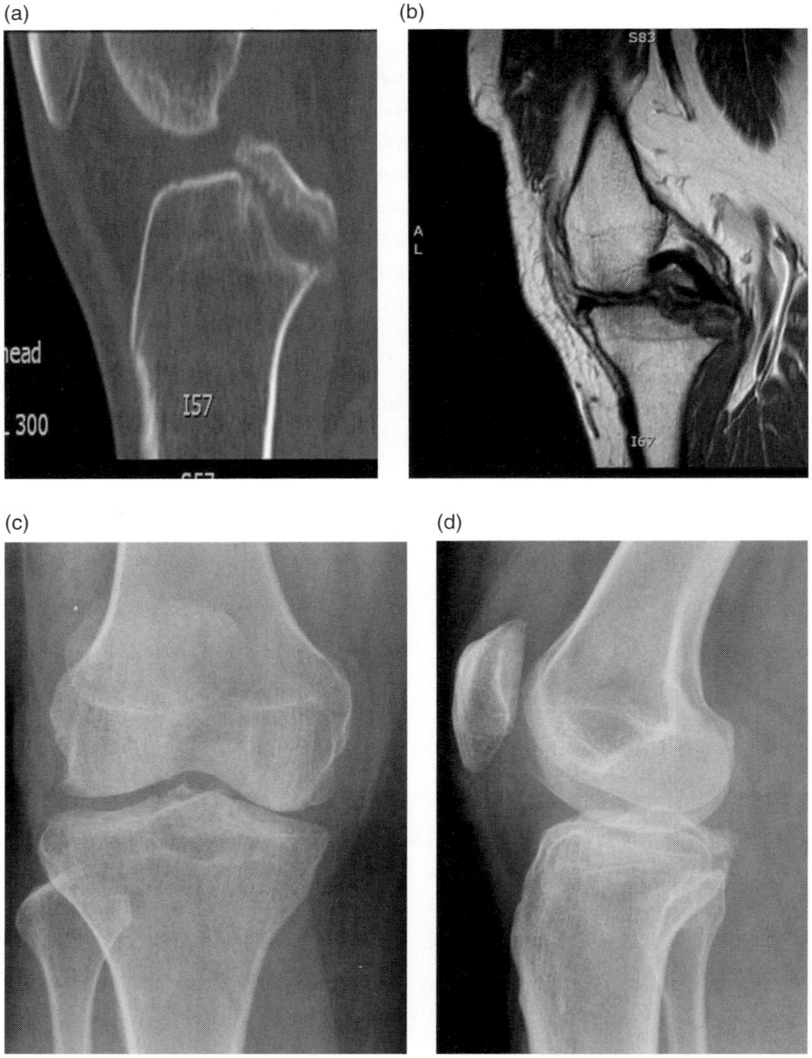

(a)

(b)

Figures 3.6a, 3.6b, 3.6c and 3.6d CT, MRI and plain radiographs of left knee.

(c)

(d)

place femoral tunnel too anterior or 'resident's ridge'. This restricts flexion of the knee and may result in elongation of graft. Similarly, too posterior tunnel placement results in excessive tightening of graft when knee is extended. It's been shown that abnormally narrow intercondylar notch correlates directly with increased incidence of ACL tears. Careful assessment of notch should be done prior to graft insertion using a pin to ensure no impingement on lateral femoral condyle. The presence of impingement with correct placement of tunnels necessitates notchplasty of the anterior portion of lateral femoral condyle.

EXAMINER: Which graft would you use and why?

CANDIDATE: I would use a hamstring four-strand autograft. The two main biological autografts used in ACL reconstruction are hamstring and bone patella tendon bone (BPTB) graft. The BPTB graft has the advantage of being easy to harvest, rigid fixation and faster integration as it uses bone to bone healing. However, it has donor site morbidity which includes anterior knee pain in 30–50%, patellar tendonitis 3–5%, patellar fracture and patella baja. The hamstring graft on the other hand has less donor site morbidity, can be harvested from a small incision and can be passed relatively easily. However it has slow healing because of tendon to bone incorporation which takes 8 to 12 weeks. It can also result in hamstring weakness and saphenous nerve injury. There are several studies comparing outcome of BPTB versus hamstring graft. Most studies show arthroscopic reconstruction with either graft results in similar functional outcome but increased morbidity in BPTB in form of early OA and increased knee laxity with radiographic femoral tunnel wide in hamstring graft.

Feller JA, Webster KE. A randomized comparison of patellar tendon and hamstring tendon anterior cruciate ligament reconstruction. *Am J Sports Med* 2003;**31**:564–573.

Howell SM, Taylor MA. Failure of reconstruction of the anterior cruciate ligament due to impingement by the intercondylar roof. *J Bone Joint Surg Am* 1993;**75**-A:1044.

Pinczewski LA, Deehan DJ, Salmon LJ, Russell VJ, Clingeleffer A. A five-year comparison of patellar tendon versus four-strand hamstring tendon autograft for arthroscopic reconstruction of the anterior cruciate ligament. *Am J Sports Med* 2002;**30**:523–536.

Debrief: With a thorough understanding of ACL reconstruction, the candidate has recovered from a bad start of this viva. Candidates should be honest and be prepared to say they have not seen some operations.

Structured oral examination question 7: Revision knee replacement

EXAMINER: Have a look at these images and tell me what you can see. (Figure 3.7.)

CANDIDATE: These are AP and lateral radiographs of failed left total knee replacement. The implants appear to be loose with widespread osteolysis and bone loss in the femur and tibia. The tibial base plate is in varus and extended. There is notching of the anterior cortex of femur. There is calcification of soft tissues including the popliteal vessels. I would like to see immediate postoperative and most recent radiographs for comparison. The radiographs are suggestive of infection until proven otherwise.

EXAMINER: Good. You investigate this patient and come up with a diagnosis of aseptic loosening. The patient is keen to consider single-stage revision surgery. What are your concerns with regards to these radiographs?

CANDIDATE: I am concerned about several factors, namely:

- The state of the collateral ligaments (stability).
- Soft tissues and vascular status of the limb.
- The extensive bone loss.

The collateral ligaments are likely to be dysfunctional and especially the MCL therefore a constrained knee replacement may be required. The soft tissues appear contracted and calcified which may lead to wound complications. The bone loss will require bone graft, augmented or stemmed implants.

EXAMINER: Are you aware of any classification system for bone loss around knee arthroplasty?

(a)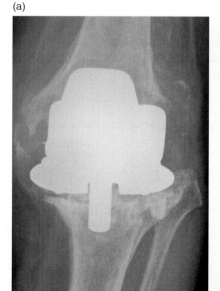

(b)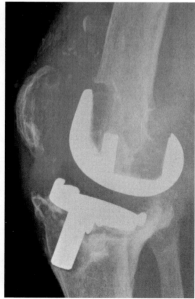

Figures 3.7a and 3.7b Anteroposterior (AP) and lateral radiographs of left TKA.

CANDIDATE: The most commonly used classification system is that of the Anderson Orthopaedic Research Institute (AORI) which classifies the femur (F) and tibia (T) separately as follows:

Type 1 – Intact metaphyseal bone with minor defects which will not compromise the stability of a revision component.

Type 2 – Damaged metaphyseal bone. Loss of cancellous bone in the metaphyseal segment which will need to be filled with cement, augments or a bone graft at revision in order to restore the joint line. Defects can occur in one femoral condyle or tibial plateau (2A) or in both condyles or plateaux (2B).

Type 3 – Deficient metaphyseal bone. Bone loss which comprises a major portion of either condyle or plateau. These defects are occasionally associated with detachment of the collateral or patellar ligaments and usually require long-stemmed revision implants with bone grafts or a custom-made hinged prosthesis.

Engh G. Bone defect classification. In GA Engh, CH Rorabeck (Eds), *Revision Total Knee Arthroplasty*. Baltimore, MD: Lippincott Williams and Wilkins, 1997, pp. 63–120.

EXAMINER: You mentioned that a constrained implant may be required. What are the levels of constraints?

CANDIDATE: The constraint ladder within knee implant design includes:

PCL retaining (cruciate retaining or CR). Rotating platform more constrained due to conformity.

↓

PCL substituting (posterior stabilized or PS).

↓

Unlinked constrained condylar implant (varus–valgus constrained or VVC) provides anteroposterior and varus–valgus stability (substitute for deficient collaterals), e.g. constrained condylar knee (LCCK, NexGen), TC3.

↓

Linked, constrained condylar implant (rotating-hinge knee or RHK). Rarely indicated. Used for global instability (total collateral disruption/recurvatum) and severe distal femoral bone loss, osteolysis/fracture.

EXAMINER: What are the indications of PCL substituting posterior stabilized (PS) implants?

CANDIDATE: Some of the indications of PCL sacrificing implants are:

- Previous patellectomy.
- Rheumatoid arthritis.

- Post-traumatic osteoarthritis with stiffness.
- Previous HTO and large deformity.
- Over-released PCL.

EXAMINER: What are the advantages of PS over CR (cruciate retaining) design?

CANDIDATE: The advantages are:

- Conforming surfaces allowing roll-back.
- No component slide.
- Provides a degree of VVC.
- The cam–post mechanism improves anterior–posterior stability.
- Facilitates any deformity correction.
- Uses more congruent joint surfaces than CR, which reduces wear.
- Better range of motion.
- Technically easier than CR and reproducible.
- Higher degree of flexion.

EXAMINER: Are you aware of any current literature regarding performance of PS and CR implants?

CANDIDATE: There are limited studies in the literature comparing the outcomes of the two designs. Most of the studies are characterized by a small number of patients, different outcome measures, poor randomization and comparing designs of different manufacturers. Range of motion appears to be the only common outcome parameter. A meta-analysis by Jacobs *et al.* showed a difference in range of motion and reproduction angle favouring posterior stabilized designs over PCL retention designs 1 year postoperatively. However, it is uncertain whether this observation is of clinical relevance. It seems that in patients with functional PCL the decision as to which design is chosen depends largely on the favour and training of the surgeon.

Jacobs WC, Clement DJ, Wymenga AB. Retention versus removal of the posterior cruciate ligament in total knee replacement. *Act Orth* 2005;**76**(6):757–768.

EXAMINER: (Going back to the radiographs.) What are the principles of management of bone loss in revision knee replacement in this patient?

CANDIDATE: The options of management of the extensive bone loss are:

1. The use of cement, either alone or combined with screws and mesh.
2. The use of bone grafting with structural or morsellized graft.
3. The use of modular augmentation of the components with wedges or blocks of metal. Recent studies show modular

porous-coated press-fit metaphyseal sleeves may be used to fill AORI type 2 and 3 defects and provide for stable ingrowth.

4. The utilization of custom-made, tumour or hinge implants.

The method of reconstruction and the materials for revision surgery are largely dependent on the potential for future further revision and the life expectancy, functional demand and comorbidities of the patient. In this patient who is reasonably young restoration of bone stock is preferable, because of likelihood of further revision surgery.

Structured oral examination question 8: Patellar instability

EXAMINER: A 17-year-old lady is referred to your Patella clinic by the GP due to recurrent bilateral patellar dislocation. How would you assess this patient?

CANDIDATE: I would start by taking a detailed history followed by clinical examination. In the history, I would enquire about age at first dislocation, frequency of dislocations, traumatic or atraumatic, any associated syndromes such as bone or connective tissue dysplasia and generalized joint laxity. I would also enquire about any mechanical symptoms, the presence and localization of pain.

EXAMINER: What are risk factors for patellar instability?

CANDIDATE: The risk factors for patellar instability are:

1. Bony factors (static)

    Trochlear dysplasia.
    Hypoplastic femoral condyle.
    Patellar shape.
    Patella alta.

2. Malalignment

    Patellar malalignment is an abnormal rotational or translational deviation of the patella along any axis.
    External tibial torsion/foot pronation.
    Increased femoral anteversion and increased genu valgum.
    Increased Q angle or abnormal tibial tuberosity–trochlear groove (TT–TG) distance.

3. Soft tissue (dynamic)

    Ligamentous laxity (medial patellofemoral ligament rupture/insufficiency).

4. Abnormal gait

    Walking with valgus thrust.

5. Genetic factors such as connective tissue disorder syndromes.

EXAMINER: Tell me about the most important static stabilizer of the patella.

CANDIDATE: The primary static restraint to the lateral patellar displacement is medial patellofemoral ligament. It provides 50% of the total medial restraining force. MPFL sectioning can lead to substantial changes in patellar tracking. It originates from the area between the medial epicondyle and adductor tubercle and inserts onto the proximal two-thirds of the patella. The average length of the ligament is 5.5 cm. During acute patellar dislocation there is a 90–95% incidence of damage to the MPFL. Femoral attachment is commonly affected. In the past 10 years, MPFL reconstruction has become a popular procedure for treatment of recurrent patellar dislocation.

EXAMINER: How would you investigate this patient?

CANDIDATE: I would perform the following investigations:

1. A lateral radiograph is the most helpful view for assessment of patellar tilt, height and trochlear depth.
2. Axial radiographs (Merchant's view) to assess patellar tilt angle (normal $< 10°$), congruence, sulcus angle (normal 138°) and trochlear dysplasia.
3. MRI for articular lesion and state of MPFL.
4. CT scan to assess:

    - Femoral anteversion (normal 5–15)
    - Tibial torsion.
    - TT–TG distance more than 15–20 mm is significant.
    - Patellar tilt.
    - Trochlear depth.

EXAMINER: What are the principles and methods of distal realignment procedures?

CANDIDATE: The three main groups of realignment procedure as determined by direction of tibial tubercle (TT) transfer are:

- Medial transfer to treat malalignment.
- Anteromedial transfer for malalignment and PFJ chondrosis.
- Anterior when there is distal PFJ chondrosis.

The methods of realignment are:

Elmslie–Trillat: Medialization without posteriorization of the tibial tubercle.

Fulkerson: Medialization with anteriorization of the tibial tubercle in the arthritic patella. The obliquity of the cut depends on the degree of malalignment and arthrosis. A steep cut up to a 60° angle maximizes anteriorization and is useful in patients who have more arthrosis than malalignment.

Hauser: Transfer of the tibial tubercle to a medial, distal and posterior position. This has been abandoned. It increases the PFJ reaction force and causes patellofemoral degenerative joint disease.

Goldthwait 1899–Roux 1888: Medial transposition of the medial half of the patellar tendon, lateral release/medial reefing. Now the lateral half is placed under the medial half and medially (historical procedure) .

Maquet: Anterior transportation of tibial tubercle, which decreases patellofemoral contact forces. Not performed nowadays (historical) as it has a high incidence of skin necrosis, compartment syndrome and no effect on the Q angle.

Structured oral examination question 9: Malalignment of total knee replacement (TKR) components

EXAMINER: Have a look at this image. What can you see? (Figure 3.8.)

CANDIDATE: This is a CT scan of the distal femur showing an axial view of the femoral component of TKR. There is a lot of metal artifact.

EXAMINER: Why do you think a CT scan was done for this patient?

CANDIDATE: CT scan can be performed following TKR to check for loosening or malalignment of the components.

EXAMINER: What do you think of the alignment of this femoral component?

CANDIDATE: The angle formed by the surgical transepicondylar axis and the posterior condylar axis show the femoral component is internally rotated.

EXAMINER: Good. What problems can arise from internal rotation of the femoral component?

CANDIDATE: Rotational alignment of the tibial and femoral component plays an important role in TKR. Once correct frontal alignment and proper soft tissue balancing have been achieved, the rotational placement of the components represents the 'third dimension' in knee TKR. Femoral component malposition has been implicated in patellofemoral

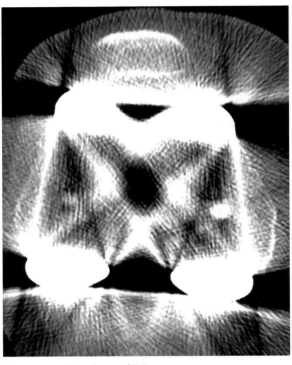

Figures 3.8 CT axial view of TKR.

maltracking following TKR, which is associated with anterior knee pain, subluxation, fracture, wear, and aseptic loosening. It has been suggested that rotating-platform mobile bearings compensate for malrotation between the tibial and femoral components and may, therefore, reduce any associated patellofemoral maltracking. Internal rotation of femoral component by resection of excessive amounts of posterior lateral femoral condyle or insufficient resection of the posterior medial femoral condyle moves the anterior femoral patellar groove portion of the femoral component medially, making it more difficult for a relatively laterally placed patella to be captured by the patellofemoral groove. In addition, internal rotation of the femoral component results in tight flexion gap on the medial side of the knee.

Nicoll D, Rowley DI. Internal rotational error of the tibial component is a major cause of pain after total knee replacement. *J Bone Joint Surg Br* 2010;**92**-B:1238–1244.

Foot and ankle structured oral questions

N. Jane Madeley and Neil Forrest

Structured oral examination question 1: Lateral ligament instability of the ankle

EXAMINER. Tell me what this diagram represents and name the structures labelled 2, 3 and 5. (Figure 4.1.)

CANDIDATE. This diagram is a representation of the lateral aspect of the ankle showing the bony and ligamentous structures. Structure 2 is the anterior talofibular ligament, structure 3 is the calcaneofibular ligament and structure 5 is the posterior distal tibiofibular ligament.

EXAMINER. What structures are injured in a lateral ligament injury?

CANDIDATE. The mechanism is usually a rotational injury with sequential failure of the ligaments from front to back, hence the anterior talofibular ligament or ATFL is most commonly injured followed by the calcaneofibular ligament or CFL and the posterior talofibular ligament is the least frequently injured.

EXAMINER. How would you go about diagnosing a lateral ligament injury to the ankle?

CANDIDATE. In the acute setting I would expect the patient to give a history of an episode of a twisting incident resulting in significant pain and swelling. There may be a history of recurrent sprains and instability. Acutely the lateral side of the ankle would be swollen and tender anterior and inferior to the tip of the fibula but discomfort may make it difficult to elicit a definite sign of instability.

In a patient with a more chronic history the clinical sign of instability would be a positive anterior drawer test or talar tilt test.

EXAMINER. Tell me more about those two tests.

CANDIDATE. The patient is examined sitting with their legs over the edge of the couch or sitting in a chair to relax the gastrocnemius soleus complex. For the anterior drawer test the distal tibia is grasped in one hand and the other hand grasps the heel and the foot is drawn anteriorly in relation to the talus. Pain or excess anterior translation or a sulcus sign developing at the anterolateral corner of the ankle are signs of an ATFL injury. The other ankle must be examined for comparison. The talar tilt test involves inversion of the ankle whist palpating the anterolateral corner of the joint to feel for movement of the talus within the mortise. A lack of firm end point or tilt in excess of the normal side would represent instability and the CFL is considered to have been injured if this test is positive.

EXAMINER: What other clinical findings may be positive in a patient with recurrent ankle sprains?

CANDIDATE: Ankle sprains are more common in patients with a cavus foot deformity or hypermobility.

EXAMINER: If you suspect a lateral ligament injury how will you proceed in managing this patient?

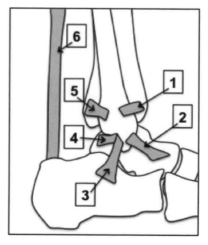

Figure 4.1
Diagram of the lateral ankle ligaments.
1, Anterior inferior tibiofibular ligament;
2, Anterior tibiofibular ligament;
3, Calcaneofibular ligament;
4, Posterior talofibular ligament;
5, Posterior inferior tibiofibular ligament; 6, Achilles tendon.

Postgraduate Orthopaedics: Viva Guide for the FRCS (Tr & Orth) Examination, ed. Paul A. Banaszkiewicz and Deiary F. Kader. Published by Cambridge University Press. © Cambridge University Press 2012.

CANDIDATE: The first step in management would be rehabilitation with physiotherapy, concentrating on peroneal strengthening and proprioceptive training. If the dynamic stabilizers of the ankle are well conditioned the majority of patients recover well from a ligament injury. Bracing may be of benefit.

EXAMINER: . . . and if the patient continues to have significant symptoms despite adequate rehabilitation?

CANDIDATE: A patient that fails to recover would need more investigation. I would begin with simple weightbearing radiographs of the ankle. Stress X-rays of the ankle may be diagnostic for diagnosing a ligament injury, however if the patient is still having significant pain and swelling I would request an MRI scan to look for additional pathology.

EXAMINER: What other conditions would you be looking for?

CANDIDATE: My differential diagnosis for an ankle sprain that doesn't get better, in addition to incomplete recovery or rehabilitation would be peroneal tendon pathology such as a split tear or subluxing tendons, intra-articular pathology such as an osteochondral defect of the talus or loose body, or non-union of an anterior calcaneal process fracture in addition to the presumed diagnosis of lateral ligament injury.

EXAMINER: What are the surgical options for management of an isolated lateral ankle ligament complex injury in a young patient who has failed to respond to non-operative treatments?

CANDIDATE: The options would be a lateral ligament repair or reconstruction of the lateral ligaments.

EXAMINER: Do you know any methods of surgical repair?

CANDIDATE: Yes, the Broström repair.[1]

EXAMINER: What are the principles of that operation?

CANDIDATE: It is an anatomical repair of the lateral ligaments. The ATFL and CFL are imbricated to re-tension them. The extensor retinaculum may then be sutured over the top of the repair for additional strength. Consideration should be given to performing an ankle arthroscopy first at the same sitting to diagnose and address any associated intra-articular pathology.

EXAMINER: Are intra-articular lesions common in this group?

CANDIDATE: Various studies have found chondral injures in a significant proportion of chronic ankle instability. In one study associated intra-articular pathology amenable to arthroscopic treatment was identified in 83% of patients undergoing Brostrom repair.[2]

EXAMINER: A patient asks how successful a ligament repair will be, what will you tell them?

CANDIDATE: I would expect a successful result in over 80% of patients.

EXAMINER: Tell me about the options available for lateral ligament reconstruction.

CANDIDATE: There are several operations described for lateral ligament reconstructions. The majority of these involve sectioning the anterior half of the peroneus brevis proximally, leaving the distal end attached and routing the free end to reconstruct a lateral ligament. The reconstruction can be anatomical or non-anatomical. I have experience of the modified Chrisman–Snook procedure which transfers the anterior half of the peroneus brevis through bone tunnels in the distal fibula and lateral calcaneum to form an anatomical reconstruction of both the ATFL and CFL. I understand that many surgeons are moving towards reconstruction using a free hamstring graft in athletes to avoid harvesting one of the dynamic ankle stabilizers.[3]

EXAMINER: Thank you.

1. Broström L. Sprained ankles VI: Surgical treatment of 'chronic' ligament ruptures. *Acta Chirurgica Scand* 1966;**132**(5):551–565.
2. Kibler WB. Arthroscopic findings in ankle ligament reconstruction. *Clin Sports Med* 1996;**15**(4):799–804.
3. Boyer DS, Younger AS. Anatomic reconstruction of the lateral ligament complex of the ankle using a gracilis autograft. *Foot Ankle Clin* 2006;**11**(3):585–595.

Structured oral examination question 2: Ankle arthritis

EXAMINER: Describe the findings on this X-ray. (Figure 4.2.)

CANDIDATE: This is an AP weightbearing radiograph of a left ankle showing narrowing of the joint space and some subchondral sclerosis consistent with post-traumatic arthritis. There is evidence of a previous fibula fracture superior to the syndesmosis and varus angulation of the ankle.

EXAMINER: Excellent, what are the most common causes of end-stage arthritis of the ankle?

CANDIDATE: Primary osteoarthritis is thought to be relatively uncommon and the most common cause of ankle arthritis is probably post-traumatic arthritis. Other causes are inflammatory arthritis and septic arthritis.

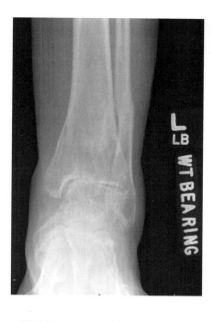

Figure 4.2 X-ray showing ankle arthritis.

EXAMINER: How is this patient likely to present?

CANDIDATE: They are most likely to complain of pain, however they may also present with restriction of movement, deformity and difficulty in performing activities of daily living (ADLs).

EXAMINER: Are you aware of any classification systems for arthritis of the ankle?

CANDIDATE: No, I am not aware of any classification systems specific to the ankle. The Kellgren and Lawrence Radiographic Criteria can be used.[1]

EXAMINER: The X-ray you have been shown belongs to a 42-year-old manual worker who had an ankle fracture 7 years ago which was managed non-operatively. Describe your management strategy for this patient.

CANDIDATE: I would first want to perform a full history and examination, and obtain a lateral radiograph.

EXAMINER: Absolutely. Tell me about the management options available for ankle arthritis.

CANDIDATE: I would start with conservative measures and optimize the patient's analgesia adding in NSAIDs, and suggest activity modification. He could try footwear modification with a cushioned sole and rocker-bottom shoe which may improve his symptoms as may use of an ankle brace or AFO. Similarly an injection of intra-articular steroid or viscosupplementation may be of symptomatic benefit. Physiotherapy could be an adjunctive treatment in patients with symptoms of instability or weakness but may aggravate symptoms.

EXAMINER: What surgical options are available?

CANDIDATE: There are two types of surgical option available, those aimed to 'buy time' or provide temporary relief and definitive treatments. The temporizing measures are debridement of the joint which can be performed arthroscopically or open depending on the extent of disease and should be aimed at treating identifiable causes of symptoms such as removing loose bodies, trimming anterior osteophytes which may give impingement symptoms, or debriding loose areas of articular cartilage and areas of synovitis. The other option is distraction arthroplasty.[2] The definitive surgical options are ankle fusion or ankle replacement.

EXAMINER: Isn't fusion an outdated treatment now that ankle replacements are available?

CANDIDATE: No, total ankle replacements are not suitable for every patient and ankle fusion is still considered the 'gold standard'.

EXAMINER: So which patients should be considered for ankle replacement surgery?

CANDIDATE: Ankle replacement surgery could be considered in low-demand patients over the age of 60 years who have inflammatory arthritis or osteoarthritis. Bilateral disease or arthritis affecting adjacent joints is a relative indication. Contraindications would include younger, more active patients, significant ankle instability, particularly deltoid ligament insufficiency, significant deformity, especially varus or valgus of more than 10°, peripheral vascular disease, a poor soft tissue envelope, marked osteoporosis or avascular necrosis of the tibial plafond or talar dome.

EXAMINER: Do you know anything about the types of ankle replacement available?

CANDIDATE: The earlier designs involved a two-component design such as the Agility total ankle replacement, which required fusion of the distal tibiofibular joint. Most modern designs are three-component uncemented mobile bearing prostheses.

EXAMINER: A patient wants to know how long an ankle replacement will last. What will you tell them?

CANDIDATE: The 10-year survival is approaching 85% but there are fewer data available than for knee and hip replacements. Many series are small.[2-5]

EXAMINER: The 42-year-old patient we began by discussing wants an ankle replacement. What would you tell him?

CANDIDATE: He is a young patient, in a manual job. He wouldn't be a candidate for total ankle replacement and I would explain to him that if his symptoms have failed to be controlled by non-operative measures and he requires definitive surgical treatment then an ankle fusion would be a better option for him.

EXAMINER: He still wants a replacement, as he is keen to get back to hill walking and sports and doesn't want a stiff ankle. What will you tell him now?

CANDIDATE: He would be at risk of early failure with an ankle replacement due to his young age and level of activity. A fusion would provide a stable pain-free ankle that would allow him to return to the majority of activities that he wishes to do. I would explain that many patients return to sports after ankle fusion. I would also explain that an ankle fusion would only sacrifice the residual movement that he has at his ankle joint and that his subtalar, midfoot and forefoot movements would still be present.

EXAMINER: What position should his ankle be fused in?

CANDIDATE: The foot should be plantigrade with a physiological 5° of hindfoot valgus and 5° of external rotation.

EXAMINER: What complications will you warn him about?

CANDIDATE: Non-union, malunion, delayed union, infection, wound-healing problems, nerve or vessel damage, DVT/PE, risk of exacerbating or developing arthritis in other joints.

EXAMINER: Thank you.

1. Kellgren JH, Lawrence JS. Radiological assessment of osteoarthrosis. *Ann Rheum Dis* 1957;**16**:494–501.

2. van Valberg AA, van Roermund PM, Marijnissen AC *et al*. Joint distraction in treatment of osteoarthritis: a two-year follow-up of the ankle. *Osteoarthritis Cartilage* 1999;7:474–479.

3. Wood PLR, Prem H, Sutton C. Total ankle replacement: medium term results in 200 Scandinavian total ankle replacements. *J Bone Joint Surg Br* 2008;**90-B**:605–609.

4. Bonnin M, Gaudot F, Laurent JR *et al*. The Salto total ankle arthroplasty: survivorship and analysis of failures at 7 to 11 years. *Clin Orthop Relat Res* 2011;**469**:225–236.

5. Mann JA, Mann RA, Horton E. STAR ankle: long-term results. *Foot Ankle Int* 2011;**32**(5):473–484.

6. Labek G, Klaus H, Schlichtherle R *et al*. Revision rates after total ankle arthroplasty in sample-based clinical studies and national registries. *Foot Ankle Int* 2011;**32**(8):740–745.

Structured oral examination question 3: The rheumatoid foot

EXAMINER: Please have a look at this radiographic print and tell me what you see. (Figure 4.3.)

CANDIDATE: This is an AP radiograph of a forefoot. There is hallux valgus with displacement of the second toe and destructive change of all the metatarsophalangeal joints. I cannot say whether this is a weightbearing film or not as it is not labelled. The intermetatarsal angle appears increased and I would normally measure this on a weightbearing film. There may be deformities of the lesser toes and I would like to see a lateral view to clarify this.

EXAMINER: Good. A lateral view would be very helpful. What do you think is the underlying diagnosis?

CANDIDATE: The destructive changes suggest that this is an inflammatory polyarthropathy such as rheumatoid arthritis.

EXAMINER: Could it be anything else?

CANDIDATE: The appearances could be secondary to a neuropathic process.

EXAMINER: What might be the commonest neuropathic process that could cause these appearances?

CANDIDATE: A peripheral neuropathy such as that associated with diabetes mellitus would be commonest.

EXAMINER: How would you confirm your diagnosis?

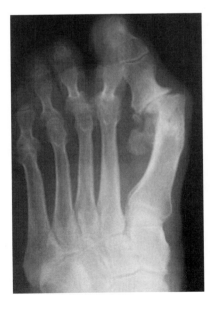

Figure 4.3
Anteroposterior (AP) radiograph of rheumatoid forefoot.

CANDIDATE: A detailed history would be most informative. Specifically, I would enquire about pain, swelling, sensory alteration and medical history.

EXAMINER: OK. This lady gives a clear history of progressive, painful, bilateral small joint swelling and post-immobility stiffness. She has great difficulty finding comfortable shoes and describes walking as if on pebbles. She is not aware of any diabetes or sensory loss. What are your thoughts at this stage?

CANDIDATE: This appears to be an inflammatory arthropathy.

EXAMINER: Yes. Her feet are making her life pretty miserable and she would like you, as an orthopaedic surgeon, to do something to make them better. Your examination finds marked active synovitis and plantar tenderness under the metatarsal heads as well as a minimally correctable hallux valgus. There is some hammering of the lesser toes with a cock-up deformity of the second toe. Sensation and perfusion appear good. What are you going to do?

CANDIDATE: First, I would want to know if she is known to a rheumatology service and has had any attempt at non-operative intervention.

EXAMINER: She has never seen a rheumatologist and has never sought help for her feet other than from you via her GP.

CANDIDATE: I would advise her that operations may be very helpful but that she should be formally assessed by a rheumatologist for diagnosis and disease control first. I would also advise review by the local podiatry and/or orthotics service as simple footwear modification may be all that is necessary to control her symptoms.

EXAMINER: I think that is appropriate advice at this stage. However, she returns to you a year later. Her synovitis is controlled by biologic agents but she has not found insoles and modified shoes helpful. How would you manage her at this point?

CANDIDATE: I would offer her a forefoot reconstruction consisting of excision of the lesser metatarsal heads, correction of lesser toe deformities and excision or fusion of the first metatarsophalangeal joint.

EXAMINER: Why?

CANDIDATE: This is a proven intervention with good results.

EXAMINER: How good?

CANDIDATE: More than 80% of patients report significant improvement.

EXAMINER: Would you fuse or excise the first metatarsophalangeal joint?

CANDIDATE: I would be guided by the age and functional demand of the patient in combination with the quality of the soft-tissue envelope. I would prefer to arthrodese the joint as I believe this aids maintenance of gait but, in a low-demand patient, excision is associated with reduced complications and more rapid rehabilitation.[1]

EXAMINER: If we say this lady is 45 years old, what would you do?

CANDIDATE: I would plan arthrodesis.

EXAMINER: How would you secure the arthrodesis?

CANDIDATE: I would use an oblique compression screw augmented by a dorsal locking plate, as biomechanical and clinical studies have shown this to be the most reliable method.

EXAMINER: Would you excise the lesser metatarsal heads in a patient of this age who now appears to have their disease under control?

CANDIDATE: If the joint surfaces were well preserved but with subluxation of the joints it might be appropriate to perform shortening metatarsal osteotomies such as Weil's osteotomies to preserve the metatarsal heads and allow reduction of the joints with soft tissue releases.

EXAMINER: Surely that just prolongs the procedure and increases the risk of complication?

CANDIDATE: Yes, but it is very difficult to salvage a rheumatoid foot without metatarsal heads if the disease progresses in subsequent years and this patient is young.

EXAMINER: Tell me about the principles of surgery in rheumatoid arthritis.

CANDIDATE: Surgery is indicated when symptoms or deformity are uncontrolled or unbraceable. The overall objective is to produce a stable, plantigrade foot. Aim for a single operation with a high rate of success. Arthrodesis is the predominant procedure. There is a high risk of complication due to osteopenia, dysvascularity, soft tissue fragility and immunosuppression.

EXAMINER: I agree. What steps can a surgeon take to minimize the risk of complication?

CANDIDATE: Biologic agents should be stopped in the run up to surgery and not resumed until there is good evidence of postoperative healing. It should go without saying that meticulous handling of soft tissues is necessary.

Incisions must be planned with care, both to maintain skin bridges and to ensure closure if significant deformities are being corrected.

EXAMINER: How long would you stop biological agents for?

CANDIDATE: Two weeks preoperatively and two weeks postoperatively.[2,3]

EXAMINER: What about other disease-modifying anti-rheumatic drugs? Which other ones would you stop?

CANDIDATE: Studies have shown that there is generally no need to stop other drugs such as methotrexate or leflunomide.

EXAMINER: I would like to backtrack a bit. Would you alter your management if she also had signs and symptoms of hindfoot arthritis?

CANDIDATE: Generally, I would plan to address the most symptomatic area first. However, a less symptomatic fixed hindfoot deformity should be corrected before proceeding to the forefoot. Flexible hindfoot deformity could be left until more symptomatic.

EXAMINER: Which hindfoot joints are most commonly affected in rheumatoid arthritis?

CANDIDATE: The talonavicular joint is most commonly affected, followed by the subtalar and calcaneocuboid joints.

EXAMINER: Can you outline the arguments for and against isolated talonavicular fusion in RA?

CANDIDATE: Isolated talonavicular fusion is a lesser procedure than triple fusion for both patient and surgeon and effectively eliminates hindfoot motion. Historically, a non-union rate of up to 37% has been reported although more recent studies suggest the non-union rate using contemporary fixation is much less. A triple arthrodesis is more reliable and allows greater deformity correction.

EXAMINER: Thank you.

1. Rosenbaum D, Timta B, Schmiegel A *et al.* First ray resection arthroplasty versus arthrodesis in the treatment of the rheumatoid foot. *Foot Ankle Int* 2011;**32** (6):589–594.

2. Lee MA, Mason LW, Dodds AL. The perioperative use of disease-modifying and biologic therapies in patients with rheumatoid arthritis undergoing elective orthopedic surgery. *Orthopedics* 2010;**33**(4):257–262.

3. Howe CR, Gardner GC, Kadel NJ. Perioperative medication management for the patient with rheumatoid arthritis. *J Am Acad Orthop Surg* 2006;**14**:544–551.

Structured oral examination question 4: Cavus foot

EXAMINER: These are pictures of the left foot of a 20-year-old man. Describe them. (Figure 4.4.)

CANDIDATE: These photographs show the anterior, medial and posterior views of a left foot with a cavus deformity. The hindfoot is in varus and there is a high arch. There doesn't appear to be any significant clawing or abnormality of the toes.

EXAMINER: What is the likely underlying cause?

CANDIDATE: A cavus foot develops a high arch as the result of imbalance in the musculature of the foot. It can be caused by a plantar flexion deformity of the forefoot or by a dorsiflexion deformity of the hindfoot known as calcaneocavus. The causes of a cavus foot may be broken down into congenital or acquired. The most common causes of congenital deformities are idiopathic, a sequela of clubfoot or due to arthrogryposis. The acquired deformities may be due to trauma or neuromuscular conditions. The neuromuscular causes may be grouped into central nervous system disease such as cerebral palsy or Friedrich's ataxia, spinal cord lesions such as spina bifida or spinal dysraphism, peripheral nervous system lesions such as an HSMN or muscular causes such as muscular dystrophy.

EXAMINER: HSMN?

CANDIDATE: Hereditary motor–sensory neuropathy. These are a group of inherited neurological conditions. Charcot–Marie–Tooth (CMT) is the most common group of these conditions.

EXAMINER: Can you go into more detail? How do these conditions lead to a cavus foot deformity?

CANDIDATE: The hereditary motor sensory neuropathies are a group of related conditions that may lead to cavus foot deformity due to muscle imbalance. The conditions are generally diagnosed by the pattern of deformity and a positive family history. The most commonly recognized is the Charcot–Marie–Tooth disease group which affects approximately 1 in 2500 people. These patients commonly have weakness of the intrinsic muscles, tibialis anterior and peroneus brevis. Type I will tend to present in the second decade, it is an autosomal dominant inheritance and patients have peroneal weakness, slow nerve conduction and absent reflexes. Type II presents later, in the third or

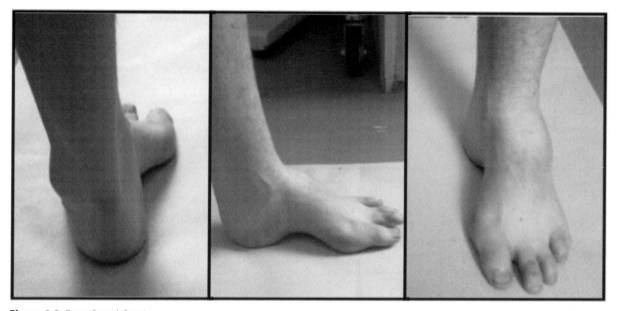

Figure 4.4 Cavus foot deformity.

fourth decade, and reflexes and nerve conduction are normal, however the foot signs may be more pronounced. Genetic analysis is able to diagnose and group these conditions more accurately and at least 17 types of CMT have been described.

EXAMINER: How would you assess this foot?

CANDIDATE: My assessment would have two components. I need to determine any underlying cause of the cavus and also evaluate the deformity itself. I would establish whether this is a unilateral or bilateral deformity and then I would begin by taking a thorough patient history. A cavus deformity is often secondary to a neurological cause so I would ask whether the foot had always been this shape and whether the deformity was progressive. I would ask what symptoms the foot causes and how it affects their function. I would also ask about any previous medical or surgical history, family history, and any previous surgical or non-surgical treatment the patient had received.

EXAMINER: What symptoms is this patient likely to complain about?

CANDIDATE: Common complaints in cavus feet are of pain, particularly forefoot pain, lateral foot pain under the metatarsal heads, or arch pain, instability of the ankle with a history of frequent ankle sprains. They may also have problems with fitting of footwear or alteration of gait.

EXAMINER: What are the main findings you would look for in the examination of a cavus foot?

CANDIDATE: On first, general inspection I would be looking to see if the deformity was bilateral and whether there were stigmata of a generalized condition such as wasting within the hands. With the patient standing I would look to see whether the heel was in varus, neutral or valgus alignment, assess the height of the longitudinal arch by inspection and also see whether I could pass more than two fingers underneath. I would look to see the posture of the toes. This would be to assess the degree of deformity. While the patient was standing I would also look at the spine for any stigmata of an underlying abnormality such as a hairy patch or scoliosis.

With the patient sitting I would inspect the soles of the feet for callosities or areas of ulceration. I would look to see whether the cavus was due to plantarflexion of the first ray or the whole forefoot. I would assess sensation, deep tendon reflexes and power of the major muscle groups, particularly the tibialis anterior and posterior and the peroneal tendons. I would assess lateral ankle ligament competence with an anterior drawer and talar tilt test and look at the active and passive range of movement and see whether the deformities were flexible or fixed.

EXAMINER: What is shown in the following two diagrams?

CANDIDATE: These diagrams show the Coleman block test. (Figure 4.5.)

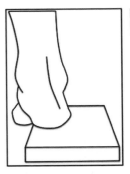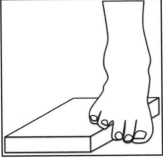

Figure 4.5 Coleman block test.

EXAMINER: And what is that?

CANDIDATE: The Coleman block test looks for flexibility of the hindfoot deformity by eliminating the deforming drive of the forefoot. In a cavus foot the first ray is plantarflexed so to place the foot stably on the ground the hindfoot has to move into varus. In the Coleman block test the foot is positioned so that the lateral border of the foot and the heel are placed on a block and the medial forefoot is allowed to hang off the edge of the block. If the heel then assumes a physiological alignment of neutral to 5° valgus when viewed from behind the hindfoot deformity is both flexible and driven by the forefoot.[1]

EXAMINER: What investigations would you use to evaluate this foot further?

CANDIDATE: In terms of evaluating the foot itself I would first obtain a series of weightbearing radiographs, a lateral of the foot and ankle, a hindfoot alignment view and an AP of the foot. If the patient had any signs or history suggesting an underlying spinal cause then radiographs or MRI scan of the spine should be considered.

EXAMINER: What information does the lateral X-ray tell you?

CANDIDATE: The magnitude of the cavus deformity can be quantified using Meary's angle, the angle between the long axis of the talus and the first metatarsal shaft. Normally this lies between +5° and −5°. Hibb's angle is the angle between the long axis of the first metatarsal shaft and the long axis of the calcaneum. This angle is normally 150° but decreases as the cavus worsens. The calcaneal pitch angle, the angle between the floor and the undersurface of the calcaneum, should be less than 30° but may be elevated in a cavus foot. The radiographs can also be used to look for signs of degenerative changes and the bones themselves may be abnormal in shape in a deformity that began early in childhood.

EXAMINER: What are the principles of managing this condition?

CANDIDATE: Firstly it is important to identify and if necessary address the underlying cause of the cavus. The patient should be examined for neuromuscular causes and investigated and referred for a neurological opinion if appropriate. The patient's current symptoms need to be understood as well as the likelihood of progression. Management can be non-operative with the use of orthotics to try and offload pressure areas and improve stability. Surgical treatment needs to be tailored to the individual patient's underlying pathology, risk of progression, level of deformity and muscular imbalance. Correction of deformity without addressing the muscular imbalance will not be successful.

EXAMINER: Thank you.

1. Coleman S, Chestnut W. A simple test for hindfoot flexibility in the cavovarus foot. *Clin Orthop Relat Res* 1977;**123**:60–62.

Structured oral examination question 5: Acquired adult flatfoot

EXAMINER: I would like you to look at this clinical photograph and tell me what you see. (Figure 4.6.)

CANDIDATE: This shows a posterior view of feet in a weightbearing stance. There is marked heel valgus and too many toes are visible. The medial longitudinal arch is not visible.

EXAMINER: How do you think the medial longitudinal arch may appear?

CANDIDATE: I would expect marked flattening of the arch.

EXAMINER: What term is used to describe this situation?

CANDIDATE: Pes planus or flatfoot.

EXAMINER: Yes. In adults, what are the causes of this condition?

CANDIDATE: Presentation in adults is usually acquired. The commonest cause is tibialis posterior dysfunction. Other causes include inflammatory arthritis, Charcot arthropathy, osteoarthritis and trauma.

EXAMINER: Good. How common is adult flatfoot?

CANDIDATE: It is commoner in females and the incidence increases with age.

EXAMINER: Okay. Let's stick with tibialis posterior dysfunction for just now. Describe a typical patient presentation.

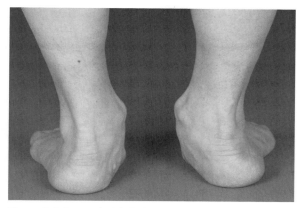

Figure 4.6 Acquired adult flatfoot.

CANDIDATE: The classic patient would be a female aged between 45 and 65 years of age. She would describe initial pain along the course of the tibialis posterior tendon. There is likely to be later development of increasing planovalgus deformity with medial deltoid ligament pain and sometimes lateral impingement pain.

EXAMINER: What are the key examination points you would look for?

CANDIDATE: I think the most useful test is the ability to perform a single heel raise. In conjunction with assessment of hindfoot flexibility, this would allow classification and guide treatment.

EXAMINER: As you have mentioned classification of tibialis posterior dysfunction, could you tell me any more about this?

CANDIDATE: Yes. Johnson and Strom proposed a three-stage classification in 1989. Myerson and Corrigan later added a fourth stage.[1] In stage I disease, there is no deformity but pain from the tendon. A single heel raise is usually possible but painful. In stage II disease, there is a flexible planovalgus deformity and weakness of single heel raise. In stage III disease, the deformity has become fixed and in stage IV, there is additional tilting of the talus in the ankle mortise. There are recommended procedures for each stage of the disease.

EXAMINER: Good. After your examination, how would you investigate this patient?

CANDIDATE: Weightbearing AP and lateral radiographs of both the foot and ankle would help to assess structural change and exclude other causes of flatfoot. They could also show associated degenerative change. The arch index could also be measured.

EXAMINER: Would the arch index influence your management?

CANDIDATE: No. I think it is mainly used as a research tool.

EXAMINER: Coming back to your classification, you suggested that there are recommended interventions for each stage of the disease. Please tell me about these.

CANDIDATE: For stage I, I would offer debridement of the tendon followed by 6–8 weeks of casting or splintage followed by provision of a definitive arch support orthosis.[2] For stage II disease I would offer either a lateral column lengthening or a medializing calcaneal osteotomy in conjunction with a FDL transfer to augment or replace the tibialis posterior.[3] In stage III disease, triple arthrodesis is recommended.[4] For stage IV disease, the management depends upon the flexibility of the ankle deformity. If it is flexible, then a triple arthrodesis combined with ankle bracing or deltoid ligament reconstruction may be adequate otherwise a triple arthrodesis combined or followed by ankle arthrodesis would be indicated.

EXAMINER: You seem very clear about surgical options. What about non-operative treatment?

CANDIDATE: I should have mentioned that. It is appropriate to offer analgesia and orthotic treatment to most patients initially. An orthotic providing medial arch support with a heel cup to control heel valgus can be helpful. There are two aims of orthotic treatment. First, this may offer adequate symptom relief. Second, it may control progressive heel valgus and flattening of the medial arch.

EXAMINER: You spoke about an FDL transfer. Tell me about this procedure.

CANDIDATE: After obtaining informed consent, anaesthesia, supine positioning, thigh tourniquet and skin prep and drape, I would make an incision over the line of the posterior tibial tendon, starting posterior to the medial malleolus. I would debride or resect the tendon according to the clinical appearances. The flexor digitorum longus sheath lies directly posterior to the tibialis posterior tendon and would be opened longitudinally as far distally as possible before the FDL tendon is divided. If there is a decent distal stump of tibialis posterior, then the FDL tendon could be sutured to this but it is probably better to pass it through a hole drilled in the navicular and suture it back to itself.

EXAMINER: In what direction would you pass FDL through the navicular?

CANDIDATE: From plantar to dorsal.

EXAMINER: What is the aim of a medializing calcaneal osteotomy?

CANDIDATE: The calcaneal osteotomy directly reduces the heel valgus and brings the weightbearing axis closer to the long axis of the leg. In addition it displaces the Achilles tendon insertion medially which stops it acting as an everter of the hindfoot.

EXAMINER: When obtaining consent, what would you advise about flexion of the toes after harvesting flexor digitorum longus?

CANDIDATE: I would expect flexion of the lesser toes to be maintained by flexor hallucis longus via the knot of Henry.

EXAMINER: Can you tell me a little more about the knot of Henry?

CANDIDATE: Flexor digitorum longus crosses flexor hallucis longus on the plantar aspect. There are a number of fibrous interconnections between the two tendons that afford a degree of cooperation in movement. This means that flexion of the digits can continue after harvest of FDL or FHL.

EXAMINER: One final question. What approach would you use for a triple arthrodesis to correct significant, fixed valgus heel deformity?

CANDIDATE: This is a potentially difficult situation. The joint preparation is most straightforward if a lateral utility approach or similar is combined with a dorsal incision over the talonavicular joint. If a significant deformity is being addressed there can be difficulty in closing the lateral incision once the deformity is corrected. There are advocates of triple arthrodesis via a single medial approach but this is difficult and not always possible.

EXAMINER: Thank you.

1. Myerson MS, Corrigan J. Treatment of posterior tibial tendon dysfunction with flexor digitorum longus tendon transfer and calcaneal osteotomy. *Orthopedics* 1996;**19**:383–388.

2. Teasdall RD, Johnson KA. Surgical treatment of stage I posterior tibial tendon dysfunction. *Foot Ankle Int* 1994;**15**(12):646–648.

3. Myerson MS, Badekas A, Schon LC. Treatment of stage II posterior tibial tendon deficiency with flexor digitorum longus tendon transfer and calcaneal osteotomy. *Foot Ankle Int* 2004;**25**(7):445–450.

4. Kelly IP, Easley ME. Treatment of stage 3 adult acquired flatfoot. *Foot Ankle Clin* 2001;**6**:153–166.

Structured oral examination question 6: Hallux valgus

EXAMINER: Please have a look at these clinical photographs and tell me what you see. (Figures 4.7 and 4.8.)

CANDIDATE: These show a frontal view of a pair of feet and an oblique view of the left foot. There is hallux valgus with the hallux over-riding the second toes. I can only count three lesser toes on the left foot and there is a scar in the webspace lateral to the hallux. The toenails appear friable and there is some excoriation around the lesser toes on the right foot. There is also a small area of scab on the dorsum of the right foot. I don't see any scars on the right foot but I think there is also a medial longitudinal scar over the left metatarsophalangeal joint.

EXAMINER: Absolutely. This 65-year-old lady had her left second toe removed some years ago for a presentation similar to that which she now has on the right. Her left-sided symptoms have also recurred. How would you assess her further?

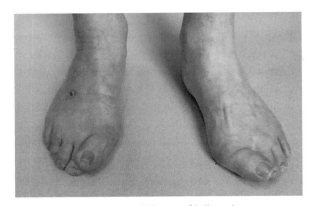

Figure 4.7 Anteroposterior (AP) view of hallux valgus.

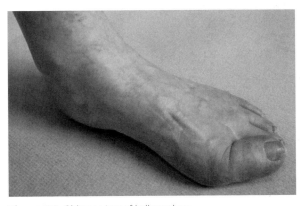

Figure 4.8 Oblique view of hallux valgus.

CANDIDATE: A detailed history should be obtained, looking to clarify the main source of her symptoms. Can I ask what symptoms she has?

EXAMINER: What do you think they are likely to be?

CANDIDATE: I would expect she has pain from her bunions and toes caused by rubbing on footwear and each other. I would be concerned to find out about symptoms suggestive of arthritic change at the MTP joint or metatarsalgia of the lesser rays.

EXAMINER: Let's say she has all these symptoms to varying degrees. Tell me about your further assessment.

CANDIDATE: I would complete the history, including questioning about relevant conditions such as diabetes, inflammatory arthritis, vascular disease and neuropathy, and proceed to examination. I would examine the gait and the posture of the weighted foot as hallux valgus is often associated with a planus foot. I would palpate for areas of tenderness, paying particular attention to the hallux MTP joint and lesser metatarsal heads. I would assess the degree of active and passive correction possible and the range of movement of the involved joints and look for gastrocnemius tightness. I would also perform a grind test to assess pain from loading the MTP joint. Neurovascular status must also be assessed.

EXAMINER: You spoke about assessing the range of movement of the involved joints. Can you be more specific?

CANDIDATE: I would want to assess the range of plantarflexion and dorsiflexion of the hallux MTP joint. It is also important to assess the movement at the first tarsometatarsal joint as excessive mobility here will influence surgical options.

EXAMINER: Okay, we might come back to that. Outline the value of plain radiographs in the management of hallux valgus.

CANDIDATE: I would routinely obtain weightbearing AP, oblique and lateral radiographs of the foot. This would allow me to objectively measure the angles, assess uncovering of the sesamoids and look for evidence of arthritic change.

EXAMINER: Keep going. What angles?

CANDIDATE: I would measure the intermetatarsal angle, hallux valgus angle and the distal metatarsal articular angulation.

EXAMINER: What is the normal range of these angles and how would these influence your management?

CANDIDATE: The intermetatarsal angle is normally less than 9°. The hallux valgus angle should be less than 15°. The distal metatarsal articular angle is normally a maximum of 15° from perpendicular to the axis of the first metatarsal. The degree of deformity largely determines the surgical management.

EXAMINER: If this lady had an intermetatarsal angle of 15° on the right with a hallux valgus angle of 35° and minimal passive correction of the hallux, what surgery would you plan?

CANDIDATE: If the first tarsometatarsal joint is normal, I would plan a scarf osteotomy combined with a lateral release and an Akin osteotomy of the proximal phalanx if necessary.

EXAMINER: Why would you choose a scarf osteotomy?

CANDIDATE: It is a very versatile procedure with stable fixation allowing postoperative mobilization without a cast. It maintains length of the metatarsal but allows translation, angulation and depression of the metatarsal head as necessary. It can also be used to shorten or even lengthen the metatarsal.[1]

EXAMINER: How would you secure the osteotomy?

CANDIDATE: With two headless compression screws.

EXAMINER: Why not use a simpler procedure such as a chevron or Mitchell osteotomy?

CANDIDATE: For the degree of deformity described, combined with the lack of passive correction of the hallux, I believe the correction that could be achieved with a distal osteotomy would be inadequate. A further disadvantage of a Mitchell osteotomy is that it produces shortening of the first metatarsal, which could lead to transfer metatarsalgia.

EXAMINER: For your proposed management, what complications would you discuss when seeking consent?

CANDIDATE: Firstly, I would advise that whilst early weightbearing is possible with a scarf osteotomy it takes up to a year for the foot to fully settle after such surgery but that typically 85% of patients are pleased with the outcome. I would advise a 1% risk of deep infection and a slightly higher risk of superficial infection. Recurrence is possible with time although the risk of this is greatest in adolescent cases. A minority of patients will have significant stiffness of the MTP joint afterwards and there can be sensory loss if the dorsomedial sensory nerve is injured. I would mention the possibility of hallux varus as a complication as this is difficult to treat. I would also mention the possibility of intraoperative and postoperative metatarsal fracture.

EXAMINER: How would you treat hallux varus?

CANDIDATE: A subtle varus may improve as the patient returns to normal foot wear. Whilst soft tissue procedures such as abductor hallucis and medial capsular release or transfer of a slip of EHL are described for flexible deformity, arthrodesis of the first MTP joint is a reliable option in the presence of significant stiffness or arthrosis.

EXAMINER: So you have successfully treated this lady's right foot and she is pleased with the result. Would you go ahead and do the same on the left?

CANDIDATE: No. The absence of the second toe predisposes to recurrence and I would propose arthrodesis of the hallux MTP joint.

EXAMINER: Thank you.

1. Barouk LS, Toullec ET. Use of scarf osteotomy of the first metatarsal to correct hallux valgus deformity. *Techniques Foot Ankle Surg* 2003;**2**(1):27–34.

Structured oral examination question 7: Hallux rigidus

EXAMINER: This 45-year-old male patient has presented with pain and stiffness of his right big toe. Describe the X-ray findings. (Figure 4.9.)

CANDIDATE: This is a radiograph of a right foot showing osteoarthritis of the first metatarsophalangeal joint (MTPJ) with loss of joint space, osteophytes and sclerosis. There is also a mild hallux valgus deformity. There is no other obvious deformity.

EXAMINER: So what is this commonly called in orthopaedics?

CANDIDATE: Hallux rigidus.

EXAMINER: Tell me the range of movement of a healthy first MTPJ.

CANDIDATE: The joint should be able to dorsiflex between 70° and 90° and plantarflex between 24° and 40°.

EXAMINER: How would you go about managing this patient?

CANDIDATE: First of all I would need to perform a full history and clinical examination on the patient. I would also obtain a weightbearing lateral and an oblique X-ray of the foot in addition to the AP view we have here.

EXAMINER: Very good. If we concentrate on the clinical examination what specific findings are you looking for to help with your management decision?

CANDIDATE: I would need to assess the integrity of the skin and the neurovascular status of the foot. I would palpate for large osteophytes and assess the range of movement of the first MTPJ and look to see whether the patient had pain limited to

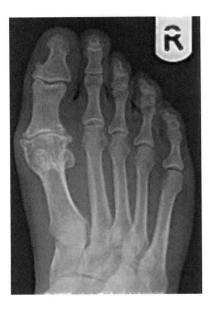

Figure 4.9 X-ray showing hallux rigidus.

the extremes of movement or throughout the arc of motion. A grind test of the joint would be informative. I also need to evaluate the motion and look for any sign of degenerative change at the interphalangeal joint (IPJ).

EXAMINER: What is the importance of the IPJ?

CANDIDATE: A fusion of the first MTPJ may accelerate degeneration in the surrounding joints so if the IPJ is already symptomatic a motion-preserving procedure at the MTPJ may be more appropriate.

EXAMINER: Right so talk me through the management options for a patient with hallux rigidus.

CANDIDATE: In the first instance, unless there is a pressing indication for surgery such as impending skin compromise, I would maximize non-operative treatment. Options here include activity modification, footwear with a stiff sole and a rocker sole to reduce MTPJ motion. NSAIDs may be useful and in some cases an intra-articular injection may provide relief.

EXAMINER: And the operative options?

CANDIDATE: That choice would depend on the grade of the disease.

EXAMINER: Can you expand on that? Are you aware of any grading systems for this condition?

CANDIDATE: The most widely used is a radiographic grading by Hattrup and Johnson in which Grade 1 has a well-preserved joint space with mild to moderate osteophytes, Grade 2 has a reduced joint space with moderate osteophytes and Grade 3 has a complete loss of joint space, marked osteophytes and there may be subchondral cysts within the metatarsal head.[1]

EXAMINER: So then, back to the operative options for treatment.

CANDIDATE: In Grade 1 or 2 disease a cheilectomy, in which the osteophytes and the dorsal 25–30% of the articular surface are resected, is widely used and gives good relief of symptoms. If there is good plantarflexion, restriction of dorsiflexion and no mid-range pain a Moberg dorsal closing wedge osteotomy of the proximal phalanx can be used to shift the arc of movement further into the dorsiflexion range to reduce symptoms.[2] For patients with severe disease and no ligamentous instability total joint replacements do exist but early loosening has been a common problem. Good results have been reported with hemiarthroplasty of either the metatarsal head or the base of proximal phalanx but few large series exist and neither is commonly used in the UK.[3,4] Arthrodesis of the first MTPJ is still the mainstay of treatment for severe disease and joint preparation with dome-shaped reamers and a lag screw and dorsal plate construct is the most biomechanically sound fixation.[5] Keller's arthroplasty is a possibility in elderly, low-demand patients, however cock-up deformities and transfer metarsarsalgia may develop.

EXAMINER: So, back to arthrodesis. What is the optimal position for fusion?

CANDIDATE: Dorsiflexion of 25° across the MTPJ, valgus of 10–15° and neutral rotation to ensure an effective plane of motion of the IPJ.

EXAMINER: How will you consent a patient for arthrodesis of the first MTPJ?

CANDIDATE: I will explain that the intentions of the surgery are to relieve pain and optimize mobility. The risks and complications include wound-healing problems, infection, damage to the medial cutaneous nerve, non-union, malunion, delayed union, metalwork irritation and accelerated degeneration in surrounding joints.

EXAMINER: If we return to the patient we started discussing. He is a 45-year-old male who is a keen walker. He has significant stiffness and pain on mobilization and dorsiflexion but a grind test is negative. He has exhausted non-operative measures. What treatment will you offer him?

CANDIDATE: His X-ray shows joint space narrowing and peripheral osteophytes, but as he is an active individual and his grind test is negative I would offer him a cheilectomy. I would also discuss fusion with him and explain to him that this may become necessary if a thorough cheilectomy failed to provide sufficient relief or he had later progression of disease.

1. Hattrup SJ, Johnson KA. Subjective results of hallux rigidus following treatment with cheilectomy. *Clin Orthop Relat Res* 1988;**226**:182–191.

2. Moberg E. A simple operation for hallux rigidus. *Clin Orthop Relat Res* 1979;**142**:55–56.

3. Taranow WS, Moutsatson MJ, Cooper JM. Contemporary approaches to Stage II and Stage III hallux rigidus: the role of metallic hemiarthroplasty of the proximal phalanx. *Foot Ankle Clin N Am* 2005;**10**:713–728.

4. Carpenter B, Smith J, Motley T *et al.* Surgical treatment of hallux rigidus using a metatarsal head resurfacing implant: mid-term follow-up. *J Foot Ankle Surg* 2010;**49**:321–325.

5. Politi J, Hayes J, Njus G *et al.* First metatarsal-phalangeal joint arthrodesis: a biomechanical assessment of stability. *Foot Ankle Int* 2003;**24**(4):332–337.

Recommended reading

1. Maffulli N, Ferran NA. Management of acute and chronic ankle instability. *J Am Acad Orthop Surg* 2008;**16**:608–615.

2. Easley ME, Adams SB Jr, Hembree WC *et al.* Current concepts review: results of total ankle arthroplasty. *J Bone Joint Surg Am* 2011;**93**:1455–1468.

3. Courville XF, Hecht PJ, Tosteson ANA. Is total ankle arthroplasty a cost-effective alternative to ankle fusion? *Clin Orthop Relat Res* 2011;**469**:1721–1727.

4. Gougoulias N, Khanna A, Maffulli N. How successful are current ankle replacements? A systematic review of the literature. *Clin Orthop Relat Res* 2010;**468**:199–208.

5. Saltzman CL, Mann RA, Ahrens JE *et al.* Prospective controlled trial of STAR total ankle replacement versus ankle fusion: initial results. *Foot Ankle Int* 2009;**30**(7): 579–596.

6. Chou LB, Coughlin MT, Hansen S Jr *et al.* Osteoarthritis of the ankle: the role of arthroplasty. *J Am Acad Orthop Surg* 2008;**16**(5):249–259.

7. Jeng J, Campbell J. Current concepts review: the rheumatoid forefoot. *Foot Ankle Int* 2008;**29**: 959–968.

8. Trieb K. Management of the foot in rheumatoid arthritis. *J Bone Joint Surg Br* 2005;**87-B**:1171–1177.

9. Younger ASE, Hansen ST Jr. Adult cavus foot. *J Am Acad Orthop Surg* 2005;**13**:302–315.

10. Schwend RM, Drennan JC. Cavus foot deformity in children. *J Am Acad Orthop Surg* 2003;**11**:201–211.

11. Haddad SL, Myerson MS, Younger A *et al.* Symposium: adult acquired flatfoot deformity. *Foot Ankle Int* 2011;**32**(1):95–111.

12. Deland JT. Adult-acquired flatfoot deformity. *J Am Acad Orthop Surg* 2008;**16**(7):399–406.

13. Coughlin MJ, Jones CP. Hallux valgus: demographics, etiology, and radiographic assessment. *Foot Ankle Int* 2007;**28**(7):759–777.

14. Easley ME, Trnka H-J. Current concepts review: hallux valgus. Part 1: Pathomechanics, clinical assessment and nonoperative management. *Foot Ankle Int* 2007; **28**(5):654–659.

15. Easley ME, Trnka H-J. Current concepts review: hallux valgus. Part II: Operative treatment. *Foot Ankle Int* 2007;**28**(6):748–758.

16. Robinson AHN, Limbers JP. Modern concepts in the treatment of hallux valgus. *J Bone Joint Surg Br* 2005; **87-B**:1038–1045.

17. Yee G, Lau J. Current concepts review: hallux rigidus. *Foot Ankle Int* 2008;**29**(6):637–646.

18. Coughlin MJ, Shurnas PS. Hallux rigidus: surgical techniques (cheilectomy and arthrodesis). *J Bone Joint Surg Am* 2004;**86-A**(S1 Part 2):119–130.

19. Coughlin MJ, Shurnas PS. Hallux rigidus: grading and long-term results of operative treatment. *J Bone Joint Surg Am* 2003;**85-A**:2072–2088.

Chapter

5

Spine structured oral questions

Alexander D. L. Baker

Introduction

What could be more central to orthopaedics than the 'orthos' (correct or straight) and 'paideion' (child) of paediatric spinal deformity surgery? Despite this, the spine viva is often an area where candidates for the FRCS (Tr & Orth) exam feel less well prepared. The subject area of orthopaedic spine surgery is broad and rapidly evolving. This makes it a fascinating area to study, but it also presents candidates for the FRCS exam with a daunting task if an exhaustive knowledge is sought. Viva questions tend to be one of two types. Either they are sufficiently 'core' that any consultant orthopaedic surgeon should know about the condition, or they are general orthopaedic questions that are being applied to the spine. In order to cover the breadth of material required this chapter will be succinct, covering core spine topics in sufficient depth to provide the candidate with a framework with which to tackle spine questions. Areas that will be covered include:

1. Tumours.
2. Infection.
3. The prolapsed intervertebral disc.
4. Scoliosis.
5. Spinal stenosis.
6. Spondylolisthesis.
7. Trauma.
8. Notes on various other viva scenarios.

Structured oral examination question 1: Spinal tumour

CANDIDATE: The images show a destructive lesion in the vertebrae which given the age (> 50) is most likely to be metastatic tumour. Breast, lung, prostate, renal, thyroid and GI malignancies are the most common sources of primary disease. (Figure 5.1.)

EXAMINER: How would you go about investigating this?

CANDIDATE: Staging and grading. Initial assessment would include a detailed history and examination, paying particular attention to any history of malignancy and asking about symptoms of altered bowel habit, respiratory problems, any prostatic symptoms or breast lumps. Examination should include breast, thyroid, respiratory, abdominal and rectal examinations (with faecal occult blood tests).

Investigations should include *local* and *distant* imaging. Local imaging should include plain radiographs and a whole spine MRI (looking at neural compression and the extent of spinal involvement). A CT may be required for detailed bony anatomy if resection is being considered. The distant imaging selected depends on the likely pathology. It might include a bone scan (looking for evidence of other skeletal metastases), a chest X-ray, or a CT chest, abdomen and pelvis to search for a primary tumour or visceral metastasis. Inflammatory markers should also be sent as well as tumour markers such as serum plasma electrophoresis or PSA.

Histological grading requires a biopsy. Following the general principles applicable to all musculoskeletal tumours this biopsy should be done within the unit that will treat the tumour and also samples sent for culture. 'Biopsy all infections and culture all tumours.'

EXAMINER: How would you decide about subsequent treatment?

CANDIDATE: The scoring system proposed by Tokuhashi is useful in establishing indications for treatment and subsequent surgical goal.[1] A poorer prognosis is correlated with a lower score. Six parameters are given a score from 0 to 2. A score of less than 5 indicates a life expectancy under 1 year and a palliative approach is suggested. A score of over 9 indicates a longer life expectancy and suggests resection/excision should be considered.

Postgraduate Orthopaedics: Viva Guide for the FRCS (Tr & Orth) Examination, ed. Paul A. Banaszkiewicz and Deiary F. Kader. Published by Cambridge University Press. © Cambridge University Press 2012.

(a)

(b)

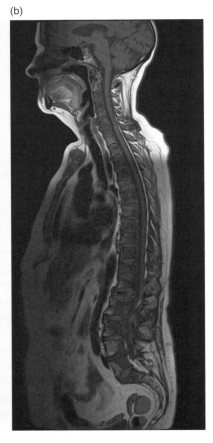

Figures 5.1a and 5.1b Sagittal T1(b) and T2(a) weighted MRI images.

General condition (Poor 0; Moderate 1; Good 2)
Number of extra-spinal metastases (3 or more scores 0; 1 or 2 scores 1; 0 scores 2).
Number of spinal bony metastases (3 or more scores 0; 2 scores 1; 1 scores 2).
Number of metastases to major internal organs (not removable 0; removable 1; no metastases 2).
Tissue of origin (lung, stomach 0; kidney, liver, uterus 1; other, breast, thyroid, prostate, rectum 2).
Spinal cord palsy (complete 0; incomplete 1; none 2).

Tumour background knowledge

Overall, metastatic disease is the most common cause of spinal involvement and primary tumours of the spine are rare. Curative resection is possible in a few cases, but palliative intervention is more common. Pain from bony destruction and resultant mechanical instability may respond well to surgical stabilization.

Decompressive surgery may prevent (or prevent progression of) neurological impairment.

Epidemiology

Vertebral body lesions are more likely to be malignant and posterior lesions benign. Under the age of 21 most spinal tumours are benign, over 21 most are malignant. Under the age of 3 metastatic malignant tumours become more common again. Breast, lung, prostate, renal, thyroid and GI malignancies are the most common sources of primary disease.

Surgical treatment

Surgery is increasingly being performed. Following surgery, patients can often expect functional improvement, pain relief, and in a few cases cure. NICE has issued guidelines on the treatment of metastatic cord compression.[2] Decompression of compressed neural structures may lead to functional improvement even with prolonged paraplegia.

Simple laminectomy to 'decompress' the tumour is rarely indicated as the presence of the tumour (most frequently found in the vertebral body) is likely to lead to mechanical instability and thus kyphosis. Instrumented stabilization is frequently undertaken.

Surgical resection of tumour is aimed at improving survival. Resection may be undertaken anteriorly, or posteriorly, or both, and depending on the size and location of the lesion. In general terms, if a curative resection is hoped for, or survival is likely to extend beyond 6 months, intervertebral bony fusion should be undertaken to avoid instrumentation failure. If life expectancy is short and a palliative procedure is being considered, fusion may not be required and posterior surgery is more commonly undertaken.

Radiotherapy

- Mainly used to reduce tumour bulk.
- Many GI and renal tumours are resistant but most breast tumours are sensitive.
- Prostate and lymphoreticular tumours respond best.
- There is an increased risk of wound problems with adjuvant radiotherapy (separate radiotherapy and surgery by a period of 6 weeks).

Minimally invasive surgery and cement vertebral body augmentation

These techniques are novel and their role is yet to be firmly established.

Some patients are too unwell or are unwilling to consider major surgery.

When pain caused by instability does not require decompression, vertebral body augmentation with high viscosity cement (PMMA) may be considered.

Minimally invasive surgery may allow the surgeon to stabilize the spine whilst minimizing soft tissue trauma facilitating a faster postoperative recovery in patients with limited life expectancy.

Specific tumours
Benign

Haemangioma – Slow growing and often asymptomatic. Often detected as an incidental finding on imaging.

Osteoid osteoma/osteoblastoma are usually found in the posterior neural arch. Most present with pain (NSAID sensitive). Excision is curative but NSAID may be all that is required.

Osteochondroma are most commonly found on the spinous process (related to the apophysis). Excision is for symptomatic treatment. Sarcomatous change has been described and excision is indicated if a large (> 10 mm) cartilage cap is seen on MRI.

Aneurysmal bone cysts typically affecting the posterior elements and giant cell tumours (affecting the vertebral body) are also seen.

Malignant

Myeloma/solitary plasmacytoma typically presents with pain and can be treated with radiotherapy (highly sensitive), or cement augmentation.

Chordoma is locally aggressive and may present with compression of pelvic contents.

Lymphoma most commonly occurs in the elderly (mean age 85) and more frequently in men than women.

Chondrosarcoma typically presents with pain and X-rays may show typical matrix calcification.

Osteosarcoma presents in the young (< 20). It is rare and survival is poor (median survival 6–10 months).

Intradural tumours

In contrast to extradural tumours most intradural tumours are not metastatic.

Extramedullary tumours occur inside the dura but outside the spinal cord. They are usually benign. They cause symptoms by compressing neural structures which can lead to pain or loss of motor function. Examples include neurofibromas, schwannoma (of dorsal sensory roots) and meningioma.

Intramedullary tumours occur within the spinal cord. Most are malignant. Examples include astrocytomas (affecting children), ependymomas (affecting adults), and rarely haemangiomas.

1. Tokuhashi Y, Matsuzaki H, Toriyama S, Kawano H, Ohsaka S. Scoring system for the preoperative evaluation of metastatic spine tumor prognosis. *Spine* 1990;**15**(11):1110–1113.

2. NICE Clinical Guideline 75. *Metastatic Spinal Cord Compression*. November 2008.

Structured oral examination question 2: Infection (epidural abscess)

EXAMINER: A 68-year-old man with a past history of a lung tumour 10 years ago presents following a fall with a 4-week history of worsening thoracic back pain. Back pain is a common presenting complaint to general practitioners and orthopaedic departments. What red flags are there to indicate possible underlying pathology?

CANDIDATE: In this individual, age, the past history of tumour, the thoracic location of his pain, and the history of trauma are all 'red flags'. Other possibilities include: fever, weight loss, night sweats, night pain, non-mechanical pain, severe intractable pain, thoracic pain, age over 55 or below 20, a history of carcinoma, steroid use, IV drug abuse, saddle anaesthesia, urinary or bowel symptoms, deformity.

EXAMINER: Here is his MRI scan. What can you see? (Figure 5.2.)

CANDIDATE: This is a sequence of MRI scans, both T1- and T2-weighted MRI scans. There is a lesion in the thoracic spine, which appears to be compressing the spinal cord. The fact that the lesion is bright on the T2 scan implies that this is likely to be fluid filled and suggests an infective aetiology.

EXAMINER: How would you proceed?

CANDIDATE: We are aware of the history of a fall and should establish this man's neurological status. I would start by obtaining a history and detailed neurological examination. His temperature, routine blood tests (WCC) and inflammatory markers (CRP, ESR) will help confirm the diagnosis of infection.

The most likely diagnosis is an epidural abscess with signs of neurological compression. I would therefore proceed to urgent surgical decompression of the abscess. I would not start antibiotics before obtaining a sample for microbiology and I would also send tissue to pathology (history of tumour).

Infection background knowledge

Spinal infection still remain a serious, potentially life-threatening problem.

Diagnosis is often delayed.

MRI is the imaging modality of choice.

The vertebral body (osteomyelitis), the intervertebral disc (discitis), or the epidural space (epidural abscess) may be affected.

In the absence of a localized collection and no neurology, initial treatment is conservative and should be treated in a similar way to osteomyelitis. (High-dose intravenous antibiotics for 6 weeks or until CRP normalizes and then oral antibiotics until there are no signs of infection.) Consider radical debridement in persistent infections.

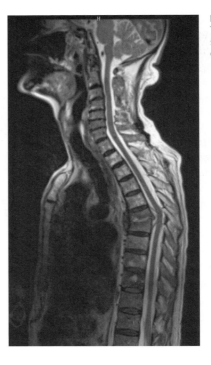

Figure 5.2
T2-weighted sagittal MRI image epidural abscess.

Discitis is more common in younger children and vertebral osteomyelitis more common in adults. The intervertebral disc is vascular in younger children.

In the neonate intraosseous, vertebral arteries anastomose with the adjoining disc through the vertebral end plate. With increasing age the disc loses its vascularity.

Risk factors for infection include intravenous drug use, diabetes, steroid use, chronic infection and other immunocompromised states. Most infections are caused by *Staphylococcus aureus* or *Streptococcus*.

Consider decompressing an abscess in the presence of neurology and/or a localized collection.

Consider radiologically guided decompression.

Structured oral examination question 3: The prolapsed intervertebral disc

EXAMINER: A 37-year-old man has been referred to your clinic with back and left lower limb pain. The general practitioner suspects a 'slipped disc'. What features in the history and on examination will you be looking for?

CANDIDATE: Dermatomal limb pain that predominates over back pain, described as burning in nature, associated with paraesthesia and numbness. Examination should reveal

(a)

(b)

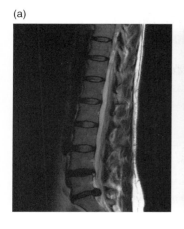
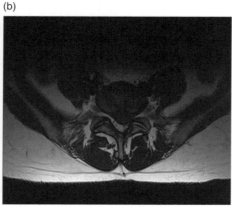

Figures 5.3a and 5.3b T2-weighted axial and sagittal MRI images showing paracentral disc L5/S1 prolapse.

positive nerve root tension signs, altered sensation in the affected dermatome and a decreased ankle jerk reflex on that side. Also, I would like to rule out serious spinal pathology or signs of a cauda equina syndrome.

EXAMINER: You request an MRI scan, here it is, what can you see? (Figure 5.3.)

CANDIDATE: This is a T2-weighted MRI scan showing the lumbar spine in coronal and sagittal section. There is a paracentral disc prolapse at the L5/S1 level.

EXAMINER: What would you expect to find in this patient?

CANDIDATE: I would expect the pain, paraesthesia and numbness to be in an S1 distribution (posterior calf, heel and lateral border of the foot) on the left. There may be an associated subjective decreased sensation in the same distribution, a decreased ankle jerk on that side, decreased straight leg raise and positive cross-over sign.

EXAMINER: How would you treat this patient?

CANDIDATE: Initially conservatively as the natural history of most lumbar disc prolapses is that they resolve with time. If it has not resolved after 6–12 weeks of conservative management I would offer the patient microdiscectomy.

Disc prolapse background knowledge

The clinical features and treatment options for disc prolapse vary depending on age and the location of the prolapsed disc.

In children the symptoms and signs of disc prolapse are less well defined and back pain is a more prominent feature. Nerve root tension signs are also less likely to be positive and spontaneous resolution is less likely.

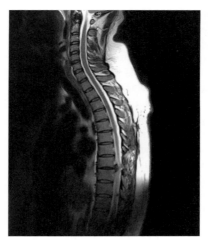

Figure 5.4 T2-weighted MRI showing a thoracic disc prolapse.

A thoracic disc prolapse (rare) will typically present with symptoms and signs of spinal cord compression associated with thoracic back pain (Figure 5.4). The discs are usually calcified and require decompression from the front. Treatment therefore is via a thoracotomy and partial vertebrectomy.

A cervical disc prolapse may present with symptoms and signs of a cervical radiculopathy or cervical myelopathy.

Cauda equina syndrome

Cauda equina syndrome caused by compression of the cauda equina (usually by a large acute disc prolapse) is characterized by some or all of the following:

Urinary retention.

Faecal incontinence.

Saddle area numbness and loss of anal tone.

Widespread neurological signs.

The importance of detecting cauda equina syndrome early is that early intervention (< 24 hours) has been shown to improve outcome. More recently the extent of the compression has also been linked to outcome and the importance of timing questioned.[1]

Exiting nerve roots in the cervical and lumbar spine

The knowledge that the L4 nerve root exits the spinal canal below the L4 pedicle may (incorrectly) lead the candidate to expect the L4 nerve root to be compressed when a disc prolapse occurs below the L4 vertebra in the L4/5 interspace. It is best to think of this nerve root as 'already having left the canal' and therefore it is the L5 'traversing' nerve root that is most commonly compressed by the common 'paracentral' disc prolapse. (It is true to say that a 'far lateral' disc prolapse may compress the exiting nerve root in the exit foramen but this is rare.) Thus an L4/5 disc prolapse commonly affects the L5 nerve root.

In the cervical spine, a prolapsed disc typically affects the exiting nerve root at that level (there is no traversing nerve root because the roots leave the spinal cord and exit the canal almost horizontally). But there is a nomenclature change in the cervical spine. Because the C6 nerve root exits above (not below) the C6 vertebra this double change means a prolapsed cervical disc at the C5/C6 level most commonly affects the C6 nerve root.

Nomenclature

A herniated disc is a localized displacement of nucleus pulposus beyond the normal limits of the disc. This can be broad-based (involves between 20% and 50% of the disc circumference), focal (involves < 25%) or symmetrical (involves 50–100% of the circumference of the disc).

A focal disc herniation may be described as a protrusion or extrusion. An extruded disc has a narrow 'neck' at its base. Extruded disc material is sequestrated if it is no longer in continuity with the disc.[2]

1. Sell P, Qureshi A. Cauda equina syndrome treated by surgical decompression: the influence of timing on surgical outcome. *Eur Spine J* 2007;**16**:2143–2151.

2. Fardon D, Milette P. Nomeclature and classification of lumbar disc pathology. Recommendations of the Combined Task Forces of the North American Spine Society, American Society of Radiology, and American Society of Neurology. *Spine* 2001;**26**(5):E930E113.

Structured oral examination question 4: Scoliosis

EXAMINER: What can you see? (Figure 5.5.)

CANDIDATE: This is an AP radiograph showing the spine, ribs and iliac crests. There is a left-sided, lumbar scoliosis.

EXAMINER: What different types of scoliosis do you know? What type of scoliosis is this?

CANDIDATE: The radiograph shows a congenital scoliosis. There is a hemivertebra within the lumbar spine producing the scoliosis.

Scoliosis occurs in different groups of patients and can be classified according to aetiology. Scoliosis may be idiopathic, congenital, neuromuscular or associated with other conditions such as Marfan's syndrome or neurofibromatosis.

EXAMINER: Why might you treat a scoliosis?

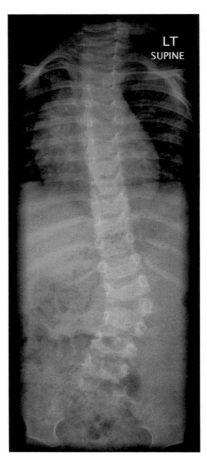

Figure 5.5
Anteroposterior (AP) radiograph of the thoracic and lumbar spine demonstrating a left-sided lumbar scoliosis.

CANDIDATE: The primary indication for treating a scoliosis is progressive deformity. Additionally, patients with 'early-onset' scoliosis and some types of neuromuscular scoliosis are at risk of progressive cardiorespiratory compromise as the curve deteriorates.

EXAMINER: How might you treat this scoliosis?

CANDIDATE: I would refer this patient to a specialist centre for treatment. I suspect that, if after monitoring the curve, it shows signs of progression they might consider excising the hemivertebra.

EXAMINER: The vertebra could be excised using an anterior, posterior or combined approach. Can you describe the thoraco-abdominal (Hodgson's) approach that might be used to approach this vertebra?

CANDIDATE: The patient is positioned in the lateral position with the limbs and trunk supported. The table is 'broken' with apex at the thoracolumbar junction. A skin incision is made over the 10th rib and curved distally to run longitudinally along the lateral border of rectus abdominus. Skin and fat are incised, as are serratus anterior, external oblique and latissimus dorsi. The rib is removed subperiosteally. The parietal pleura is incised exposing the lung and diaphragm.

A key step in this procedure is splitting the costal cartilage to enter the retroperitoneum. Retroperitoneal fascia is swept away with swabs. The diaphragm is divided 2 cm from its origin down to the vertebrae using marking stitches. Segmental vessels are ligated and the discs above and below the vertebrae excised.

Scoliosis background knowledge

Scoliosis is defined as a lateral curvature of the spine in the coronal plane that measures more than 10° using the Cobb method. When present it usually forms part of a three-dimensional spinal deformity. It is sometimes described as a four-dimensional deformity (the fourth dimension being time, emphasizing the progressive nature of the condition).

The key to treating scoliosis is knowledge of the natural history of the condition in order to predict curves that are likely to deteriorate rapidly so that they can be detected and treated at an early stage. Scoliosis has been classified according to severity, location, aetiology and age of onset.

Severity – The Cobb angle also defines the magnitude of the curve with minor (small) curves measuring between 10° and 25°, moderate curves between 25° and 50° and severe (large) curves measuring over 50°.

Location – The 'side' of a scoliosis is the side of the patient to which the spine deviates away from the midline, it is the side of the convexity of the curve. A scoliosis is also described by the region of the spine that it affects. The Scoliosis Research Society have defined a 'thoracic' scoliosis as having its apex between T2 and the T11–T12 disc, a 'thoracolumbar' curve as having its apex between the T12 and L1 vertebrae and a lumbar scoliosis as having its apex between the L1–2 disc space and L4. The apex of the curve is located by the most laterally deviated vertebra. Curves can be single, double or triple 'major' curves depending on whether the curves above and below the main curve are flexible or structural (flexible curves reduce to less than 25° on lateral bending).

Aetiology – Scoliosis is classified according to its aetiology and pathogenesis.

- **Idiopathic** (the largest group – 70%). In this group the scoliosis is produced by an imbalance in the growth of the spine with the convexity of the curve growing at a faster rate than the concavity.
- **Congenital scoliosis**. In this group abnormalities of one or more vertebrae are present at birth. The subsequent growth of these abnormal vertebrae cause the scoliosis. (The name might be confusing as it is the vertebral abnormalities that are present at birth and the scoliosis develops later with growth.)
- **Neuromuscular** (cerebral palsy, Duchenne muscular dystrophy, spinal muscular atrophy). In this group the scoliosis is produced by a lack of support to the spine causing the spine to collapse to one side.
- **Miscellaneous conditions associated with scoliosis** (5% – e.g. Marfan syndrome, neurofibromatosis).

Age of onset – Idiopathic scoliosis has been classified by age into infantile (age 0–3 years), juvenile (3–10 years) and adolescent (10–maturity) idiopathic scoliosis. An alternative classification divides scoliosis into early-onset scoliosis (associated with a high risk of cardiorespiratory compromise as the developing heart and lungs may be affected) which has its onset before the age of 7 and late-onset scoliosis which has its onset after the age of 7. (The age of 7 is used by the AO group – others have suggested 5.)[1,2]

The assessment of a spinal deformity

The assessment of spinal deformity should aim to detect conditions that might mimic (leg length discrepancy, disc prolapse) or be associated with a scoliosis. It should also characterize the patient in terms of skeletal maturity and fitness for anaesthetic as well as characterizing the scoliosis itself. Finally it should formulate a treatment plan.

History – key features

Curve onset and progression.

Maturity (age, menarche, height relative to parental height, recent growth).

General health/fitness for anaesthesia (especially in neuromuscular group). Although patients with scoliosis do experience back pain, scoliosis is not typically thought of as a painful condition. Severe pain may indicate the possibility of an underlying cause (prolapsed disc, osteoid osteoma, spondylolisthesis).

Examination – key features

Height, arm span, weight and assessment of maturity (secondary sexual characteristics).

Assessment of the curve (location and severity).

Common associated problems (rib prominence, shoulder height, pelvic asymmetry, skin creases, hairline and neck shape).

How flexible is the curve and the remainder of the spine?

Features of spinal dysraphism such as hairy patches on the back overlying the spine.

Neurological examination – abnormal abdominal reflexes are most commonly associated with intraspinal anomalies.

Adam's forward bend test.

Investigations

X-ray: Full-length standing AP and lateral plane radiographs showing the ribs, iliac crests and hip joints. Risser's sign grades the progression of development and fusion of the iliac apophysis, is visible on plain X-rays and is a useful indication of maturity.

MRI scanning of the spine can be used to detect underlying intraspinal anomalies such as diastomatomyelia, syringomyelia and Arnold–Chiari malformations (particularly in atypical curves).

Surface topography is also frequently used to assess scoliosis. This can produce an objective assessment of the results of surgery but in some circumstances can also be used instead of frequent X-ray when following up the progression of curves.

Pattern recognition

The most common type of curve seen is a late-onset adolescent idiopathic scoliosis with a 'right thoracic' curve presenting in a girl just after menarche. Atypical features indicate possible underlying pathology (e.g. left-sided curves, severe pain, rapid progression and short angular deformities.)

Late-onset (adolescent idiopathic) scoliosis

Late-onset (adolescent) idiopathic scoliosis is the most common form of scoliosis (70%).

Prevalence of curves over $10°$ is 2% (female 1:1 male).

Prevalence of curves over $20°$ is 0.2% (female 5.4:1 male).

There is a genetic tendency to develop scoliosis with 20% of affected individuals having at least one affected family member.

The development and progression of scoliosis is related to skeletal growth, typically deteriorating most rapidly during the adolescent growth spurt. Features that indicate an increased likelihood of curve progression are therefore associated with but not limited to immaturity. They are:

- Young age at onset.
- Premenarchal status.
- Physical immaturity.
- Large curves.
- Female gender.

Once skeletal maturity is reached the scoliosis tends to stabilize and progress less rapidly ($1°$ per year).

Treatment

Bracing

- Applied for progressive curves measuring $25–40°$.
- Not thought of as corrective but aims to prevent progression of the curve whilst growth continues aiming to reduce the need for surgery.
- To be effective, a brace needs to be worn 23 hours a day.
- Not without morbidity.

Surgery

The aim of surgery is to (partially) correct and stabilize the curve, reducing the deformity and the risk of further progression. Instrumentation is used to correct and stabilize the curve whilst bone graft stimulates fusion of the spine.

Indications:

- Unacceptable deformity.
- Progressive curves.
- Usually reserved for curves with a magnitude > 50°.
- Earlier intervention is indicated in curves with greater potential for progression.

Approaches:

- With 'third-generation' instrumentation (segmental pedicle screws), there has been a recent trend towards the posterior approach.
- Consider anterior approach for thoracolumbar curves.

When selecting which levels to fuse, the first question to ask is, is there just one curve to fuse or more than one? This is the same as asking: are the curves above and below the primary curve sufficiently correctable/flexible? If on the lateral bending X-ray the 'compensatory' curve bends down to less than 25°, it does not need to be included in the construct.

Early-onset scoliosis

Applies to patients under the age of 7 years with an idiopathic scoliosis.

The developing heart and lungs may be affected by the scoliosis.

Cardiorespiratory compromise may result from a progressive curve resulting in decreased life expectancy.

Patients that present with an idiopathic scoliosis below the age of 3 (infantile scoliosis) have the most heterogeneous prognosis. A significant number (80–90% of curves) will resolve before the age of 2 years. However, those that do not resolve go on to develop extremely severe curves that cause major deformity and affect cardiac and respiratory function leading to death in early adult life. Treatment is problematic and prolonged. The most common forms of treatment are serial plaster jackets (localizer casts), subsequently bracing and eventually growing rods.

Neuromuscular scoliosis

Occurs in association with a neuromuscular condition.

Typical collapsing long 'C' shaped curve (other patterns have been described).

Classified into upper motor neurone, lower motor neurone and myopathic.

The two most frequently encountered neuromuscular conditions causing scoliosis are cerebral palsy and Duchenne muscular dystrophy.

Duchenne muscular dystrophy: In almost all patients with Duchenne muscular dystrophy (90%) a scoliosis will develop 1–2 years after the loss of ambulatory function.

Cerebral palsy: The likelihood of developing a curvature is related to its severity. Overall 25–30% of patients with cerebral palsy develop a scoliosis but in four-limb cerebral palsy the incidence of scoliosis increases to 75%. In cerebral palsy the average age of onset of a scoliosis is approximately 10 years.

In this group the problems associated with scoliosis include:

- Pressure sores.
- Pain from costo-pelvic impingement.
- Problems with sitting balance causing patients to become hand-dependent sitters, which in turn limits upper limb function.
- Reflux and swallowing difficulty and associated chest complications.

Treatment

The goals of treatment in neuromuscular scoliosis are improved quality of life, maintenance of function, maintenance of respiratory function and sitting balance. Treatments include:

- Bracing/total contact orthoses (permanent/continuous).
- Wheelchair modifications.
- Surgery – posterior spinal fusion.

In cerebral palsy high levels of care-giver satisfaction following surgery have been reported.[3] Similar benefits are seen in Duchenne muscular dystrophy and surgery may also allow patients to live for longer, having an additive effect with nocturnal ventilation in delaying the deterioration of respiratory function.

Congenital scoliosis

- Scoliosis develops as a result of the growth of vertebral anomalies present at birth.
- The vertebral anomalies may be part of the VATER or VACTERL associations.
- Multiple vertebral anomalies are often hereditary.
- Isolated anomalies are mostly sporadic.
- No single genetic or environmental cause has been identified.

Classification: Anomalies present can be failures of formation or segmentation. More common congenital vertebral anomalies include the unilateral unsegmented bar, the hemivertebra (either fully segmented, semi-segmented or incarcerated), wedge vertebra and block vertebra. A fully segmented hemivertebra is one that has growth plates cranial and caudal to it.

Progression of congenital curves depends on growth potential and whether that growth is balanced. Thus a fully segmented hemivertebra in connection with a contralateral unsegmented bar has the least balanced growth and the worst prognosis. A block vertebra on the other hand has benign prognosis rarely leading to a curve beyond 20°.

1. Aebi M, Arlet V, Webb J. *AO Spine Manual*. New York: Theime Publishing, 2007.
2. Dickson RA. Early-onset scoliosis. In Weinstein SL (Ed.), *The Paediatric Spine: Principles and Practice*. New York: Raven Press, 1994.
3. Tsirikos AI, Chang WN, Dabney KW *et al*. Comparison of parents' and caregivers' satisfaction after spinal fusion in children with cerebral palsy. *J Ped Orthop* 2004; **24**(1):54–58.

Structured oral examination question 5: Lumbar spinal stenosis and cervical myelopathy

EXAMINER: A 70-year-old lady has been referred to your clinic having been seen by one of your arthroplasty colleagues. Her walking distance had reduced significantly but no abnormalities of her hips had been found and this MRI scan had been requested. Can you see anything that might cause this lady's symptoms? (Figure 5.6.)

CANDIDATE: Yes. The images are T2-weighted MRI scans showing the lumbar spine in axial and sagittal section. Both sagittal and axial scans show significant narrowing of the spinal canal, judging from the sagittal scan this appears to be at the L4/5 level.

EXAMINER: Yes, there is a very significant spinal stenosis at that level with obvious compression of the thecal sac surrounding the cauda equina and significant reduction of the CSF signal on the axial scan. How does this kind of stenosis arise and what neurological abnormalities are you like to find on examination?

CANDIDATE: Neurological examination of patients with lumbar spinal stenosis is often remarkably normal. The stenosis arises as a consequence of dehydration of the intervertebral disc leading to bulging of the disc, overload and hypertrophy of the facet joints, segmental instability and hypertrophy of the ligamentum flavum and osteophyte formation.

EXAMINER: Okay, so how do these patients typically present, and what will you be looking for on examination?

(a)

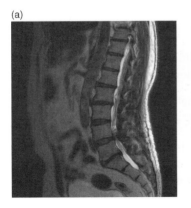

(b)

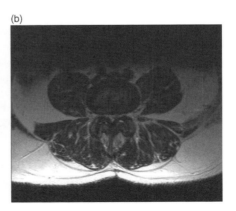

Figures 5.6a and 5.6b T2-weighted MRI axial and sagittal images of lumbar stenosis.

CANDIDATE: Patients with symptomatic lumbar spinal stenosis typically present with neurogenic claudication. Neurogenic claudication is a reduction in walking distance as a result of bilateral aching leg pain, a feeling of heaviness, fatigue, numbness and unsteadiness in the lower limbs. Symptoms are frequently reduced by rest and bending forward. Bending forward flexes the lumbar spine, reducing the lumbar lordosis, and increases the space available for the cauda equina within the spinal canal. Activities that involve flexion of the lumbar spine (e.g. walking uphill, upstairs, pushing a shopping trolley and cycling) are frequently found to be easier than less arduous tasks that extend the lumbar spine (increasing the lordosis).

The most common differential diagnosis is vascular claudication. Clinical examination with palpation of peripheral pulses as well as ankle–brachial pressure measurement is required. Standing relieves vascular claudication whereas neurogenic claudication may be made worse.

EXAMINER: Here is an MRI scan showing severe narrowing of the cervical spinal canal. Is this likely to present in the same way? (Figure 5.7.)

CANDIDATE: No, in this case we are at the level of the spinal cord rather than the cauda equina. There is a bulging cervical disc at the (most common) C5/6 level and the patient will present with symptoms of cervical myelopathy.

EXAMINER: What are the typical features of cervical spondylotic myelopathy and what would you expect to find on examination?

CANDIDATE: Cervical myelopathy presents with upper motor neurone signs and symptoms in both upper and lower limbs. Symptoms include decreased coordination, loss of fine dexterity (e.g. buttoning a shirt, handwriting, manipulating small objects), balance and gait problems, and problems with bowel and bladder function. Typically symptoms follow a slow, progressive course deteriorating in a stepwise manner with stable periods and periods of rapid deterioration. Balance and walking problems may lead to patients complaining of frequent trips, falls or bumping into things.

Associated (upper motor neurone) signs include: a wide based unsteady gait, upper and lower limb weakness, hyper-reflexia, intrinsic muscle waiting in the hand, positive Babinski and Hoffman signs and an inverted radial reflex.

Stenosis background knowledge

Lumbar spinal stenosis can occur within the spinal canal, the lateral recesses or the intervertebral (neural exit) foramen. Central stenosis may be asymptomatic

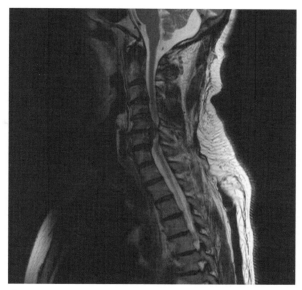

Figure 5.7 T2-weighted sagittal MRI image demonstrating cervical stenosis.

or it may give rise to the symptoms of neurogenic claudication. Lateral recess stenosis or foraminal stenosis may lead to unilateral or dermatomal symptoms. Stenosis is frequently associated with a degenerative spondylolisthesis (which will be discussed in more detail in the next section).

Distinguishing between neurogenic claudication and vascular claudication:

	Type of claudication	
Symptom	**Neurogenic**	**Vascular**
Pain	Worse on standing	Relieved by standing
Numbness	Present	Absent
Site of pain	Buttock/thigh	Calf (rarely anterior)
Relieving factors	Bending forward	Standing
Walking distance	Reduced and variable	Reduced and fixed
Worse going	Downstairs	Upstairs

Hoffman's sign – Flicking the distal phalanx of the middle finger produces reflex contraction of thumb and index finger.

Babinski's sign – Extension of the toes on scraping/firmly stroking the sole of the foot.

Anterior approach to the cervical spine

Many right-handed surgeons prefer the right-sided approach. The left-sided approach has been reported as having a lower rate of recurrent laryngeal nerve injuries. Consider using a foot rest and tapes over the shoulders (acromion) to allow as much of the cervical spine to be exposed as possible for lateral imaging. The head is positioned on a horseshoe ring and neck is in slight extension (towel roll between shoulders). The skin crease incision is made in line with the following landmarks.

C3/4 – Hyoid bone
C4/5 – Laryngeal prominence
C5 – Thyroid cartilage
C6 – Cricoid cartilage

Platysma is incised in line with the skin incision and the fascia dissected to expose the medial border of sternocleidomastoid. The plane between the larynx and oesophagus medially and the carotid sheath laterally is dissected using blunt dissection. The omohyoid muscle is retracted or divided. Pre-cervical fascia is divided medial to the neurovascular bundle and further blunt dissection exposes the longus colli muscles. These are elevated and a retractor placed. The intended spinal procedure can then be undertaken.

Anterior cervical decompression and fusion provides excellent results and has a low complication rate. The anterior approach allows access to the cervical disc that can be removed along with osteophytes at the posterior aspect of the vertebral body. It allows removal of most lesions causing myelopathy or radiculopathy. Placement of anterior bone graft between the vertebral bodies in the excised disc space helps to decompress the exit foramen indirectly and facilitates fusion.

Complications include pseudarthrosis (increased in smokers), hoarse voice and swallowing problems caused by retraction or injury to the recurrent laryngeal nerve (2–5%). This may also be caused by placement of the ET tube (more common). Graft complications also include the graft loosening and migration. Fusion alters the mechanics of the cervical spine, increasing the lever arms of forces acting at adjacent levels, and there is a significant rate of adjacent level degeneration.

One contributing cause of cervical stenosis may be ossification of the posterior longitudinal ligament, particularly in Japanese individuals.

Cervical disc replacement

Cervical disc replacement is a newer technique which treats similar pathologies through the same anterior approach but attempts to preserve motion in the cervical spine by replacing the cervical disk with materials similar to those used in large joint arthroplasty. Initial results are encouraging.[1]

1. Murrey D, Janssen M, Delamarter R *et al.* Results of the prospective, randomized, controlled multicenter Food and Drug Administration investigational device exemption study of the ProDisc-C total disc replacement versus anterior discectomy and fusion for the treatment of 1-level symptomatic cervical disc disease. *The Spine J* 2009;**9**:275–286.

Structured oral examination question 6: Spondylolisthesis

EXAMINER: What is this? (Figure 5.8.)

CANDIDATE: I can see T2-weighted sagittal and coronal MRI images showing the lumbar spine and there is a spondylolisthesis at L5/S1.

EXAMINER: What grade is it and what types of spondylolisthesis do you know?

CANDIDATE: Spondylolisthesis is graded according to Meyerding's grading system which is graded I–IV according to how far from posterior to anterior the more cranial vertebral

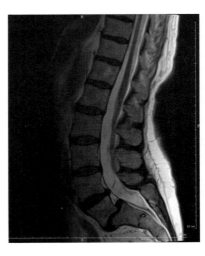

Figure 5.8
T2-weighted MRI sagittal demonstrating L5/S1 spondylolisthesis.

body has slipped forward. Grade I is less than a ¼ (25%), grade II is ¼ – ½ (25–50%), grade III is ½ – ¾ (50–75%) and grade IV is > ¾ (>75%). A spondyloptysis is a slip greater than 100% where the more cranial vertebral body lies anterior to the more caudal one (grade V).

Five different types of spondylolisthesis were described by Wiltze

I. Dysplastic – Congenital abnormalities of the sacrum or L5 allow the slip to occur.
II. Isthmic – Here the defect is in the pars and it is subdivided into a lytic failure, an acute fracture, or an elongated but intact pars.
III. Degenerative – This is due to degenerative change that produces intersegmental instability (due to changes in disc, joint capsules and facet joints).
IV. Traumatic – Due to a fracture (but not of the pars, e.g. pedicle).
IV. Pathological – Caused by local bone disease (disease may not be localized).

Spondylolisthesis background knowledge

Note: When considering an isthmic (spondylolytic) spondylolysis the 'step' in the spinous processes posteriorly the step in the posterior elements will occur one level above that of the pars defect. The posterior element step is at L4/5 in an L5 spondylolysis (the spondylolisthesis being at L5/S1).

In children spondylolytic (isthmic) spondylolisthesis at the L5/S1 junction is more common. Approximately 50% of spondylolyses have a spondylolysis without the associated slip. It is twice as common in men as in women. Typically it first occurs during or just before adolescence and may progress until skeletal maturity. There is a genetic component with between one-third and two-thirds having a family member affected. It may also be associated with spina bidifa (up to 40%). The main symptoms are usually a dull aching pain in the low back and buttocks exacerbated by activity; this may be associated with an L5 radiculopathy. Many are asymptomatic. Of symptomatic children the majority (90%) also become symptomatic again in adult life. Hamstring shortening is a common finding on examination. In high grade slips adolescents may present with a 'spondylolytic crisis' in which pain, neurological compromise and the Phalen–Dickson sign of flexed hips and knees and a waddling gait when walking may all be present.

Conservative management (activity modification, +/− bracing) may allow healing of the pars defect. Core stability exercises, hamstring stretching and bracing all have a role. Surgical stabilization may be considered if conservative management fails or a progressive slip is identified. Patients should be followed up until skeletal maturity after which it is unlikely that the slip will progress.

Degenerative spondylolisthesis most commonly occurs at the L4/L5 level and is frequently associated with stenosis at that level. There is an intact neural arch and the slip is caused by instability of the motion segment, in turn caused by dehydration of the disc and loss of disc height as well as facet joint degeneration. This type is five times more common in women than in men. Symptoms may be of back pain radiating into the thighs, radicular symptoms (50%), or symptoms of neurogenic claudication.

Structured oral examination question 7: Spinal trauma

EXAMINER: A 26-year-old man crashes his motor-bike and sustains the fracture shown. How would you go about assessing a patient with a suspected spinal injury? (Figure 5.9.)

CANDIDATE: The assessment of seriously injured patients begins with the Airway (with cervical spine control), Breathing and Circulation. Circulation assessment includes assessment for neurogenic shock. Then comes neurological disability assessment using the Glasgow Coma Scale followed by a log roll (looking for steps, swelling or bruising indicating posterior injury), rectal examination and neurological examination (using an ASIA chart). Initial imaging will include the trauma series (chest, c-spine and pelvis) X-rays. If a fracture is identified, imaging of the whole spine is required as there is a significant chance of a second fracture (10%). Once a fracture has been identified further imaging with a CT scan is indicated. MRI may also be required to assess disc and spinal cord injuries. Spine fractures are often associated with other injuries. Cervical spine fractures may be associated with vascular injuries, thoracolumbar fractures with visceral injuries and lumbar fractures with lower limb (calcaneal) fractures.

EXAMINER: What is neurogenic shock?

CANDIDATE: Neurogenic shock should be distinguished from hypovolaemic shock. Relative bradycardia and warm peripheries indicate the cause of shock is loss of sympathetic tone secondary to spinal cord injury (SCI).

(a)

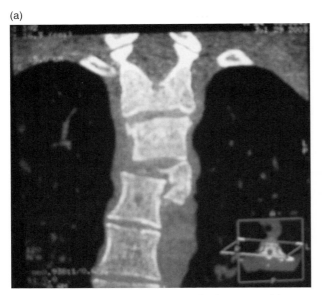

(b)

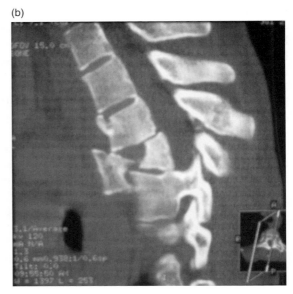

Figures 5.9a and 5.9b CT scan images of a thoracic spinal fracture.

Spinal shock is transient neurological dysfunction that is caused by a contusion or oedema of the spinal cord that usually resolves over 24–72 hours. The bulbocavernosus reflex (usually tested by pulling on an indwelling catheter) is the first reflex to return.

EXAMINER: Would you give this person steroids?

CANDIDATE: No. The current (2006) BOA guidelines on the initial care of patients with spinal cord injuries states 'the use of high dose steroid in the management of acute spinal cord injury could not be recommended or supported on the current evidence'.[1]

EXAMINER: How do you classify thoracolumbar fractures?

CANDIDATE: I would use the AO classificatn. This divides thoracolumbar fractures into three types: A, B and C based on the mechanism of injury. Type A fractures are compression type injuries and are subdivided into three subtypes (type 1 – wedge, type 2 – pincer and type 3 – burst fractures). Type B fractures are distraction injuries associated with a fracture or ligamentous injury to the posterior column (flexion–distraction or hyper-extension injuries). They are subdivided into three types: type 1 – posterior ligamentous injury with anterior injury, type 2 (chance type) fractures of both anterior and posterior elements with distraction posteriorly, type 3 are associated with anterior distraction. Type C injuries are injuries that occur with rotation. The subtype C1 are A type fractures with rotation, C2 are B type fractures with rotation and C3 injuries are injuries with rotation and shear. Fractures become more unstable as type progresses from A to C and subtype from 1 to 3.

EXAMINER: What role does spinal surgery have and what factors do you know that indicate prognosis?

CANDIDATE: Incomplete spinal cord injuries are more likely to recover than complete injuries. Sacral sparing implies an incomplete lesion and improved prognosis. Spinal surgery attempts to decompress the injured spinal segment and stabilize the injury. Decompression aims to remove compression (either direct or indirect) but currently there is limited evidence showing improved neurological outcome. Stabilization of the spine reduces pain, facilitates patient handling and allows earlier mobilization helping prevent the complications associated with recumbency. Surgical stabilization prevents further displacement in unstable fractures preventing further injury and late deformity with better posture and balance. (A stable fracture is one that will not displace under normal physiological loads.)

1. *The Initial Care and Transfer of Patients with Spinal Cord Injuries.* London: British Orthopaedic Association, 2006.

Spinal trauma background knowledge

Vaccaro and colleagues have devised the TLICS system (thoracolumbar injury classification and severity score) for decision making in spinal trauma,[1] based on the configuration of the fracture, neurological state of the patient and the integrity of the posterior ligamentous complex. Compression fractures score 1, burst fractures 2, translational/rotation injuries 3 and distraction injuries 4. Patients that are neurologically intact score 0, nerve root or complete spinal cord injuries 2 and incomplete injuries 3. The posterior ligamentous component scores 0 if the ligament is intact, 2 if it is suspected and 3 if it is confirmed.

Patients with a score of < 3 are considered not to be operative candidates, and those with scores > 5 are considered for surgery.

1. Lee JY, Vaccaro A, Lim MR *et al.* Thoracolumbar injury classification and severity score: a new paradigm for the treatment of thoracolumbar spine trauma. *J Orthop Sci* 2005;**10**(6):671–675.

Neurological injury

Neurological injury can be classified as 'complete' or 'incomplete'. Incomplete injuries have a better potential for recovery. Various patterns of incomplete injury have been described:

Anterior cord syndrome – Loss of motor function with sparing of proprioception and pressure sensation (poor prognosis).

Posterior cord syndrome – Rare, there is loss of proprioception and pressure sensation but no motor loss (prognosis for recovery is relatively good).

Central cord syndrome – This is the most common with mixed motor and sensory loss typically greater in upper than lower limbs (prognosis for recovery is fair).

Brown–Sequard (hemicord) syndrome – Ipsilateral motor function and contralateral pain and temperature sensation. Commonly caused by penetrating injury and carries the best prognosis.

Complete injuries have no function below a certain level. The 'level' of the injury is determined by distal-most level with intact motor and sensory function (power 3/5, sensation 2/2 – intact light touch).

Frankel grading system:

A – Complete paralysis.

B – Sensory preservation below level of injury – no voluntary motor function.

C – Sensory preservation below level of injury – useless motor function.

D – Sensory preservation below level of injury – useful voluntary motor function.

E – Normal function.

Specific fractures

Occipital condyle fractures: Rare, mostly detected on CT, associated with cranial nerve dysfunction. Classified by Anderson and Montesano (Type I comminuted axial impact fracture, Type II continuous with base of skull fracture, Type III avulsion at the attachment of the alar ligament). Treatment for types I and II is a cervical collar. Type III treated with halo vest or with occipito-cervical fusion.

Atlanto-occipital joint subluxation: Rare, Powers' ratio defines subluxation (> 1 anterior subluxation < 1 posterior). Treatment is with halo-vest.

C1 (Atlas) fractures: Commonly associated with other injuries. Widening of lateral masses on 'open-mouth' view or CT. Classified by Levine and Edwards into Type I posterior arch fractures, Type II lateral mass fractures and Type III burst fractures (also known as Jefferson fractures). Treatment is with halo-vest immobilization.

C2 (Axis) fractures: two main groups

Anterior odontoid peg (Dens) fractures have been classified by Anderson and D'Alonzo into three types that guide treatment.

1. Fracture of the tip – treat symptomatically.
2. Fracture of the base of the odontoid. High rate of non-union. Treatment is either posterior stabilization or odontoid screw fixation. (Consider halo-vest immobilization if minimally displaced.)
3. Fracture through vertebral body. Management is usually with a halo vest.

The second group of C2 fractures are the pars (Hangman's) fractures that represent a traumatic spondylolisthesis. Some are associated with facet joint dislocations which require reduction (open or closed), otherwise treat in halo vest.

C3 to C7 (subaxial) fractures

These comprise 80% of cervical spine fractures. Treatment of these injuries is guided by the Allen and Fergusson classification and is based on the mechanism of injury.

Vertical (axial) compression injuries

Stage 1 – Compression only – treat with a cervical collar.

Stage 2 – Compression and fracture with minimal displacement – treat with cervical collar or halo vest.

Stage 3 – Fracture with displacement or fragmentation – may require surgery

Flexion–compression injuries

Stage 1 – Blunting of superior endplate – treat in cervical collar.

Stage 2 – Vertebral body beaking – treat in cervical collar.

Stage 3 – Beak fracture – consider surgery.

Stage 4 – Retrolisthesis < 3 mm – consider surgery.

Stage 5 – Retrolisthesis > 3 mm – consider surgery.

Flexion–distraction injuries

This mechanism frequently causes facet joint dislocations as a result of failure of the posterior tension band. Diagnosed on oblique radiographs. Treat with reduction (skull traction up to one-third body weight) and subsequent fusion.

Note: With reduction there is a risk of further injury that can be caused by an associated disc injury anteriorly. An MRI scan prior to reduction is required.

Extension–compression injuries

These injuries cause failure of the posterior elements in compression. Minor (minimally displaced) injuries can be treated in a cervical collar; posterior fusion surgery is considered for more severely displaced or comminuted fractures.

Extension–distraction injuries

The anterior column fails under distraction with anterior longitudinal ligament injuries associated with a vertebral body fracture. Displaced fractures require surgical stabilization. Minimally displaced injuries may be treated in a halo vest.

Lateral flexion injuries

Lateral flexion injuries typically either cause a unilateral compression fracture or a unilateral compression fracture with a distraction injury on the contralateral side. Displaced fractures associated with a contralateral injury require surgical stabilization. Minimally displaced injuries may be treated in a halo vest.

Sacral fractures

Denis Classification:

Zone 1 injuries lateral to the sacral foramina (L5 may be injured).

Zone 2 injuries through the sacral foramina (15% have sacral root injuries).

Zone 3 injuries medial to the foramen (30–50% have sacral root injuries).

Surgical treatment is indicated for fractures with neurological injury of displaced fractures.

Notes on various other viva scenarios

Structure of the intervertebral disc

Draw the structure of the intervertebral disc and describe the biochemical changes within the disc with ageing (Figure 5.10).

Increasing age is associated with progressive dehydration of the intervertebral disc. Histologically, the boundary between the nucleus pulposus and the annulus fibrosus becomes less distinct. There is a progressive loss of agrecan and water from the extracellular matrix and an increase in proteases. There is an increase in the keratin to chondroitin sulphate ratio.

Paget's disease

Paget's disease is a disorder of metabolism affecting the turnover of bone. Local exaggeration of osteoclastic resorption of bone is followed by exaggerated deposition of bone resulting in deformed and misshapen bones. A third of patients with Paget's disease have spinal involvement. In the spine it may give rise to symptoms as the result of stenosis or localized compression of a nerve, giving rise to radiculopathy (serum alkaline phosphatase is elevated, calcium is normal, urinary hydroxyproline is elevated). Conservative management is with NSAIDs and bisphosphonates. Surgery is rarely undertaken because of a significantly increased risk of bleeding.

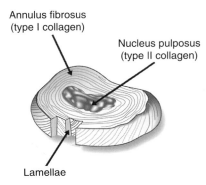

Annulus fibrosus (type I collagen)

Nucleus pulposus (type II collagen)

Lamellae

Figure 5.10 Diagram of intervertebral disc structure.

Diffuse idiopathic skeletal hyperostosis (DISH)

Also called Forestier's disease this idiopathic condition most commonly affects the thoracic region and there is a progressive ('flowing') ossification of the spinous ligaments. The ossification is defined as 'non-marginal' syndesmophytes to distinguish it from ankylosing spondylitis. It is associated with chronic back pain and is more common in patients with diabetes and gout and an increased risk of heterotopic ossification after hip arthroplasty.

Ankylosing spondylitis

Ankylosing spondylitis is a systemic inflammatory arthropathy that affects the spine. It is associated with HLA-B27 in 90% of cases and affects men and women equally although men are typically more severely affected. Onset is usually between 15 and 35 years of age and diagnosis is often delayed. Physiotherapy and anti-inflammatory medication is the mainstay of treatment. Physiotherapy and postural exercises aim to prevent deformity. Surgery in the form of spinal osteotomy may be considered to correct fixed deformity.

Spinal fractures in these patients are often unstable because of the long lever-arms generated by the fused segments and involvement of all columns.

Minimally displaced fatigue fractures or fractures as the result of minor trauma are easily missed. Fractures that correct pre-existing deformities are associated with a high (30–75%) rate of neurological injury. Because fractures are more likely to be unstable surgery is more often required and decompression with long (rather than short) segment stabilization is required.

Bone grafting techniques

Spinal fusion procedures play an integral role in many aspects of spine surgery and a picture of a spinal fusion may lead on to questions about the biology of bone grafts. Different regions that can be fused are:

Within the facet joints (Moe 'interfacetal' fusion).
Between the transverse processes – 'Intertransverse' or 'posterolateral' fusion.
Between the vertebral bodies – PLIF – posterior lumbar inter-body fusion.
ALIF – anterior lumbar inter-body fusion.

Both PLIF and ALIF aim to fuse the vertebral bodies but the surgical approach is either through a posterior or anterior approach.

Autograft, allograft and bone graft substitutes, and bone morphogenic protein are all available to facilitate spinal fusion. Autograft (typically from the iliac crest) is regarded as the 'gold standard' but there is associated donor site morbidity.

Chapter

6

Shoulder and elbow structured oral questions

Asir Aster

Introduction

Viva is like playing a game. The candidate should know the subject well, have a game plan and should know the opponent (who has been bored by the previous unchallenging candidates). A candidate who asks clever questions and answers appropriately will gain control (over the examiner) making it a rewarding 5 minutes (for both examiner and candidate) and more importantly will score highly in the viva. An examiner relishes a candidate who takes control and makes his life easy.

Avoid guess work. Avoid talking generally about the shoulder conditions to fill the time if your aim is to score well. A targeted question or answer will take you far.

Again I must stress the importance of time management in viva, as you have got only 5 minutes to score either 8 or 4.

The main aim of this chapter is to express the importance of the viva techniques and therefore it is not written as a textbook. Analyse the good as well as the poor techniques illustrated in the scenarios and follow the ones you find useful.

Shoulder

In a shoulder structured oral question try to analyse the question according to its presentation. Broadly, the shoulder pathology could be classified as painful, weak, stiff or unstable conditions. Shoulder pathology varies with different age groups and therefore you should have a list of age-related diagnoses clear in your mind, which will be helpful in the viva. There can be overlaps of these conditions, for example a painful stiff shoulder may represent frozen shoulder or acute calcific tendonitis. Therefore candidates should have a list of conditions and one or two classic

questions to differentiate one from another, to lead into the scenario comfortably right from the start.

Structured oral examination question 1

EXAMINER: This is a radiograph of the left shoulder of an 84-year-old lady. Describe the radiograph please. (Figure 6.1.)

CANDIDATE: Well . . . Good morning.
This is the plain radiograph of an 84-year-old lady's left shoulder . . . anteroposterior (AP) view. There is evidence of joint destruction with loss of articular anatomy.

EXAMINER: What do you think is wrong with this shoulder?

CANDIDATE: Well, to be certain I need to ask a few questions and examine the patient.

EXAMINER: Go on then and ask some questions.

CANDIDATE: Is she right handed or left handed?

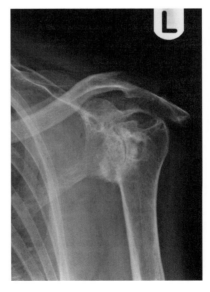

Figure 6.1
Anteroposterior (AP) radiograph left shoulder.

Postgraduate Orthopaedics: Viva Guide for the FRCS (Tr & Orth) Examination, ed. Paul A. Banaszkiewicz and Deiary F. Kader. Published by Cambridge University Press. © Cambridge University Press 2012.

EXAMINER: Right handed.

CANDIDATE: How long has she had a problem with this shoulder?

EXAMINER: 70 years.

CANDIDATE: How did the problem start?

EXAMINER: It started as a painless lump when she was 14 and a few months later she began to have a discharging sinus that required several joint washouts and medication.

CANDIDATE: Does she have an active sinus now?

EXAMINER: No, the sinus healed after she underwent the washouts and started the medication and has never recurred.

CANDIDATE: That is good. What are her current problems?

EXAMINER: Well, she has some restriction of movements and therefore visited her GP who performed this X-ray and sent her to you for your opinion.

CANDIDATE: Then I would examine the patient.

EXAMINER: She has 60° of abduction and forward elevation and has very restricted rotations.

CANDIDATE: I would like to know the power of her cuff muscles.

EXAMINER: It is not possible to assess the power as she has very restricted range of movements.

CANDIDATE: Now . . .

TRING. . . . . .

EXAMINER: Thank you.

Did this candidate do well? Was there a diagnosis? Was there a discussion about the management? Only a 4 or 5 score would be given as the candidate did not even arrive at a diagnosis and missed all the clues.

A different candidate with the same scenario:

EXAMINER: This is a radiograph of left shoulder of 84-year-old lady. Describe the X-ray please.

CANDIDATE: This radiograph of shoulder anteroposterior (AP) view shows evidence of joint destruction and loss of articular cartilage.

EXAMINER: What do you think is wrong with this shoulder?

CANDIDATE: This appearance suggests several possible causes such as previous joint infection, trauma or a neurogenic cause. May I know how the problem started?

EXAMINER: Problems started as a painless lump when she was 14 and a few months later she began to have a discharging sinus for which she had several joint washouts and medication.

CANDIDATE: The presentation sounds like she had a low-grade joint infection. Was there any microbiological investigation performed at the time of the joint washouts?

EXAMINER: Yes, it was diagnosed as acid-fast bacillus and now what will be your management?

CANDIDATE: Well, I would like to know if she had any reactivation of infection in the last 70 years.

EXAMINER: No.

CANDIDATE: In that case what is the expectation of the patient?

EXAMINER: The patient does not want any surgical treatment. She wants to know if she can have some injections into her shoulder which can prevent the pain at the extremes of movements.

CANDIDATE: I will be cautious about the intra-articular injections as it can trigger the dormant bacillus and rekindle the infection.

EXAMINER: The patient does not want to take this risk and wants to be left alone.

Thank you.

Although the viva questions started in the same manner, this candidate with his or her knowledge took the viva to a good level of demonstration of his or her clinical judgement by asking specific questions and had control over the situation. Certainly this candidate deserves a good score.

Structured oral examination question 2

EXAMINER: Good afternoon. Can you tell me what is going on in this radiograph of the right shoulder (Fig. 6.2.)? This patient had anterior dislocation 2 years ago and has on-going problems.

CANDIDATE: Well this shoulder is reduced congruently. I cannot see any interposition of bony fragments. And I would like to investigate this shoulder with MR arthrogram.

EXAMINER: !! What do you want to rule out?

CANDIDATE: Well the risk of re-dislocation of the shoulder is much higher with anterior dislocation due to labral detachment in younger patients and it could be treated successfully if identified with MR arthrogram.

EXAMINER: This gentleman is claustrophobic!

CANDIDATE: I would talk to the radiologist and anaesthetist to find out if it could be done under sedation.

EXAMINER: The anaesthetist is not happy! And your radiologist suggests an ultrasound examination of the shoulder.

CANDIDATE: Ultrasound examination is not the gold standard examination for labral pathology.

EXAMINER: Well, the patient had only ultrasound examination and it shows a subscapularis tear!

CANDIDATE: There is then a high risk of having damaged the anterior labrum also . . . I think I have to speak to the anaesthetist again . . .

Another candidate follows this miserable viva of negotiations between anaesthetist and radiologist in the FRCS ortho exam (by the candidate's own fault).

EXAMINER: Good afternoon. Can you tell me what is going on in this radiograph of the right shoulder? This patient had anterior dislocation 2 years ago and has on-going problems.

CANDIDATE: Thanks. May I know the age of the patient and the nature of the ongoing problem please?

EXAMINER: This 76-year-old gentleman dislocated his shoulder 2 years ago. Now he has got difficulties in overhead activities and we found out that he is claustrophobic!

CANDIDATE: I suspect rotator cuff tear in this age group following dislocation and also there is a risk of infra-clavicular plexus injury following the dislocations, therefore I would like to assess his cuff muscles clinically.

EXAMINER: He has got weakness on internal rotation and the rest of the cuff power is good. Neurologically he is intact.

CANDIDATE: I suspect subscapularis tendon tear from this clinical assessment and I would investigate this shoulder with an ultrasound examination.

EXAMINER: The ultrasound examination shows subscapularis tear, with proximal migration of the tendon by 4 mm.

CANDIDATE: I would like to know, what has been done so far? And what are his expectations?

EXAMINER: Nothing has been done so far. He wants to play golf, which he has not been able to in the last 2 years.

CANDIDATE: Well, I would assess his shoulder arthroscopically and repair his cuff.

EXAMINER: Would you call this a cuff arthropathy as it is going on for 2 years?

CANDIDATE: No. The radiograph does not show any evidence of proximal migration of the humeral head. And the ultrasound scan shows intact supra- and infraspinatus tendons. To develop cuff arthropathy at least two of the three supports should have been lost.

TRING . . .

This candidate knew the importance of age-related pathophysiology and succeeded well in the viva.

Structured oral examination question 3

EXAMINER: This is a radiograph of right shoulder of a lady who has got severe pain in her shoulder. Anything you find interesting? (Figure 6.2.)

CANDIDATE: Well . . . No not really . . . I cannot see any abnormal or disease process in this radiograph.

EXAMINER: She is in your clinic referred by her GP. What would you like to do for her?

CANDIDATE: I want to get history . . . then to examine the patient . . . to decide on the management plan.

EXAMINER: Go ahead.

CANDIDATE: In the history I will first find out her age, job and dominant side . . . and how and when the problem started.

EXAMINER: She is 45, right-hand dominant and does clerical work. The pain started 8 months ago when she was reaching out for the seat belt in her car.

CANDIDATE: The age and history suggest probable frozen shoulder . . . I will proceed with the examination.

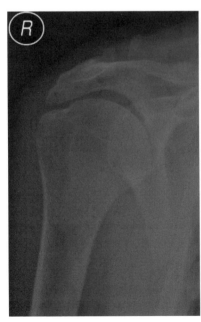

Figure 6.2
Anteroposterior (AP) radiograph right shoulder.

EXAMINER: She has got global restriction of her movements.

CANDIDATE: That confirms frozen shoulder. So . . .

EXAMINER: What do you want to do?

CANDIDATE: I would offer intra-articular steroid injection for her shoulder and also advice on stretching exercises by physiotherapists.

EXAMINER: She has already had three intra-articular steroid injections and regular physiotherapy from her GP practice.

CANDIDATE: Well in that case I would advise her to have manipulation under anaesthesia or arthroscopic arthrolysis.

EXAMINER: What will you specifically offer the patient?

CANDIDATE: mmm . . . MUA.

EXAMINER: The patient wants to know the risks associated with MUA.

CANDIDATE: Well apart from the anaesthetic risks, there is a risk of fracturing the humerus as it can be osteopenic from disuse . . . also the risk of recurrence.

EXAMINER: If the bone fractures, what will be the management?

CANDIDATE: It is like any fracture. Can be treated in a cast or operated.

EXAMINER: The patient decides now to leave it alone.

CANDIDATE: I will then convince her to have an injection today and review her situation in 12 weeks.

Do you think this candidate impressed the (patient) or the examiner, with this simple shoulder scenario? Before we look at the next candidate, think how you would approach this differently!

EXAMINER: This is a radiograph of right shoulder of a lady who has got severe pain in her shoulder. Anything do you find interesting?

CANDIDATE: Yes, this radiograph is essentially normal. May I know the age of this patient and does she suffer from diabetes or thyroid-related problems?

EXAMINER: Well she is 45 and she has hypothyroidism. Is there anything else would you like to examine other than her ‚shoulders?

CANDIDATE: Yes, I would like to look at her hand to see if she has any evidence of Dupuytren's contracture as it has some association with frozen shoulder.

EXAMINER: She is in your clinic referred by her GP. What would you like to do for her?

CANDIDATE: I want to know the history and examination findings.

EXAMINER: She is right-hand dominant and does clerical work. The pain started 8 months ago when she was reaching out for the seat belt in her car. She has got global restriction of her movements.

CANDIDATE: Does this pain affect her sleep? What is the range of her external rotation?

EXAMINER: Yes, she struggles to sleep at night and her ER is only to neutral position. What would you like to do for her?

CANDIDATE: I want to know what has been done to her so far and what is her expectation?

EXAMINER: She has had three intra-articular injections and physiotherapy from her GP practice. She wants to be able to wash and dress herself independently.

CANDIDATE: Well, I would like to offer her either manipulation under anaesthesia or arthroscopic capsular release, explaining the advantages and disadvantages of both procedures and the importance of immediate post-intervention physiotherapy, and make her understand the disease process of frozen shoulder so that the patient could have a realistic expectation of the treatment process.

EXAMINER: The patient understands your explanation very well and wants to have the key-hole surgery. What will you do in arthroscopic capsular release?

CANDIDATE: The anterior capsule release especially at the rotator interval, followed by middle glenohumeral ligament release and the release of coracohumeral ligament. Inferior capsule will be stretched by manipulation . . . this is my preference as the arthroscopic release of inferior capsule carries a small risk of damaging axillary nerve.

EXAMINER: Thank you.

When the examiner sensed an ability, a small extra challenge was given – anywhere else you want to examine? And the candidate was able to demonstrate his or her knowledge – association with Dupuytren's contracture – the candidate would have been given an extra point for these smart moves.

Structured oral examination question 4

EXAMINER: This is a radiograph of a 63-year-old gentleman's right shoulder. Proceed.

CANDIDATE: This plain AP radiograph shows normal glenohumeral joint and acromioclavicular joint, well-maintained subacromial space but the undersurface of the acromion is sclerotic suggesting possibility of him suffering from subacromial impingement. Can I see an axillary view please?

EXAMINER: Yes.

CANDIDATE: There are deposits of calcium in the supraspinatus tendon . . .

EXAMINER: What is your opinion about his pain in the shoulder?

CANDIDATE: Well, he could be struggling with calcific tendonitis.

EXAMINER: What do you want to do?

CANDIDATE: I would like to know the patient's symptoms, examination findings, the treatments he had so far and his expectations.

EXAMINER: He is a keen golfer and gradually over the last 2 years he has developed the pain on over-head activities. He has not had any interventions so far. He wants to continue playing golf without pain. He has got positive impingement signs.

CANDIDATE: Well, I would inject his subacromial space with steroid today to relieve the bursitis secondary to the calcific tendonitis, which is causing impingement symptoms and review him in 8 weeks in clinic with repeat X-rays to assess the calcium deposits.

EXAMINER: Incidentally there is also another X-ray of his right shoulder which was performed 2 years ago when he started to have the pain, which shows the same calcium deposits. Does it change your plan?

CANDIDATE: . . . Well, I would then book him now for arthroscopic excision of the calcium deposits.

EXAMINER: Will you perform any other procedures during the surgery?

CANDIDATE: I will consent him for arthroscopy and proceed . . . so that I can assess the shoulder and perform the necessary at the time of the surgery.

Did he not start well? Did this candidate proceed well – with diagnosis and management plan? Did he pick up the clues by the examiners and correct himself? What will be your scoring for this candidate? Will you diagnose and manage this problem differently like the next candidate?

EXAMINER: This is a radiograph of a 63-year-old gentleman's right shoulder. Proceed.

CANDIDATE: This plain AP radiograph shows normal glenohumeral joint and acromioclavicular joint, well-maintained subacromial space but the undersurface of the acromion is sclerotic suggesting possibility of him suffering from subacromial impingement. Can I see an axillary view please?

EXAMINER: Yes.

CANDIDATE: There are deposits of calcium in the supraspinatus tendon . . .

EXAMINER: What is your opinion about his pain in the shoulder?

CANDIDATE: Looking at the radiographs, duration of his problem . . .

(*EXAMINER*: 2 years) and his age I feel he has got degenerative calcification in his cuff and subacromial impingement.

EXAMINER: What do you want to do?

CANDIDATE: I would like to know the patient's symptoms, examination findings, the treatments he had so far and his expectations.

EXAMINER: He is a keen golfer and gradually over the last 2 years he has developed the pain on over-head activities. He has not had any interventions so far. He wants to continue playing golf without pain. He has got positive impingement signs.

CANDIDATE: I want to know if he had any X-rays in the past and would like to assess the status of his cuff with an ultrasound scan.

EXAMINER: This is the X-ray taken 2 years ago – showing the same calcification. The ultrasound scan shows intact cuff.

CANDIDATE: Well I would inject the subacromial bursa today with steroid and review the patient in 8 weeks to see if the injection has helped his pain as a diagnostic test for impingement.

EXAMINER: He comes back in 8 weeks saying the pain was well controlled for 3 weeks and now the pain is back. What will you do?

CANDIDATE: This proves the pathology of subacromial impingement and I am going to talk to the patient about the subacromial decompression.

EXAMINER: Will you perform excision of the calcium deposits?

CANDIDATE: No, not necessarily. This degenerative calcification is a chronic one. It is not acute calcific tendonitis. Therefore I will perform only the subacromial decompression.

EXAMINER: Thank you.

This second candidate was much clearer about the pathology and management plan, which will be rewarded by a better score. He did not have to be prompted by the examiners regarding the calcium deposit which was there 2 years ago suggesting the degenerative calcification. The previous candidate failed to understand these prompting clues.

Structured oral examination question 5

EXAMINER: Good afternoon. Can you tell me the findings from this radiograph of the left shoulder of a 76-year-old left-handed fit gentleman? (Figure 6.3.)

CANDIDATE: This anteroposterior view of left shoulder shows no evidence of glenohumeral joint or acromioclavicular joint arthritis. The subacromial space is narrowed with sclerosis of the undersurface of the acromion.

EXAMINER: Would you like any other investigations . . . prior to committing yourself with a diagnosis?

CANDIDATE: I would like to have ultrasound of his shoulder . . . and may I know his symptoms please?

EXAMINER: The ultrasound, which was requested by his GP, shows torn subscapularis and supraspinatus with massive retraction of the tendons. He has difficulties with overhead activities. Can you tell me what is wrong with this shoulder?

CANDIDATE: From the X-ray . . . which shows evidence of impingement by narrowing of the subacromial space, from the ultrasound scan . . . which shows evidence of torn subscapularis and supraspinatus tendons and clinically he has got difficulties in overhead activities . . .

EXAMINER: Yes, it is a nice summary of the situation (wasting time)

CANDIDATE: I think he has severe subacromial impingement and secondary cuff tear.

EXAMINER: What would you do for this gentleman?

CANDIDATE: Well, first I would perform a steroid injection into his subacromial space.

EXAMINER: Can you tell me the landmarks and how will you perform the injection?

CANDIDATE: Yes, 2 cm inferior and medial to the posterolateral corner of the acromion, I will direct the needle towards the anterolateral corner of the acromion to be specific into the bursa.

EXAMINER: Is it necessary to be specific in this patient . . . he has got a massive cuff tear?

CANDIDATE: ??

EXAMINER: Well, he comes back to clinic in 8 weeks with no difference to his symptoms. Do you have any management plans?

CANDIDATE: I will then perform an arthroscopic debridement of the cuff and bursa and a subacromial decompression.

EXAMINER: !! Thank you.

Do you recognize the candidate's mistakes? What will you do differently? Did he treat the patient or the investigations? Did he interpret the investigations appropriately? Now the last candidate of the day arrives for the same scenario.

EXAMINER: Good afternoon. Can you tell me the findings from this radiograph of the left shoulder of a 76-year-old left-handed fit gentleman?

CANDIDATE: This anteroposterior view of the left shoulder shows proximal migration of humeral head with narrowing of the subacromial space and there is no evidence of glenohumeral joint or acromioclavicular joint arthritis.

EXAMINER: Would you like any other investigations . . . prior to committing yourself with a diagnosis?

CANDIDATE: I would like to have an axillary view of his shoulder.

EXAMINER: Yes, we have axillary view. What are you looking for?

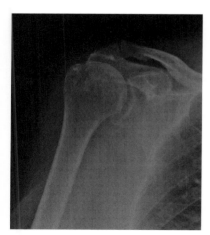

Figure 6.3
Anteroposterior (AP) radiograph left shoulder.

CANDIDATE: I am looking for anteroposterior subluxation of the humeral head in the axillary view ... yes, there is anterior subluxation, suggesting torn anteriorly placed subscapularis and from the AP view, the proximal migration of the humeral head suggesting supraspinatus tear ... this gentleman has got established cuff arthropathy.

EXAMINER: What would you do for him?

CANDIDATE: I need to know the patient's symptoms, what has been done to the patient so far and what are his expectations?

EXAMINER: He has got difficulties in overhead activities. He has had three injections by his GP which has made no difference and being an artist he would like to have reasonable ability to abduct his shoulder to reach for the top of the canvas during painting.

CANDIDATE: Could you please tell me if he has any pain associated with his shoulder abduction?

EXAMINER: No ... not at all

CANDIDATE: I would then offer a reverse-polarity shoulder replacement if he is otherwise healthy and fit for surgery.

EXAMINER: He is very fit. Why do you prefer reverse shoulder to a total shoulder replacement?

CANDIDATE: The reverse shoulder although non-anatomical brings the centre of rotation of the glenohumeral joint medially and thereby increases the moment arm of the deltoid, allowing good abduction of the shoulder.

EXAMINER: Would you not try to repair the cuff prior to this major surgery?

CANDIDATE: No. The radiographs show an established cuff arthropathy and in this situation a rotator cuff repair is not possible.

EXAMINER: Well, we will move on to the next scenario.

Whom do you think played the game well in this scenario? Analyse the candidate's ability to show their knowledge to the examiner. Learn how not to waste time and not to lower the expectations of the examiner. When the examiner's expectations go down, the questions may become simpler and the score becomes lower. Show the knowledge appropriately to please the examiner. Make the game interesting for the examiners and you walk away with a good score. Treat each scenario as a separate exam to reach a good overall score. Remember the examiners do not know your previous performance – either good or bad. Therefore forget the previous performance – either good or bad – and move on.

Elbow

Make a list of conditions causing painful, locking, stiff, flail and unstable elbow. Painful elbow pathology could be best remembered by its anatomical position – anterior, medial, posterior and lateral. Do not forget the nerves around the elbow while making your list.

Structured oral examination question 1

EXAMINER: A 36-year-old right-hand dominant manual worker, referred by GP with painful right elbow. His elbow radiograph is essentially normal. What would you like to do?

CANDIDATE: Well, I need to assess the patient's elbow ... after I had asked the history of his pain.

EXAMINER: Pain is on the lateral side, started gradually 3 months ago ... no history of injury, aggravated by using hammer and was initially relieved by rest. Now it is constant. He has normal range of movements. The point of tenderness is just around the lateral epicondyle.

CANDIDATE: From history and examination I think he has got tennis elbow ...

EXAMINER: What do you do to confirm the diagnosis?

CANDIDATE: I will test if the pain is reproduced by resisted wrist extension.

EXAMINER: Well, he has more pain on resisted finger extension than wrist extension. Does it make you think more specifically?

CANDIDATE: ...

EXAMINER: Which tendons are involved in tennis elbow?

CANDIDATE: ECRB ...

EXAMINER: Can EDC also be affected?

CANDIDATE: ...

EXAMINER: Well, tell me the pathophysiology of tennis elbow.

CANDIDATE: It is termed angiofibroblastic hyperplasia, which is ... hyperplasia of the angiofibroblasts ...

EXAMINER: Do you know any other similar pathology around the elbow?

CANDIDATE: Golfer's elbow, which is tendonitis of the common flexor origin.

EXAMINER: Why do you say tendonitis? What is the difference between tendonitis and tendonosis?

CANDIDATE: . . .

EXAMINER: Going back to the provocation test, if he had tenderness over the lateral proximal forearm on resisted finger extension, what does it tell you?

CANDIDATE: Maybe the disease process is extensive into the common extensor muscle belly.

EXAMINER: We'll move onto the next scenario.

How easy it is to mess up a simple scenario? Is the candidate a classic example for tennis elbow misdiagnosis? Does the candidate deserve anything above a score of 4? Will you approach this subject differently? Think and analyse before looking into the performance of the next candidate.

EXAMINER: A 36-year-old right-hand dominant manual worker, referred by GP with painful right elbow. His elbow radiograph is essentially normal. What would you like to do?

CANDIDATE: I want to know the history of his right elbow pain please.

EXAMINER: It is on the lateral side, started gradually 3 months ago . . . no history of injury, aggravated by using hammer and was initially relieved by rest. Now it is constant.

CANDIDATE: I will proceed with his examination . . . posture of elbow, range of movements especially looking for the lack of full extension and rotation . . . proceed to examine the specific site of tenderness on the lateral aspect.

EXAMINER: He has normal range of movements. The point of tenderness is just around the lateral epicondyle.

CANDIDATE: I would like to know if he has tenderness anterior or posterior to the lateral epicondyle and also any tenderness just distal to the lateral epicondyle.

EXAMINER: What does it tell you?

CANDIDATE: Anterior and distal to lateral epicondyle – ECRB tendonosis. Posterior and distal to lateral epicondyle – EDC tendonosis.

EXAMINER: It is anterior and distal to lateral epicondyle. Tell me the provocation test for ECRB tendonosis.

CANDIDATE: Pain on elbow extension/forearm pronation/fingers flexion/wrist in extension against resistance.

EXAMINER: What is the test for EDC?

CANDIDATE: EDC tendonosis should have pain on elbow extension/forearm pronation/wrist neutral/fingers extension/ long finger extension against resistance.

EXAMINER: Does the EDC provocation test tell you anything else?

CANDIDATE: Yes. If EDC provocation test produces pain over EDC origin, it suggests EDC tendonosis. Pain over radial tunnel – radial tunnel syndrome.

EXAMINER: What do you understand by tennis elbow?

CANDIDATE: It is the tendonosis and not tendonitis of ECRB/ EDC tendons.

EXAMINER: Tell me the histological appearance of tendonosis.

CANDIDATE: Histologically, there are no acute inflammatory cells. There is granulation-like tissue consisting of immature fibroblasts and disorganized non-functional vascular elements called angiofibroblastic hyperplasia. It is theorized to result from an aborted healing response to repetitive micro-trauma. Pain arises possibly from tissue ischaemia. Electron microscopy has shown that these vascular elements do not have lumina. Essentially the repetitive tensile overload, which exceeds tissue stress tolerance, causes tissue damage. If the tissue damage occurs at a rate which exceeds tissue's ability to heal, this causes tissue degeneration.

EXAMINER: Lastly, do you know any other tendonosis around the elbow other than golfer's elbow?

CANDIDATE: Yes, the posterior tennis elbow, which is triceps tendonosis.

If you were the examiner, what score would you give this candidate?

Structured oral examination question 2

EXAMINER: Look at these radiographs of of the right elbow of a 33-year-old patient and tell me the findings.

CANDIDATE: This plain radiograph of a right elbow shows one loose body in the anterior aspect of the joint.

EXAMINER: What would you like to know if you are allowed to ask only one question?

CANDIDATE: I want to know his presenting symptoms.

EXAMINER: He gets intermittent painful locking symptoms. What is the diagnosis here?

CANDIDATE: Well, he has a loose body in the elbow . . .

EXAMINER: Tell me the conditions which produce loose bodies in a joint.

CANDIDATE: Could be post-traumatic, secondary to osteoarthritis, osteochondritis dissecans (OCD) or synovial chondromatosis.

EXAMINER: Now again . . . What would you like to know if you are allowed one more question?

CANDIDATE: Did he have any injury in the past?

EXAMINER: No, never . . . What is your diagnosis here, keeping in mind that there is only one loose body in the elbow?

CANDIDATE: It could be either secondary to osteoarthritis or OCD and I could rule out post-traumatic cause as he had no injury.

EXAMINER: Can you look at the radiographs again and be more specific? (Showing the X-ray again to the candidate.)

CANDIDATE: I can see only one loose body. There is no calcification in the muscle or capsule.

EXAMINER: What does it tell you?

CANDIDATE: It helps me to rule out myositis ossification and synovial sarcoma.

EXAMINER: I want you to concentrate in the intra-articular pathology and try to narrow down your diagnosis between OCD and osteoarthritis.

CANDIDATE: I would like to know the history of his symptoms and have more investigations to be more specific.

EXAMINER: Well he had unexplained painful elbow which lasted for about 18 months when he was 17 years of age. What do you think is going on with this elbow?

CANDIDATE: It sounds like it may not be osteoarthritis . . . it could be OCD.

EXAMINER: If you had been consulting him at the time of initial presentation 16 years ago, what will be your concern?

CANDIDATE: I would . . .

TRING. . .

Was the candidate a happy customer at the end of this viva? Did he lack the knowledge of this subject of loose bodies? Did he use his knowledge appropriately?

EXAMINER: Look at these radiographs of the right elbow of a 33-year-old patient and tell me the findings.

CANDIDATE: This plain radiograph of a right elbow shows well-maintained joint space with evidence of one loose body in the anterior aspect of the joint.

EXAMINER: What would you like to know if you are allowed to ask only one question?

CANDIDATE: I want to know if this patient had any problem with this elbow in the past.

EXAMINER: Yes, this patient had unexplained painful elbow which lasted for about 18 months when he was 17 years of age. What do you think is going on with this elbow?

CANDIDATE: Well, he could have had osteochondritis dissecans when he was 17, which explains the unexplained pain he had for 18 months and the OCD segment must have separated to form the loose body.

EXAMINER: Do you know a name for OCD of elbow?

CANDIDATE: Yes, Panner's disease.

EXAMINER: If you had consulted him at the time of initial presentation of OCD, what would you have done and why?

CANDIDATE: I would have performed an MRI scan.

EXAMINER: MRI was not widely available then.

CANDIDATE: Well, I would have performed an elbow arthrogram with contrast to assess if the segment had separated from the base. Also the age at which he presented was not in the favourable range . . . that is after the closure of the physis . . . therefore I would have followed him clinically more closely.

EXAMINER: This patient unfortunately had only one X-ray at the start of the presentation and as it did not show any obvious pathology, he was discharged from follow-up. What would you like to do now?

CANDIDATE: I would like to know his presenting symptoms. Has he had any treatment so far and what are his expectations?

EXAMINER: He has had no treatment so far. And can you tell me what would be his presenting symptom?

CANDIDATE: I would expect him to have intermittent painful locking of the elbow.

EXAMINER: Yes, that is his symptom. He wants to have something done to prevent these unexpected painful locking episodes.

CANDIDATE: I would perform an arthroscopic removal of the loose body.

EXAMINER: Can you tell me another cause for one or two loose bodies in a joint?

CANDIDATE: In osteoarthritis the osteophytes can break and present similarly. But the radiograph will show evidence of osteoarthritis.

EXAMINER: If you see multiple loose bodies, what is the diagnosis?

CANDIDATE: Synovial chondromatosis.

This is a good example of using your knowledge appropriately. Compare these two candidates. Candidate 2 has made life easier by being specific and appropriate on every opportunity available.

Structured oral examination question 3

EXAMINER: What do you see in this radiograph of a 67-year-old lady's right elbow? (Figure 6.4.)

CANDIDATE: This radiograph shows extensive erosion of the articular cartilage which has involved both ulnohumeral and radiocapitellar joints. The radial head is dislocated and the elbow articulation is aligned only with ulna and humerus. There is peri-articular osteopenia. There is no subchondral sclerosis or osteophytes.

EXAMINER: What could be the cause?

CANDIDATE: It is characteristic of inflammatory arthropathy and I suspect rheumatoid arthritis. It is a flail elbow.

EXAMINER: Indeed this lady has had RA for the last 34 years. What would you like to do for her?

CANDIDATE: I want to know her presenting symptoms from this elbow. What has changed now to think about doing something about this elbow now? What has been done to this elbow so far? What are her expectations?

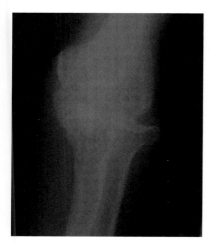

Figure 6.4
Anteroposterior (AP) radiograph right elbow.

EXAMINER: As an RA patient she has many joint problems and recently she is finding lack of strength in her right upper limb to do day-to-day activities. She has had no specific elbow treatments. She wants to do her normal household activities.

CANDIDATE: I would specifically assess her elbow stability and range of movements. And more importantly check her hand function with regards to any tendon ruptures and posterior interosseous nerve function.

EXAMINER: She has no valgus and varus stability but good range of active and passive movements. Hand function is also good. Now how will you differentiate between PIN palsy and extensor tendon rupture?

CANDIDATE: Well if there is no active extension of the fingers at MCP joint and tenodesis test is showing no passive extension of finger at MCP joint on passive flexion of wrist, then the diagnosis is extensor tendon rupture. If the tenodesis test produced passive extension at MCP joint then the diagnosis is PIN palsy. But I will cautiously assess the other tendons supplied by PIN prior to making final diagnosis as in RA patients both can exist together.

EXAMINER: What will be your management plan?

CANDIDATE: It is a multidisciplinary approach with re-consultation with rheumatologists and assessment by occupational therapists. I would initially offer her an elbow brace.

EXAMINER: She comes back after 3 months and says the brace has improved her life quality to some extent but finds it difficult as it gets wet in the kitchen and she still has difficulties in the shower as she could not wear it in the shower.

CANDIDATE: If she is fit for a general anaesthetic, I will do a cemented linked/semi-constrained total elbow replacement for her as this elbow is unstable. I would perform a c-spine X-ray to assess the atlanto-axial joint and obtain an anaesthetic opinion.

EXAMINER: Finally, what happens to juvenile rheumatoid joints?

CANDIDATE: Contrasting to adult RA, juvenile RA produces stiff joints.

Who had the control in this viva? Did this candidate get the questions he played for? Was his technique good? Did he not manage to get a bonus question? Would you be happy if you were the candidate of this scenario? Would you have played it any better? Now the next candidate approaches this table.

EXAMINER: What do you see in this radiograph of a 67-year-old lady's right elbow?

CANDIDATE: This radiograph shows extensive erosion of the articular cartilage which has involved both ulnohumeral and radiocapitellar joints. The radial head is dislocated and the elbow articulation is aligned only with ulna and humerus.

EXAMINER: What could be the cause?

CANDIDATE: It is characteristic of inflammatory arthropathy and I suspect rheumatoid arthritis. It is a flail elbow.

EXAMINER: Indeed this lady has had RA for the last 34 years. What features in the radiograph made you rule out osteoarthritis?

CANDIDATE: In osteoarthritis there will be joint space narrowing, subchondral sclerosis, subchondral cysts and osteophytes. This radiograph does not show these features.

EXAMINER: What is the bone quality here?

CANDIDATE: . . . The bone appears to be osteopenic . . . could be disuse from pain or the disease process itself.

EXAMINER: Now, what would you do for her?

CANDIDATE: I need to know the history of presenting complaints and I would examine the elbow.

EXAMINER: She recently finds her right upper limb weak affecting her day-to-day activities. In the examination there is valgus/varus instability.

CANDIDATE: It is an unstable elbow from advanced RA. Therefore I would do a total elbow replacement for her.

EXAMINER: Is there anything you would consider prior to surgery?

CANDIDATE: Well, I can try a splint if she is willing to try . . .

EXAMINER: She comes back after 3 months and says the brace has improved her life quality to some extent but finds it difficult as it gets wet in the kitchen and she still has difficulties in the shower as she could not wear it in the shower.

CANDIDATE: Then I will proceed with the total elbow replacement.

EXAMINER: Which nerve specifically would you like to assess in the RA elbow especially prior to total elbow replacement?

CANDIDATE: Posterior interosseous nerve as it can be affected by the synovial swelling/dislocation of the radiocapitellar joint.

EXAMINER: What would be the findings if she has PIN palsy?

CANDIDATE: There will be no active extension of the fingers at the level of MCP joints.

EXAMINER: Do you know any other cause for the inability to extend MCP joints?

CANDIDATE: Yes, progressive rupture of extensor tendons called Vaughn–Jackson syndrome.

EXAMINER: Is there any concern regarding this RA patient undergoing general anaesthesia?

CANDIDATE: These patients can have lung fibrosis . . . apart from this, yes . . . of course I will perform a c-spine X-ray to see the stability of atlanto-axial joint.

EXAMINER: Thank you.

Did he not answer all the questions? Did he not possess the knowledge of the subject? But, did he gain the control of this viva? Did he ever lead the examiner to the next question? Or did the examiner have to guide him with leading questions? Would he ever get a score of 8?

Structured oral examination question 4

EXAMINER: Good morning. Here are the radiographs of a right-hand dominant 43-year-old man's right elbow. Tell me the findings. (Figure 6.5.)

CANDIDATE: Good morning. These radiographs show narrowing of joint space on both ulnohumeral and radiocapitellar joints with subchondral sclerosis and cysts and medial, anterior and posterior osteophytes suggesting osteoarthritis. Has he had any previous injury to this elbow?

EXAMINER: Well he had a dislocation of this elbow 8 years ago which was reduced in A&E and as he improved to full function in 8 weeks he was discharged from the fracture clinic. Now over the last 3 years he has got problems with this elbow. What would you advise for this patient?

CANDIDATE: I want to know his present symptoms. How much does it affect his job? What are the treatments he has had so far? And what is his expectation?

EXAMINER: This elbow is affecting his job as he has got restricted movements – flexion extension from 50° to 110° and supination is only to 40°. He had a few intra-articular injections by his GP. He wants to have more movement in the elbow.

CANDIDATE: He has got post-dislocation osteoarthritis with stiffness. He is not presenting with pain as a main symptom. Therefore I would like to perform an arthroscopic debridement/arthrolysis of his elbow.

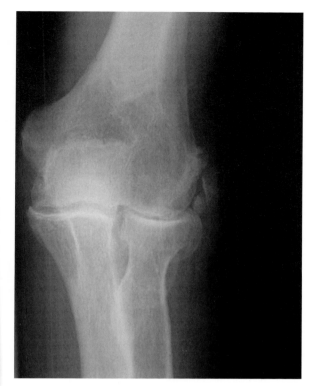

Figure 6.5 Anteroposterior (AP) radiograph right elbow.

EXAMINER: Can you show me the arthroscopic portals in this elbow picture?

CANDIDATE: (Marking and talking to the examiner.)

Direct lateral portal:	At the centre of a triangle defined by the lateral epicondyle, the radial head and the olecranon. This is frequently used as the initial entry portal to inflate the joint with saline.
Anterolateral portal:	1 cm distal and 1 cm anterior to the lateral epicondyle, between the radial head and the capitellum. This gives good access to the anterior aspect of the joint.
Anteromedial portal:	2 cm distal and 2 cm anterior to the medial epicondyle. This is often created using an 'inside out' technique by cutting down onto the tip of the arthroscope inserted using the anterolateral portal.
Proximal medial portal:	2 cm proximal to the medial epicondyle along the anterior surface of the humerus towards the radial head.
Direct posterior portal:	1.5 cm proximal to the tip of the olecranon. Access to olecranon fossa.
Posterolateral portal:	Access to radiocapitellar joint.

EXAMINER: Is the benefit of the debridement permanent?

CANDIDATE: No, it is not … and varies between individuals.

EXAMINER: Patient wants to know if there is any procedure which can provide long-lasting benefit.

CANDIDATE: The longer-lasting result can be achieved by a total elbow replacement … But as this patient is only 43 and he is a manual worker and his dominant elbow is affected with osteoarthritis, I would not advise a total elbow replacement at this moment as the TERs do not have long life expectancy in young osteoarthritic patients.

TRING …

Would you handle this scenario differently? How much will you score this candidate? Was his knowledge sufficient and well presented? Now a confident-looking candidate approaches the table.

EXAMINER: Good morning. Here are the radiographs of a right-hand dominant 43-year-old man's right elbow. Tell me the findings.

CANDIDATE: The radiographs show advanced osteoarthritis of his dominant elbow.

EXAMINER: Correct. What would be your advice to this patient?

CANDIDATE: It depends on if he has pain, stiffness, difficulty with his job and also depends on his expectations.

EXAMINER: Pain is not a main issue here. This elbow is affecting his job as he has got restricted movements – flexion extension from 50° to 110° and supination is only to 40°. He wants to have more movement in the elbow.

CANDIDATE: I will initially inject his elbow with steroids and send him for stretching physiotherapy.

EXAMINER: Patient has had a few injections already and also physiotherapy from his GP and therefore he prefers to have a more definitive procedure.

CANDIDATE: Well, if the injections have been tried without any success, I would advise a total elbow replacement.

EXAMINER: Is there anything you could offer prior to TER?

CANDIDATE: (Suddenly losing confidence.) Probably an attempt at manipulation under anaesthesia …

EXAMINER: Is MUA and passive stretching of a stiff elbow good advice?

CANDIDATE: … perhaps not … as there is a small risk of myositis ossification.

EXAMINER: In the last 30 years . . . the number of implanted TERs is in decline. Why?

CANDIDATE: . . .

EXAMINER: Well, 20 to 30 years ago the TER was commonly used for which group of patients?

CANDIDATE: Rheumatoid patients, and it has declined as rheumatoid patients are better treated now and we do not see advanced joint pathology in this group of patients.

EXAMINER: What is the clinical finding in an advanced RA elbow?

CANDIDATE: Arthritis affects the entire joint, the ligament stability is also lost as RA is primarily a soft tissue problem and the radial head dislocates and the elbow becomes flail.

EXAMINER: Have you seen flail RA elbow recently?

CANDIDATE: No, I haven't seen any which have progressed to radial head dislocations . . . instead the appearance we see now is more like osteoarthritis.

EXAMINER: Does this modification of disease pathology have anything to do with declining number of implanted TER?

CANDIDATE: Yes, the TER failed earlier in this group.

EXAMINER: This is because we are treating stable disease-modified osteoarthritic RA elbows, with the implant designed to treat flail elbows.

CANDIDATE: . . .

EXAMINER: Would you like to offer anything else prior to TER for this young manual worker?

CANDIDATE: An arthroscopic washout?

EXAMINER: Is there any . . .

TRING . . .

Did the confident start last long? Was the knowledge adequate to handle this scenario? Would you like to be this candidate on the day of exam?

Structured oral examination question 5

EXAMINER: I have a problem with my left elbow. Proceed.

CANDIDATE: Well, I want to know your age, hand dominance, your occupation and the nature of your problem please.

EXAMINER: I am 47, a right-hand dominant mechanic and in certain positions my elbow pops which is painful.

CANDIDATE: Is the popping sensation on the inner side or outer side of your elbow?

EXAMINER: The outer side . . . yes, my thumb side.

CANDIDATE: Did you ever have any problem in your elbow as a child?

EXAMINER: I had problems as a child in my right elbow, but now my right side is fine. My left side, although I did not have any problem as a child, 3 years ago I had a simple dislocation.

CANDIDATE: What problem did you have on the right side?

EXAMINER: My older sister pulled me by my right hand and my elbow became painful and the doctor had manipulated my elbow and told my parents not to let anyone pull me by my hand. And he said it was a pulled elbow . . . where the radial head pops out.

CANDIDATE: I want to check if you have general joint laxity.

EXAMINER: No I am rather stiff. What do you think is wrong with my left elbow?

CANDIDATE: I think radial head dislocations . . . probably secondary to annular ligament insufficiency secondary to the dislocation. In what position do you get this popping sensation?

EXAMINER: Whenever I push myself off the chair with my arm.

CANDIDATE: I would like to perform an X-ray of your elbow to assess the radial head.

EXAMINER: The X-ray is normal. Can you tell me about the ligaments around the elbow?

CANDIDATE: Sure. There are two main groups of ligaments, medial and lateral collateral ligaments. MCL has three bundles: anterior, posterior and transverse bands. LCL has lateral ulnar collateral ligament (LUCL), annular ligament, radial collateral ligament and accessory collateral ligament.

EXAMINER: Have you heard of postero-lateral rotatory instability of the elbow?

CANDIDATE: . . .

Did the candidate reach the diagnosis? Did he understand the clues given by the examiner? The next candidate arrives.

EXAMINER: I have a problem with my left elbow. Proceed.

CANDIDATE: Well, I want to know your age, hand dominance, your occupation and the nature of your problem please.

EXAMINER: I am 47, a right-hand dominant mechanic and in certain positions my elbow pops with pain.

CANDIDATE: Have you ever injured your left elbow in the past? And in what position are you feeling the popping sensation in the elbow?

EXAMINER: Well, I had a simple dislocation of my left elbow 3 years ago which was reduced in A&E. Now whenever I push myself off a chair using my arm I get this sensation.

CANDIDATE: I would like to have a quick assessment of your elbow.

EXAMINER: What would you like to test?

CANDIDATE: I want to perform the pivot-shift test to assess the lateral ulnar collateral ligament.

EXAMINER: If the pivot-shift test is positive, what is your diagnosis?

CANDIDATE: Postero-lateral rotatory instability of the left elbow.

EXAMINER: I had been told that I had 'pulled elbow' on the other side as a child. Could this be the same?

CANDIDATE: No, usually the pulled elbow settles as the child grows and you had a definite injury to the left elbow.

EXAMINER: What could you do to me to prevent these unpleasant episodes?

CANDIDATE: I need to perform an MRI scan to confirm injury to LUCL and to see if the injury to the ligament is intra-substance or from the origin to decide on the treatment. And did you have any recent X-rays?

EXAMINER: My X-rays were normal. If the MRI scan shows injury to the LUCL, how will you manage this problem?

CANDIDATE: If the LUCL is avulsed from the origin or insertion and the ligament itself is healthy, it could be re-attached to the bone using bone anchors. It may not be possible in your case as the injury was 3 years ago. My main inclination is to reconstruct the LUCL using palmaris longus tendon or triceps fascia.

Did this candidate manage to please the examiner? Which candidate you would prefer to treat your elbow?

The examiner's aim is all about finding out, can I let this candidate be my consultant. As you would like to win the patient's confidence while consulting in the clinics, it is vital to win the examiner's confidence in each and every scenario by showing adequate knowledge expressed with correct technique.

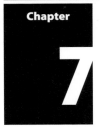

Chapter

7

Orthopaedic oncology

Thomas B. Beckingsale

Definitions

As in all other areas of the viva examinations, knowing basic definitions gives you an easy starting point when answering questions and gives the impression to the examiners that you have both a logical and clear thought process, and are in command of the subject matter.

Neoplasm/tumour: A growth or swelling, which enlarges by cellular proliferation more rapidly than surrounding normal tissue and continues to enlarge after the initiating stimuli cease. Usually lacks structural organization and functional coordination with normal tissues and serves no useful purpose to the host.

Malignant tumour: Malignant tumours have a predisposition to invasive and destructive local growth, and to distant metastasis usually via the vascular or lymphatic systems.

Benign tumour: Benign tumours do not metastasize, but can still exhibit locally aggressive behaviour.

Sarcoma: A diverse and rare group of malignant tumours of mesenchymal/connective tissue origin. Tumours of peripheral nerves are often included in this group.

Generic structured oral examination question 1: Biopsy

EXAMINER: So how would you obtain a tissue diagnosis?

CANDIDATE: A tissue sample can be obtained by biopsy. In general terms this can be performed by excisional, incisional or percutaneous means, but I would not perform a biopsy without first having discussed the case with a bone tumour multidisciplinary team (MDT).

EXAMINER: Good. Let's suppose you are the bone tumour surgeon now. When might you perform an excision biopsy?

CANDIDATE: The indications for an excision biopsy are narrow. The entire lesion is removed and the margins are often marginal. Hence, this type of biopsy is really only applicable to benign lesions where the imaging has been diagnostic, for example lipomas, or where the lesion is small and superficial such that excision biopsy would not compromise later re-excision. However, if there is any doubt about the diagnosis I would perform a percutaneous or incisional biopsy first.

EXAMINER: Ok, tell me how you would perform an incisional biopsy.

CANDIDATE: I would perform the procedure through a short longitudinal incision. I would plan the incision using the imaging, and position it such that the entire biopsy tract could be excised *en bloc* during the definitive resection, and such that it does not contaminate more than one compartment or key neurovascular structures. I would pay close attention to haemostasis and use minimal tissue dissection in order to minimize local tissue seeding.

EXAMINER: We perform most of our biopsies percutaneously now. Do you know any advantages or disadvantages to doing it this way?

CANDIDATE: I've seen biopsy performed by Tru-Cut needle. The procedure can be performed easily in clinic under local anaesthetic, which removes delay and the requirement for theatre time. Welker *et al.* have shown that it is safe, has a low complication rate and reliably provides enough tissue for diagnosis and treatment planning.[1] Other advantages are that it can be combined with imaging modalities, for example ultrasound for soft tissue lesions and CT for bony lesions. The disadvantage is that necrosis and mitotic rate is less reliable on core needle but this rarely affects management, and an incisional biopsy can always be performed subsequently if more information is required.

Postgraduate Orthopaedics: Viva Guide for the FRCS (Tr & Orth) Examination, ed. Paul A. Banaszkiewicz and Deiary F. Kader. Published by Cambridge University Press. © Cambridge University Press 2012.

1. Welker JA, Henshaw RM, Jelinek J, Shmookler BM, Malawer MM. The percutaneous needle biopsy is safe and recommended in the diagnosis of musculoskeletal masses. *Cancer* 2000;**89**(12):2677–2686.

Generic structured oral examination question 2: Margins

EXAMINER: What do you understand by a marginal margin?

CANDIDATE: A marginal margin, as described by Enneking, is when the resection line passes through the reactive zone of the tumour being excised.[1]

EXAMINER: Explain to me what you mean by the reactive zone.

CANDIDATE: Tumours grow in a centifugal fashion and this leads to compression and subsequent atrophy of the surrounding tissue forming a pseudocapsule. Outside the pseudocapsule is an area of oedema where inflammatory cells and micronodules of tumour are present. This is the reactive zone. Hence, if a resection line passes through this reactive zone, as in a marginal margin, then micronodules of tumour are likely to be left behind, increasing the risk of a local recurrence.

EXAMINER: So what other margins did Enneking describe and what do you understand by them?

CANDIDATE: Enneking described three other possible margins. He described intra-lesional margins, where the resection line passes through the tumour leaving macroscopic deposits of tumour in the surgical wound. He described wide margins, where the resection line passes outside the reactive zone and the tumour is excised with a surrounding cuff of normal tissue. In wide margins it is still possible that tumour will remain in the form of skip lesions. Finally, he described the radical margin, where the entire compartment in which the tumour resides is excised *en bloc*, in theory removing the entire tumour.

1. Enneking WF, Spanier SS, Malawer MM. The effect of the anatomic setting on the results of surgical procedures for soft parts sarcoma of the thigh. *Cancer* 1981;**47**(5):1005–1022.

Generic structured oral examination question 3: Staging

EXAMINER: So what stage is this tumour?

CANDIDATE: I would stage this tumour using the Musculoskeletal Tumour Society staging system as described

Table 7.1 Enneking/MSTS staging system.[2]

Stage	Description	Grade	Site	Metastases
IA	Low-grade, intracompartmental	G_1	T_1	M_0
IB	Low-grade, extracompartmental	G_1	T_2	M_0
IIA	High-grade, intracompartmental	G_2	T_1	M_0
IIB	High-grade, extracompartmental	G_2	T_2	M_0
III	Any grade, metastatic	G_{1-2}	T_{1-2}	M_1

by Enneking.[1] We have discussed that it is a high-grade osteosarcoma, which makes it at least Stage II. It's an intramedullary tumour that has invaded the surrounding soft-tissues making it extracompartmental, and upstaging it to IIB. We've not discussed whether there is any evidence of metastasis yet, but, if there is, that would immediately make it a Stage III, regardless of the other features we've talked about.

General advice: This question will usually follow a discussion about a malignant tumour, for example osteosarcoma as in this example. The Enneking system (Table 7.1) is the easiest to remember and can be applied equally to bony and soft-tissue sarcomas.[2] The other commonly used system is the American Joint Committee on Cancer (AJCC) system, which is more complicated. The AJCC also have separate systems for bony and soft-tissue tumours.

1. Enneking WF, Spanier SS, Goodman MA. Current concepts review. The surgical staging of musculoskeletal sarcoma. *J Bone Joint Surg Am* 1980;**62**-A:1027–1030.
2. NCCN. *National Comprehensive Cancer Network Clinical Practice Guidelines in Oncology: Soft Tissue Sarcoma. V.2.2008.* National Comprehensive Cancer Network, 2008.

Structured oral examination question 1: Osteochondroma

EXAMINER: This young lad has been referred to you urgently by his GP after his mum brought him in with a firm lump on the front of his left thigh. Tell me about his X-ray. (Figure 7.1.)

CANDIDATE: This is a lateral radiograph of his left femur including the knee joint but not the hip joint. There is a bony

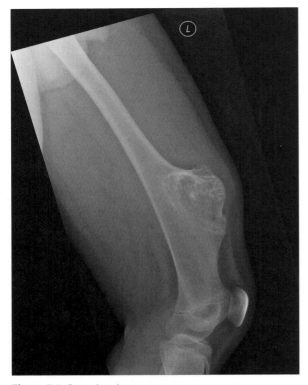

Figure 7.1 Osteochondroma.

growth on the anterior aspect of the femur, which looks like a large osteochondroma.

EXAMINER: What makes you think it's an osteochondroma?

CANDIDATE: Well, the cortices are in continuity with the bone as is the medullary cavity, and the lesion is extending out from the metaphyseal region of the distal femur, which is the most common site for these (25%). This is a sessile lesion rather than the pedunculated variety and appears to be a solitary lesion, although I'd want to examine the child to look for other lumps. It is quite a large lesion and there is some slightly atypical sclerosis within it so I would definitely get an MRI scan.

EXAMINER: OK, so you get an MRI, which shows a nice thin cartilage cap and no worrying features. How are you going to treat it?

CANDIDATE: First I'd take a history and examine the child. I'd want to know if it is tender or symptomatic before I decide what to do.

EXAMINER: It's not tender and it only bothers him occasionally if he knocks it, but his mother is adamant she wants it removed.

CANDIDATE: I would suggest a period of watchful waiting to see if it continues to grow or becomes more symptomatic. Removing it would carry risks of recurrence and neurovascular damage. There is also a chance of fracture, during the operation and afterwards as it's a large sessile lesion and removing it will weaken the anterior cortex of the femur considerably.

EXAMINER: His mum still wants it removed and she's worried that it's going to become cancer.

CANDIDATE: If this is a solitary lesion then malignant change is very rare indeed. If the child has multiple hereditary exostoses the risk is a bit higher. The textbooks often quote figures of 10% but it is probably more like 1–5%.

General advice: Examiners may show an example of a solitary osteochondroma in an area that is difficult to access for the purposes of excision, but then insist that the patient wants it removed, e.g. posterior, proximal tibia. The resultant discussion is then used to assess knowledge of anatomy and approaches, e.g. posterior approach to the knee. If the MRI has shown no sinister features, and the lesion is asymptomatic, then you can have a reasoned discussion with the examiner about watchful waiting versus removal, i.e. both answers are perfectly acceptable.

Other points:

- Continued growth after physeal closure raises the suspicion of malignant transformation.
- EXT gene mutation is the genetic abnormality in multiple hereditary exostoses. It is an autosomal dominant condition.

Structured oral examination question 2: Enchondroma

EXAMINER: Tell me about these radiographs of this chap's right foot. (Figure 7.2.)

CANDIDATE: Well they're AP and oblique views and they show an expansile, lytic lesion in the proximal phalanx of his second toe.

EXAMINER: What do you think it is?

CANDIDATE: The radiographs show features consistent with an enchondroma. It has a short zone of transition and appears quite well defined. There's also some stippled calcification within the substance of the lesion, which suggests a chondroid matrix.

EXAMINER: How would you treat this lesion?

CANDIDATE: Well, I would want to get more information so I would take a full history and examination. I would also want to get more imaging of the lesion with an MRI and discuss the pictures with a bone tumour MDT. If there's any doubt about the diagnosis they may want to do a biopsy, but in general the surgical treatment of an enchondroma is with curettage, with or without grafting.

General advice: Even if the diagnosis appears obvious and is of a benign lesion, don't be rushed into offering surgical treatment. Always work through history, examination and imaging. You will never be criticized for discussing the diagnosis with a bone tumour MDT, but you will end up in a very tricky discussion with the examiners and fail if you have made the wrong diagnosis, it turns out to be malignant, and you've not discussed it with an MDT first.

Other points:

- 50% of solitary enchondromas arise in the hands.
- Malignant transformation is very rare, but when it does occur it is usually in large lesions of long bones.
- Enchondromatosis = Ollier's disease (risk of bone malignancy is 10%, but if visceral and brain malignancies are included then the overall risk is 25%).
- Enchondromatosis + haemangiomas = Maffucci syndrome (risk of malignancy approaching 100%).

Structured oral examination question 3: Non-ossifying fibroma

EXAMINER: Tell me about this radiograph. (Figure 7.3.)

CANDIDATE: This is an AP radiograph of a left lower leg of a child, which includes both the ankle joint and the knee joint. There is a lucent lesion, eccentrically placed in the metaphyseal region of the tibia. The lesion is well-demarcated and its margin is slightly sclerotic. These features are typical of a non-ossifying fibroma.

EXAMINER: Good. What else can you tell me about this lesion?

CANDIDATE: Non-ossifying fibromas are developmental or hamartomatous lesions. They are actually very common and some have suggested an incidence of up to 35% in normal

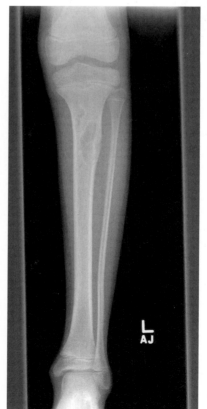

Figure 7.3
Non-ossifying
fibroma.

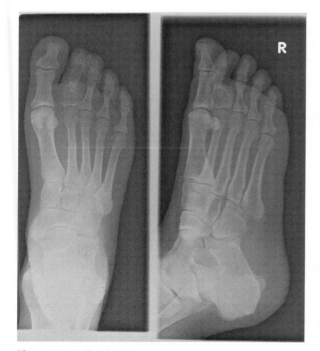

Figure 7.2 Enchondroma.

children. They are usually asymptomatic and are often discovered as an incidental finding. Occasionally they can present after a pathological fracture, after which they tend to heal up.

EXAMINER: How would you treat this lesion?

CANDIDATE: I can't see any evidence of fracture. I would take a history and examine the patient to ascertain whether the lesion is painful or symptomatic and I would discuss the images with our local tumour MDT to make sure that they were in agreement with the diagnosis. That being the case this can be treated with observation only as these lesions normally resolve by adulthood. I would plan to keep the patient under review with surveillance radiography.

General advice: Again, you will not be criticized if you say that would take advice from the bone tumour MDT. You will, however, be in a very difficult situation if you have not stated that you would take their advice and your diagnosis is wrong.

Structured oral examination question 4: Chondrosarcoma

EXAMINER: This 60-year-old lady presented with pain and swelling around her lower back. What can you see on this CT scan? (Figure 7.4.)

CANDIDATE: This is an axial section showing the sacrum and iliac wings. There is an expansile lesion in the left iliac wing, which has extended into the soft tissues. The lesion has both lytic and sclerotic elements to it.

EXAMINER: What do you think the diagnosis might be?

CANDIDATE: The expansile nature, as well as the permeative margin and local invasion suggest a malignant process. Malignant tumours of bone can then be broken down into primary, metastatic, or immunohaematopoietic lesions. Metastatic and immunohaematopoietic tumours tend to produce lytic lesions within bones, whereas this lesion has areas of sclerosis and is much more expansile. Primary bone tumours can be classified according to their matrix as either bone-producing, cartilage-producing, fibrous tissue-producing or non-matrix producing. The patchy sclerosis within this lesion is in keeping with either a bone- or cartilage-producing primary tumour, although I would not rule out other diagnoses without further investigations.[1]

EXAMINER: You're right to suggest a primary lesion in this case. You've suggested bone- or cartilage-producing

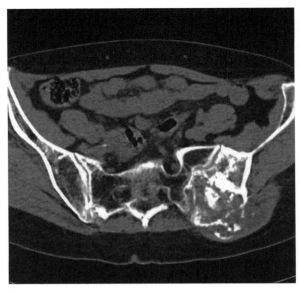

Figure 7.4 Chondrosarcoma.

as the likely matrix. Which do you think is more likely here?

CANDIDATE: It is most likely to be a chondrosarcoma. The incidence of chondrosarcoma increases with age. This lady is 60 and although there is a second peak in the incidence of osteosarcoma in elderly patients, the majority of cases occur in adolescents around the growth spurt. The site of the tumour also makes chondrosarcoma the more likely diagnosis. Only around 5% of osteosarcomas occur in the pelvis, whereas up to 30% of chondrosarcomas are pelvic in origin. Finally, there is the appearance on the CT. It is not the clearest image but I'm trying to convince myself that there's stippled calcification, which would indicate a chondroid lesion.

EXAMINER: Very good. What treatment options are there for an aggressive-looking chondrosarcoma like this is?

CANDIDATE: Chondrosarcomas are poorly chemo- and radio-sensitive so the only treatment option is wide local excision plus or minus reconstruction. However, despite surgical excision, longer-term survival is dependent on the presence or absence of metastases.

EXAMINER: So what do you think the prognosis is for this high-grade lesion?

CANDIDATE: The key is the presence or absence of metastasis and the patient needs staging investigations. In general, low-grade, or grade I, lesions are rarely metastatic and have a better than 90% 5-year survival. High, Grade III, lesions, as you've intimated this one is, are metastatic in over 70% of cases and have only a 30% 5-year survival.

1. Bullough PG. *Orthopaedic Pathology*. Fourth Edition. Edinburgh: Mosby, 2007.

Structured oral examination question 5: Chondrosarcoma

EXAMINER: This is a very fit and well 50-year-old chap, who has come into A&E after falling down the stairs at home, sustaining this injury to his left leg. Tell me how you are going to manage this. (Figure 7.5.)

CANDIDATE: I would manage this patient initially using the principles of ATLS [Airway and protect cervical spine, Breathing, Circulation, Disability, Exposure and environment control].

EXAMINER: Fine. No issues with ABC and the patient is alert and orientated.

CANDIDATE: Moving on I want to assess whether the patient has any other injuries, and regarding this injury I want to know whether it is open or closed and whether the limb is neurovascularly intact.

EXAMINER: Okay. This is his only injury. It's an open fracture with a 1 cm wound on the lateral thigh. The limb is neurovascularly intact. How are you going to manage this?

CANDIDATE: If it's an open injury then I would take a picture of the wound and cover it with a betidine-soaked swab. The patient

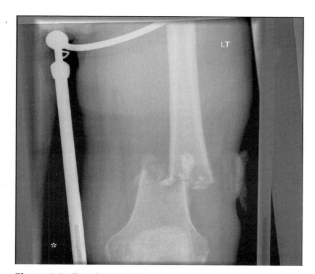

Figure 7.5 Chondrosarcoma.

needs IV antibiotics and coverage for tetanus, depending on their vaccination history. Some form of immobilization is also important for patient comfort and nursing care. In this case I can see that a Thomas splint has been applied.

EXAMINER: Good. So shall I book this patient for theatre with a plan to perform a debridement of the wound and nailing of the fracture?

CANDIDATE: Well, I know it's an open fracture but I have some concerns about the X-ray. There's some odd calcification within the medullary cavity, so I'm worried that this is a pathological fracture through a bony lesion.

EXAMINER: Why does that make a difference?

CANDIDATE: It's a rare situation, but if this is pathological fracture through a bone tumour, and we open up the fracture site and nail it, we would spread tumour the length of the femur and might convert a resectable tumour into one that is unresectable.

EXAMINER: But doesn't the open fracture need washing out?

CANDIDATE: It's a small puncture wound and I've put the patient on IV antibiotics so I think the infection risk is low. In this case I would arrange some urgent investigations, get more information and discuss the case immediately with the bone tumour MDT before rushing the patient to theatre.

General advice: Always look at the available evidence carefully and look out for any atypical features. If in doubt, say so! You will never be criticized for taking advice, but you will fail if you have blazed on with treatment and taken this patient to theatre for wash-out and nailing. If there is no threat to life or limb, then there is always time for further investigations, and to seek further opinions.

Always take time to look carefully before answering, especially if a question on a fracture comes up in the adult and pathology viva station.

Structured oral examination question 6: Osteosarcoma

EXAMINER: This young lad presented with a painful knee and a lump after a football injury. What do you think of the X-ray? (Figure 7.6.)

CANDIDATE: [*When I was shown the X-ray I immediately thought that the diagnosis was an osteosarcoma and described the X-ray changes that supported my initial*

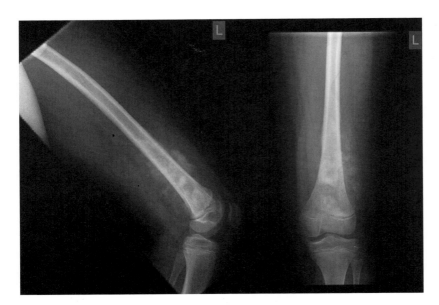

Figure 7.6 Osteosarcoma.

reaction.] There is an intramedullary sclerotic lesion with a wide zone of transition and there is extension through the cortices and into the soft tissues. There is sunray spiculation but at this resolution I can't see an obvious Codman's triangle.

EXAMINER: What's a Codman's triangle?

CANDIDATE: [*I knew what a Codman's triangle was but I did not have a clear definition at my fingertips (a triangle of reactive bone at the edge of the tumour where the periosteum is elevated). I struggled for a few seconds but managed to explain that it is indicative of a periosteal reaction.*]

EXAMINER: So what do you think the diagnosis is?

CANDIDATE: I think the diagnosis is an osteosarcoma.[1] The imaging shows an osteogenic tumour in an adolescent male. It is also in a classical position in the metaphyseal region of the distal femur, where about 35% of these tumours occur.

EXAMINER: So how would you investigate it further?

CANDIDATE: I would take a history and examine the patient. I would refer the child on to a bone tumour MDT immediately rather than delay the process by organizing more investigations locally.

EXAMINER: Okay, so you're working for the bone tumour MDT, what further investigations would you request?

CANDIDATE: I would request investigations to further delineate the tumour itself and I would arrange tests to assess for metastatic disease.

An MRI scan is the best modality for investigating the tumour itself and will delineate the local extent of the tumour, its relationship to key neurovascular structures, and the presence or absence of skip lesions. A CT scan can also be helpful as these lesions are osteogenic and therefore show up well on CT. These investigations can also be used to plan a biopsy. To stage the tumour one might initially get a chest X-ray but CT scan of the chest is mandatory to look for metastases and these are sadly found in about 30% at diagnosis. Other investigations you might use are blood tests, for example alkaline phosphatase and lactate dehydrogenase, which, if elevated, are associated with a poorer prognosis.

EXAMINER: Tell me about the general principles of treatment in cases like this.

CANDIDATE: Before commencing treatment, a confirmatory tissue diagnosis is made by biopsy and staging investigations are completed. Treatment for osteosarcoma then follows four distinct phases: neo-adjuvant chemotherapy, surgical excision and reconstruction, adjuvant chemotherapy and follow-up with clinical examination and imaging to look for recurrent disease or distant metastases.

EXAMINER: Why does the treatment start with neo-adjuvant chemotherapy? Why don't we start by excising the tumour and then start chemotherapy?

CANDIDATE: There are three main reasons for beginning treatment with neo-adjuvant chemotherapy rather than primary surgery. Firstly to treat occult micrometastases, which are likely to be present in a much greater proportion of patients than the 30% who present with radiologically detectable metastases at diagnosis; secondly to reduce the inflammation around the primary tumour, aiding later surgical resection; and finally to allow assessment of response to the neo-adjuvant chemotherapy, determine prognosis and direct adjuvant chemotherapy.

EXAMINER: You mentioned assessment of response to neo-adjuvant chemotherapy. Why is this important?

CANDIDATE: Response of the tumour to chemotherapy treatment is measured as a percentage necrosis on histology of the resected specimen. A greater than 90% necrosis is considered a good response and this carries a better prognosis than poor or non-responders. The reason for this is that if the tumour has a good response to chemotherapy then occult, but clinically undetectable, micrometastases are more likely to be eliminated by treatment, reducing the risk of them enduring and developing into detectable metastases, and ultimately fatal disease.

EXAMINER: Do you know of any novel treatments?

CANDIDATE: I have read about muramyl-tripeptide. It is not directly tumouricidal but works by stimulating the immune system, causing macrophages to exhibit cytotoxic anti-tumour activity. In a randomized trial, Meyers *et al.* showed that, when MTP was added to the standard chemotherapy regime of cisplatin, doxorubicin and methotrexate, 6-year overall survival improved from 70% to 78%.[2] At the current time, NICE have not permitted its use for osteosarcoma, but this decision is under further discussion and appraisal.

1. Beckingsale TB, Gerrand CH. Osteosarcoma. *Orthopaed Trauma* 2010;**24**(5):321–331.

2. Meyers PA, Schwartz CL, Krailo MD *et al.* Osteosarcoma: the addition of muramyl tripeptide to chemotherapy improves overall survival – a report from the Children's Oncology Group. *J Clin Oncol* 2008;**26**:633–638.

Structured oral examination question 7: Aneurysmal bone cyst

EXAMINER: This is a 20-year-old man who presents with pain in his proximal left tibia. What do you make of his MRI scan? (Figure 7.7.)

CANDIDATE: This is an axial T2 image, which shows a lesion in the postero-lateral tibia. It appears well circumscribed with a sclerotic margin, is eccentrically placed, and there are multiple

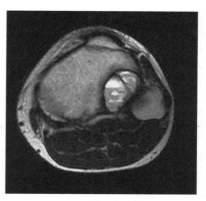

Figure 7.7
Aneurysmal bone cyst.

septations and loculations with fluid levels. These appearances would be in keeping with an aneurysmal bone cyst.

EXAMINER: That's right. What's the normal management for these?

CANDIDATE: Firstly it's important to confirm the diagnosis and I would always discuss bony lesions of this type with a bone tumour MDT. Aneurysmal bone cysts can often form as a reactive change to another benign lesion, for example an osteoblastoma or giant cell tumour, which needs to be ruled out. The differential diagnosis of an aneurysmal bone cyst also includes a telangiectatic osteosarcoma, which would require very different management. In general, treatment of aneurysmal bone cysts is with curettage and grafting, but the recurrence rate can be as high as 50%.

Structured oral examination question 8: Ewing's sarcoma

EXAMINER: This is a histology slide taken from a biopsy of a tumour in the femoral diaphysis of a 16-year-old boy. What does this slide show? (Figure 7.8.)

CANDIDATE: This picture shows a magnified view of a stained histology slide. I'm no expert at histology, but I would describe the cells' appearance as small, round and blue, and given the brief history you provided I suspect this may represent a Ewing's sarcoma.[1]

EXAMINER: Excellent. What other features might this patient have presented with?

CANDIDATE: Patients usually present with pain and swelling related to the tumour. They usually present around the knee, with 25% occurring in the distal femur. Frequently, erythema, systemic pyrexia, a leukocytosis and a raised ESR are also presenting features, which can incorrectly lead the unwary to a diagnosis of infection. Hence, it is mandatory to obtain radiographs when patients present with any unexplained pain or swelling. Patients can occasionally also present with pathological fracture through the lesion or with symptoms related to metastatic disease, such as bone pain in other sites or respiratory symptoms.

EXAMINER: And what would be the characteristic features you'd look for on an X-ray?

CANDIDATE: Ewing's sarcoma leads to a lytic, moth-eaten appearance to the bone. The classic finding, described as onion peel, is seen as a laminated periosteal reaction and probably reflects phases of tumour growth.

EXAMINER: How would you investigate this further?

CANDIDATE: I would start with a full history and examination. MRI scan is essential to delineate the local extent of the tumour and any involvement of key neurovascular structures. It can also be used to plan the biopsy. Other investigations aim to root out any evidence of metastatic disease. A CT chest is required to look for lung metastases, but, in Ewing's sarcoma, a bone scan and bone marrow biopsy are also required to look for widespread bony metastases. Distant bone marrow involvement carries a significantly poorer prognosis.

EXAMINER: In general terms, what is the management for Ewing's sarcoma?

CANDIDATE: There is a national videoconference MDT for all cases of Ewing's sarcoma, which recommends on management. In broad terms, Ewing's sarcomas are both chemo- and radio-sensitive and hence these modalities form

part of the management protocol. Neo-adjuvant chemotherapy is the first-line treatment and usually precedes surgery, which involves wide excision and bony reconstruction where required. Occasionally lesions are treated solely with chemotherapy and radiotherapy, usually in surgically inaccessible lesions around the pelvis. The response to chemotherapy, like in osteosarcoma, is key to prognosis. The 5-year survival is 75% with a good response but only 20% with a poor one.

1. Bullough PG. *Orthopaedic Pathology*. Fourth Edition. Edinburgh: Mosby, 2007.

Structured oral examination question 9: Lipoma

EXAMINER: This is an MRI of a patient who has presented with a painless mass on the lateral aspect of his right elbow. To orientate you the round structure (labelled A) is the radial head. Tell me about the lesion adjacent to it, which is labelled B. (Figure 7.9.)

CANDIDATE: There is an intramuscular mass in the extensor compartment adjacent, and lateral, to the radial head. The mass itself appears bland and is of the same intensity as the subcutaneous fat, suggesting a diagnosis of an intramuscular lipoma.

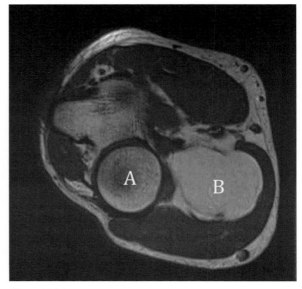

Figure 7.9 Lipoma.

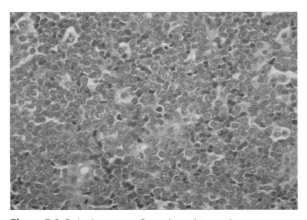

Figure 7.8 Ewing's sarcoma. See colour plate section.

EXAMINER: What is a lipoma?

CANDIDATE: A lipoma is a benign tumour of mature adipocytes, identical to the surrounding adipose tissue, and showing little variation of cell size or shape.

EXAMINER: And how would you treat this lesion?

CANDIDATE: I would want to start by taking a history and examination, in particular looking for any abnormal features like pain or distal neural compromise, which might suggest a more aggressive lesion than a simple lipoma, and alter my management. Also, this is only a single image of the lesion and I would want to see the rest of the scan and discuss it with the sarcoma MDT. Bland, innocent-looking lesions are usually treated with excision biopsy with a marginal margin. If there is any doubt then a biopsy should be taken prior to excision. Histology of lesions below the fascia, like this one, often come back labelled as atypical lipomas by the histologist, despite very bland appearance on MRI.

EXAMINER: What do you mean by an atypical lipoma?

CANDIDATE: The term is quite controversial and the literature often refers to them as lipoma-like liposarcomas. In essence, an atypical lipoma is a lipoma with some slightly atypical features but no evidence of malignancy. The histology of such lesions shows variation of adipocyte size, in contrast to the bland adipocytes of a simple lipoma, and nuclear atypia, as well as the presence of lipoblasts. These lesions are benign and management is still with marginal excision but they do have a low rate of local recurrence.[1]

1. Beckingsale TB, Gerrand CH. The management of soft-tissue sarcomas. *Orthopaed Trauma* 2009; **23**(4):240–247.

Lower limb trauma

8

Mohammed Al-Maiyah and Ali S. Bajwa

Introduction

As far as the exam is concerned, it is very similar to a chess match. It ought to be treated with respect, but played in a clever fashion. As soon as you try to think of the exam as a wrestling match pitfalls for failing are plentiful. In the orals, just like chess, you have to preempt the move of your opponent, which in this situation is the examiner. It is a time-dependent chess match where every move must be undertaken in a specified time. Keep this analogy as you attempt different clinical scenarios. It is not only knowledge of the subject that is important, but to impart it in an appropriate fashion, which is inherently more important in the orals.

Treat each subject as a chess game that is going to last 5 minutes.

Structured oral examination question 1

A 35-year-old motorcyclist came off his bike yesterday; he has been resuscitated and has an isolated closed injury of the knee. (Figure 8.1.)

Minute 1

EXAMINER: What are your views?

Here the next 1 minute belongs to the candidate and you can take it whichever way you want to. However, there are essentials to be covered. In the first 30 seconds you are expected to comment on the following:

- Name of the patient.
- Site of radiograph.
- Fracture through the tibia with depression of the lateral tibial plateau and always ask for a lateral radiograph.

In the next 30 seconds the candidate is expected to comment on the exact nature of the injury, such as Schatzker III fracture with more than 10 mm depression of the articular surface, comminution, concern about the fracture going through the tibial spines and whether the medial side is involved. A candidate should end the 30 seconds by mentioning they would assess the whole patient for any co-existing injuries,

(a)   (b)

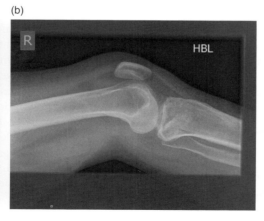

Figures 8.1a and 8.1b Anteroposterior (AP) and lateral radiographs of right knee demonstrating tibial plateau fracture.

Postgraduate Orthopaedics: Viva Guide for the FRCS (Tr & Orth) Examination, ed. Paul A. Banaszkiewicz and Deiary F. Kader. Published by Cambridge University Press. © Cambridge University Press 2012.

the whole lower limb for other injuries and then arrange further imaging studies.

Minute 2

EXAMINER: What further imaging studies would you arrange?

CANDIDATE: A CT scan to evaluate the fracture pattern and plan surgery.

The examiner is likely to produce promptly two slices of the CT, in sagittal and coronal.

Note: Do not make a stupid remark 'do you want me to comment on this?'! But it is useful to correlate that it is the same patient's CT. Describe the findings and end up by offering to discuss the findings with the patient (Brownie points). As well as offering in the closing comments about management options. (Let the examiner ask you about the management options rather than carrying on.)

You should be at this stage by 90 seconds.

EXAMINER: What are the management options?

CANDIDATE: [Take the next 30 seconds to describe operative and non-operative options.] Non-operative management is a poor choice because of the patient's young age and amount of articular segment depression. Operative management would require a non-compromised soft tissue envelope and exclusion of lower limb neurovascular injury. Assessment of the injury pattern and of any significant knee ligament damage needs to be done prior to surgical intervention.

Minute 3

At the 2-minute mark you should have committed yourself to operative intervention. Before the examiner asks, offer your management option because it annoys them to keep asking again and again: what will you do? Stick with the principles.

The principles of management are to restore the articular surface, stabilize and hold the fracture in such a fashion as to allow early mobilization. The aim of the treatment is to have a mobile, pain-free and functional joint.

The options of surgical treatment include direct or indirect reduction, percutaneous or open fixation augmented with plate osteosynthesis or external fixation. Before being prompted, suggest your preferred option, which in the authors' opinion is indirect reduction using a cortical window in the proximal tibia, restoration of articular surface with a raft of

screws augmented with a buttress plate. Suggest at this stage you will perform an assessment under X-ray control for a ligamentous stability and if needed an arthroscopic assessment.

Minute 4

The examiner can lead the viva along two aspects:

EXAMINER: What is a buttress plate?

CANDIDATE: A plate applied perpendicular to the force that it resists.

EXAMINER: What is the role of knee arthroscopy?

CANDIDATE: It is threefold. Firstly, to assess the reduction of articular surface. Secondly, to check that soft tissues are not trapped in the fracture such as lateral meniscus. Thirdly, to assess intra-articular ligament damage. Pressure pumps are not to be used to avoid iatrogenic compartment syndrome due to extravasation of fluid. I will use a bladder syringe through the arthroscopy cannula to wash out the haemarthrosis before viewing the joint. [This gives the examiner the impression that you have done the procedure before.]

EXAMINER: What surgical approach will you use?

CANDIDATE: Anterolateral approach with the skin incision being longitudinal and if needed muscle retraction with a reverse L-shaped incision inside.

The examiner can also talk about a posterolateral approach and a fibula osteotomy for posterolateral fractures. Whilst discussing these issues you should be at the 4-minute stage.

Minute 5

With 1 minute left and if the examiner is discussing rehabilitation and weightbearing status, you know that you are probably winning. Talk about range of motion and protected weightbearing. Assessment of weightbearing will be based on stability of the fracture, strength of the fixation, stiffness of the construct and the quality of the host bone plus reliability of the patient. Do not, repeat do not, use absolute numbers such as 20 kg for each patient on day 1. Tailor the management for each individual patient based on host quality of bone, fracture pattern and construct stability.

Warning: Be prepared to be shown a radiograph of metalwork failure with screws cut out into the articular surface. Stay calm. Assess the patient clinically, radiologically (including CT), rule out infection, soft tissue problems, patient compliance and then proceed from the start, take out the metalwork, align the articular surface, stabilize the fracture and mobilize again. It is the same story all over.

Structured oral examination question 2

A 79-year-old woman fell in her garden sustaining this injury. She is generally quite independent, has a history of angina which is controlled and likes meeting her friends at the local social club every Wednesday.

Minute 1

In the first 30 seconds you are expected to comment on the name of the patient, site of radiograph and the exact nature of the injury:

EXAMINER: Please comment on the radiograph. (Figure 8.2.)

CANDIDATE: She has got a left-sided intracapsular neck of femur fracture in the presence of early degenerative changes of the hip joint. [Always ask for the lateral radiograph.]

EXAMINER: How will you manage this patient?

CANDIDATE: I'd like to assess the whole patient. The degree of mobility prior to injury, comorbidities, any systemic illness, red flag signs for any pathological lesions, drug history, cause of fall and appropriate investigations. In addition, I would perform a full clinical examination of the patient including the left lower limb. [Be a safe surgeon but not hesitant.]

Minutes 2 and 3

EXAMINER: She has well-controlled angina and is otherwise independent.

CANDIDATE: In this patient group surgery would be my preferred option so as to avoid the known complications of non-operative management. These include the risks from a period of bed rest (HEAD TO TOE: depression, confusion, chest infections, pnuenomia, constipation, ileus, urinary tract infection, renal calculi, pressure sores, DVT/PE, muscle wasting, osteoporosis, joint contractures) and a probable painful non-union of the fracture. We can perform either an uncemented or cemented hip hemiarthroplasty. I would generally only use an uncemented hemiarhroplasty in very frail high risk patients as the implant can work loose in the femur, rattle around and cause pain. Cement allows a firm fixation of

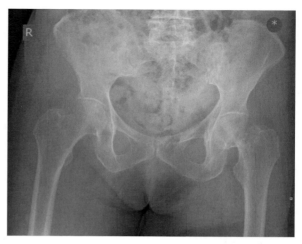

Figure 8.2 Anteroposterior (AP) pelvis radiograph demonstrating intracapsular fractured left neck of femur.

implant to bone, reduces the need for revision surgery and allows better mobility with less thigh pain. My choice [authors' opinion] in this situation would be a total hip arthroplasty rather than a cemented hemiarthroplasty in line with current NICE guidelines.

EXAMINER: Why do you prefer a THA rather than hemiarthroplasty? It is more expensive!

CANDIDATE: [At this stage you should take the presented opportunity to talk and cover the whole subject!] The THA has a better functional outcome than hemiarthroplasty and has better survivorship results. My choice will be a cemented double-tapered polished stem with long-term proven results (such as Exeter) with a cemented highly cross-linked PE and a relatively large head (such as 32 mm). We have data from the Swedish hip registry favouring THA for functional results. Recent NICE guidelines have endorsed such a practice in the selected population, which include mentally alert patient with good pre-injury mobility levels and who are relatively healthy. This patient ticks all the criteria and will benefit from THA. My practice is to use a relatively larger head such as 32 mm, to reduce the risks of dislocation. I would aim for correct orientation of components, good soft tissue balancing and restoration of leg length. The management would continue with aggressive rehabilitation including early mobilization with full weightbearing and repatriation to the place of usual abode. It also includes addressing any underlying metabolic abnormalities such as osteoporosis, risk assessment for falls and nutritional deficiency. Ideally the management will be carried out by a multidisciplinary team.

Minute 4

EXAMINER: She arrives at 18:00 to your ward. When will you undertake the surgery?

CANDIDATE: The surgery should be undertaken as soon as safely possible. It should not be rushed in the middle of the night, however, so if the patient is fit for anaesthesia then aim for surgery on the next morning's trauma list with the necessary theatre staff, kit and consultant cover available. It is important to optimize any correctable causes prior to surgery. This should be undertaken in an objective and efficient manner to avoid 'unnecessary' delay.

Minute 5

The examiner may talk about the potential complications of THA in this patient group, which may include higher risk of dislocation due to a previously mobile hip as opposed to stiff arthritic hip with capsular fibrosis, leg length discrepancy, cement reaction, infection, early loosening etc.

Structured oral examination question 3
Minutes 1 and 2

EXAMINER: A 49-year-old lady fell on the stairs. Her foot is very painful, bruised, swollen and she can't bear weight. The CT1 went to see her in A&E, but he is not sure what the problem is, what do you think? (Figure 8.3.)

CANDIDATE: AP and oblique radiographs of left foot. There is diastasis of > 2 mm between the base of the first and second metatarsals, features suggestive of Lisfranc tarsometatarsal fracture dislocation. There is a small avulsed fragment of bone in that interval. This avulsion fracture could be from the insertion of the Lisfranc ligament into the base of the second metatarsal, called a 'fleck sign'. [Always ask for the lateral radiograph.]

EXAMINER: Okay, how will you manage this patient?

CANDIDATE: I would start with assessing the patient as a whole, following ATLS protocol. I would take relevant history: mechanism of injury, patient's general condition, past medical history, allergies, smoking as well as occupation and previous level of activity.

EXAMINATION OF THE INJURED FOOT:
- Soft tissue status, swelling, pain, tenderness and ecchymosis.
- Painful passive abduction/pronation.

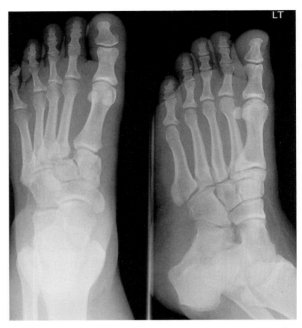

Figure 8.3 Anteroposterior (AP) and oblique radiographs left foot.

- Neurovascular status, dorsalis pedis pulse.
- Compartment syndrome must be excluded.

Following assessment, my initial management includes analgesia, elevation and splinting using below-knee backslab. On admission to hospital I would arrange for regular clinical examinations and monitoring in order not to miss an early developing compartment syndrome.

EXAMINER: What would you do if the radiographs were inconclusive in diagnosing this condition?

CANDIDATE: I would consider further radiographic imaging, oblique and lateral view, stress views and a CT scan or may opt for an MRI scan.

Minute 3

EXAMINER: How do you treat Lisfranc tarsometatarsal fracture dislocation?

CANDIDATE: This depends on severity of injury and degree of displacement of fracture. There is a role for non-operative management of an undisplaced stable injury or sprain which includes a non-weightbearing cast for 6 weeks and regular clinical and radiological review. However, in the presence of subluxation or dislocation, accurate reduction and stable fixation is essential. In this case, I would consider open reduction and internal fixation with screws and possible plating, as required. With a severely comminuted fracture, primary arthrodesis of tarsometatarsal joints may be required.

Informed consent should be taken. The management options, postoperative rehabilitation, outcome and potential complications should be discussed in detail with the patient and documented in medical records.

Minute 4

EXAMINER: What prognosis will you give this patient?

CANDIDATE: This is a serious injury with potentially a poor outcome. Post-traumatic osteoarthritis may occur in more than 50% of cases despite surgical intervention. Residual pain and stiff foot are not uncommon complications of this injury. What makes the outcome of a serious condition even worse is that up to 20% of tarsometatarsal joint complex injuries are missed on initial examination. Patients must be informed about the length of treatment, recovery period and future implications for work and lifestyle.

Minute 5

EXAMINER: If this patient developed compartment syndrome, then how would you manage it?

CANDIDATE: Once compartment syndrome has been diagnosed clinically, emergency decompression is required. Theatre staff and anaesthetic on call team should be informed, informed consent must be obtained. I will take patient to theatre as soon as it is safe to do that. There is more than one technique described to decompress compartment syndrome of the foot, but I have been trained to decompress the nine compartments of the foot through three incisions, two dorsal over the second and third metatarsals and one on the medial side, just under the medial border of the first metatarsal. The patient will need to go back to theatre to have the wounds closed, once the soft tissue swelling has gone down.

Structured oral examination question 4

A 33-year-old roofer fell from a height of 20-feet, when scaffolding collapsed under him, landing on his feet. (Figure 8.4.)

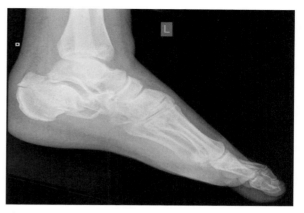

Figure 8.4 Radiograph left lateral foot.

Minute 1

EXAMINER: This is a radiograph of his foot. What are your thoughts?

CANDIDATE: This is a radiograph of left foot, lateral view. It shows a displaced intra-articular fracture of calcaneus with reduced calcaneal height. There is flattening or even reversal of Bohler's angle and a fracture of the calcaneal tuberosity.

A fall from a 20-feet height is a serious injury, so initially I would assess the patient as a whole following ATLS protocol (Airway and protect cervical spine, Breathing, Circulation, Disability, Exposure and environment control).

I will exclude potential associated injuries. These include compression fractures of the spine (10–15% of cases), fracture of proximal femur, fractures around the knee, ankle and other foot injuries, open fractures and neurovascular deficit.

Minute 2

EXAMINER: Assume that there are no other injuries, how would you manage this closed calcaneal fracture?

CANDIDATE: My management would start with initial management, followed by further investigation, planning and then definitive management.

Initial management includes analgesia, splinting, foot elevation and monitoring for compartment syndrome of foot and status of the soft tissue envelope as well as patient reassessment. The key is to manage the soft tissue envelope, which may require cryotherapy and use of foot pumps to reduce the swelling. CT scan would be arranged to plan definitive management. Patient's factors including medical

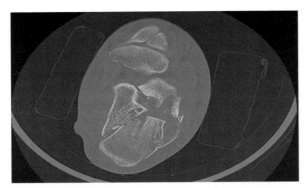

Figure 8.5 CT scan axial view left foot demonstrating calcaneal fracture.

conditions such as diabetes and peripheral vascular disease as well as smoking and occupation.

EXAMINER: Okay, this is the CT scan you requested, what can you see and what would you do next? (Figure 8.5.)

CANDIDATE: This CT scan section in axial view shows shorting of the calcaneus, varus deformity with a comminuted displaced fracture. There is a large sustentacular fragment, depressed middle fragment and blow-out of lateral wall. It also shows considerable heel widening.

I would discuss management options with the patient including open reduction and internal fixation once the soft tissue envelope has settled and swelling gone down. I would base the decision on the fracture pattern, soft tissue status and patient factors. This fracture pattern would benefit from surgical intervention but the decision will depend on factors such as smoking, drinking pattern, occupation, systemic illnesses and expectations of the patient.

Minute 3

EXAMINER: Following discussion with the patient you have decided to proceed with internal fixation. How will you do it?

CANDIDATE: I would take informed consent from the patient. General anaesthesia, prophylactic antibiotics, tourniquet, lateral decubitus position and fluoroscopy control. I would use an L-shaped lateral incision taking care to avoid any damage to the sural nerve. I would keep full thickness flap by taking the incision down to the bone, I would use K-wires bent over themselves to act as retractors, take off the lateral wall, manipulate the fracture fragments to restore length and height of calcaneum as well as correction of varus deformity and

reconstruct the articular surface and then reapply the lateral wall. I would use K-wire for temporary fixation and definitively fix using screws and a calcaneal plate. My preference is a low-profile lateral calcaneal plate, the size of which depends on the patient's calcaneus and I would contour the plate prior to application. The key is to capture the sustantacular fragment under fluoroscopy. Postoperatively, the patient should mobilize non-weightbearing for 6 weeks and then a further 6 weeks of partial weightbearing.

EXAMINER: What prognosis will you give for this patient?

CANDIDATE: A calcaneal fracture is a significant injury with a high incidence of long-term pain and disability. Thordarson & Krieger and Buckley et al. reported a more favourable outcome associated with open reduction and internal fixation, compared to non-operative treatment.[1,2] Similar findings were also reported by Potter & Nunley.[3] Management of calcaneum fracture is an ongoing controversial issue and attracts a lot of debate.

In other vivas, candidates were asked about associated injuries, Sanders' classification and dealing with complications.

1. Thordarson DB, Krieger LE. Operative vs. nonoperative treatment of intra-articular fractures of the calcaneus: a prospective randomized trial. *Foot Ankle Int* 1996; **17**(1):2–9.

2. Buckley R, Tough S, McCormack R et al. Operative compared with nonoperative treatment of displaced intra-articular calcaneal fractures: a prospective, randomized, controlled multicenter trial. *J Bone Joint Surg Am* 2002;**84-A**:1733–1744.

3. Potter MQ, Nunley JA. Long-term functional outcomes after operative treatment for intra-articular fractures of the calcaneus. *J Bone Joint Surg Am* 2009; **91-A**:1854–1860.

Structured oral examination question 5

A 21-year-old motorcyclist was involved in a road traffic accident. He was brought to A&E fully conscious and alert, and formal assessment following ATLS protocol showed that this was an isolated closed injury. (Figure 8.6.)

Minute 1

EXAMINER : Tell me how would you manage this injury?

CANDIDATE: This is an intra-articular fracture, around the right ankle, as a result of high energy trauma. There is a pilon fracture, fractured fibula, disruption of the syndesmosis and possibly a fractured talus.

(a)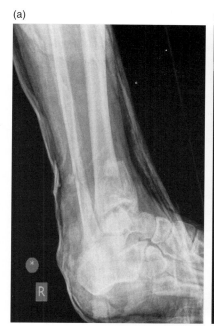

(b)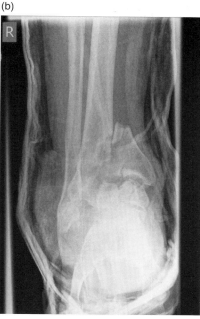

Figures 8.6a and 8.6b Anteroposterior (AP) and lateral radiographs right lower leg.

I will take a relevant history and perform a detailed clinical examination, including the skin and soft tissue condition, realign the foot into a better position, relieve pressure on the skin to avoid skin necrosis, perform a neurovascular assessment of the involved limb and exclude compartment syndrome. The limb should be splinted and elevated. Regular monitoring of neurovascular status and detection of a developing compartment syndrome is of paramount importance.

Minute 2

CANDIDATE: My principles of treatment are 'Span–Scan–Plan'.

- Span: to reduce fracture and joint, and immobilize the injured limb using spanning external fixator. This will restore alignment and allow soft tissue resuscitation and monitoring. This will also give us time to plan definitive surgery.
- Scan: CT scan will provide more details of fracture type and pattern, therefore allowing for informed planning of definitive treatment.
- Plan: Definitive treatment in details; approach, how to fix the fragments, what implant to use, timing of surgery, obtaining consent from the patient and to get an indication of what can be achieved and possible outcome.

Minute 3

EXAMINER: When are you going to fix this fracture?

CANDIDATE: There are many factors to be considered, this is a serious injury and it must be treated properly in one operation. The patient needs to be resuscitated; the soft tissue envelope needs to be in a good condition (this may take 2–3 weeks to settle), a CT scan needs to be performed and the required surgical expertise and implant should be available.

EXAMINER: How are you going to fix this fracture?

CANDIDATE: Principles of intra-articular fracture fixation are anatomical reduction, fracture stabilization and early mobilization. My approach would be tailored depending on fracture configuration, which would identified by a CT scan prior to surgery and with fluoroscopy during surgery. Looking at the fractures in the radiographs provided, I would favour an anterolateral approach that will allow me to reduce the pilon fracture, and approach the fibula as well as the talus. I would aim for anatomical reduction of the pilon fracture and stabilization using an anterolateral plate and then go on to address the fibula and talus on their relative merits. Exposure of the talus can be improved by extending the release of the ATFL through a subperiosteal approach. I would anatomically reduce and fix the talus fracture with screws making sure any loose debris is removed from the joint.

Minutes 4 and 5

EXAMINER: What is the functional outcome following a pilon fracture?

CANDIDATE: Well, generally a poor outcome. A patient may end up with a stiff ankle with a poor soft tissue envelope and there is considerable risk of post-traumatic osteoarthritis which may require an ankle arthrodesis or ankle arthroplasty.

EXAMINER: What is Hawkins' sign – is it a good or bad sign?

CANDIDATE: It is the appearance of osteopenia in subchondral bone of the talar dome, 6–8 weeks following a talar neck fracture. It is a good sign and means that the talar dome is well perfused and has a viable blood supply. It indicates that bone healing is likely to occur without the development of avascular necrosis.

Structured oral examination question 6

A 50-year-old woman, front-seat passenger, was involved in a head-on high speed car collision. In A&E she was diagnosed with a right hip dislocation.

Minute 1

EXAMINER: What will be your management?

CANDIDATE: I would assess and resuscitate the patient along ATLS principles, exclude any associated injuries. I would examine the lower right leg looking at alignment, position and document neurovascular status especially of the sciatic nerve. With the mechanism of injury it is likely to be posterior dislocation with often an associated acetabular rim or femoral neck fracture. In a posterior dislocation the leg is usually shortened and internally rotated, whilst with anterior dislocations the leg is externally rotated and abducted.

EXAMINER: It appears to be an isolated injury with paraesthesia in the sole of the foot, however motor function is intact. How will you manage this further?

CANDIDATE: A traumatic hip dislocation is a surgical emergency because of the risks to the vascularity of the femoral head, danger of chondrolysis as well as pressure effects on the surrounding soft tissues especially neurovascular structures. The paraesthesia in the foot is an indication of pressure or traction involving the sciatic nerve. I would arrange urgently for the patient to go to the theatre the same night. I would get an urgent CT scan performed provided it did not delay surgery; inform theatres, the anaesthetic team and the ward. I would arrange for haematological and biochemical investigations including crossmatch. I would take an informed consent for a closed or open reduction under general anaesthesia.

Minute 2

EXAMINER: There is delay in getting the CT scan and you take her to the operating theatre. How will you reduce the hip?

CANDIDATE: I would attempt closed reduction under general anaesthesia. I would position her supine on the table with the table height as low as possible. I would request the anaesthetist to use muscle relaxant to make it easier to reduce the hip. I would stand on the side of the dislocated hip and have the image intensifier (II) come in from the opposite side. My assistant would be on the opposite side towards the head end of the patient to hold down and stabilize her pelvis when I attempt manipulation. I would screen her first before attempting reduction to exclude a femoral neck fracture and assess the acetabulum using Judet views. If it is a posterior dislocation, I would gently apply traction on the hip (in-line) and then gradually flex the hip and the knee maintaining traction. I would check reduction under II and also check once again for any associated fractures.

EXAMINER: You manage to reduce the hip and get this radiographic image. What are your thoughts? (Figure 8.7.)

CANDIDATE: In this II view of the right hip, the femoral head appears to be in the acetabulum but is incongruent. I would like to confirm this on lateral radiograph. The femoral head is inferiorly subluxed and there appears to be a bony fragment in the hip joint superiorly and another one inferiorly. There is

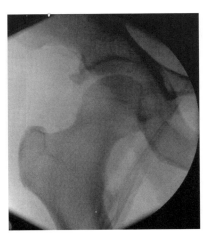

Figure 8.7 Image intensifier (II) image right hip.

one more fragment on the superolateral lip of the acetabulum. The bony fragments are most likely to be from the acetabulum, however femoral head fragments need to be ruled out.

Minute 3

EXAMINER: How will you assess this hip further?

CANDIDATE: Peroperatively I would screen the hip in AP and lateral views as well as obtaining Judet views to assess the anterior and posterior walls and columns. In addition, I would assess the hip for stability. A CT scan will be useful to delineate this further, if it has not already been done.

EXAMINER: You obtain a CT scan in the morning and this is one of the sections. What do you think? (Figure 8.8.)

CANDIDATE: [Note: just comment on what you have rather than ask for more images.] In this axial section of the pelvis at the level of the hip joints, I note that the femoral head on the injured side is at a different height to the opposite hip. There is a bony fragment trapped in the hip joint as well as a bony fragment lying posterior to the hip. It looks like a fracture dislocation with compromise of the acetabular wall postero-superiorly. I would need to study the whole CT sequence to ascertain the extent of damage.

EXAMINER: How will you deal with the bony fragment in the hip joint?

CANDIDATE: This depends on a number of factors including the exact original site of the bony fragment, the size of it, weightbearing dome state and the stability of the hip. The options for a bony fragment trapped in the hip joint are to remove it or to retrieve and fix it. If the fragment is quite small and does not affect hip stability or the weightbearing dome then it can be removed arthroscopically. However, if it compromises the weightbearing area of the hip or stability then I would retrieve it and fix it. It will have to be an open procedure though reports of arthroscopic intervention have been published. [Note: If the candidate does not have sound hip arthroscopy knowledge, then the safe option is open procedure and stay clear of hip arthroscopy.]

Minute 4

EXAMINER: You find that it is the postero-superior lip of the acetabulum. Which approach will you use to fix the fracture?

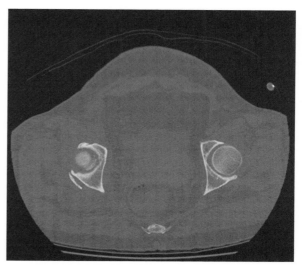

Figure 8.8 CT axial view pelvis.

CANDIDATE: The approach depends on where the bony fragment is arising from. If it is postero-superior or posterior, I would use a posterior approach. I would position the patient on the fracture table in lateral decubitus. To preserve the blood supply to the femoral head, I would remove the fractured loose body arthroscopically [however, see the argument above]. In the posterior approach to the hip one needs to respect the blood vessels supplying the femoral head and therefore not take down the quadratus or the short rotator muscles. I would retract the gluteus medius superiorly, identify the capsule and dissect superiorly to identify the fractured rim of the acetabulum. I would reduce the fragment anatomically under image intensifier screening and secure it with 2–3 partially threaded cannulated screws making sure that the screws do not penetrate the hip joint.

Minute 5

EXAMINER: What are the risks with posterior dislocation of the hip?

CANDIDATE: Immediate complications are neurovascular damage (10% with posterior dislocation), fractures and haemorrhage. Intermediate risks are chondrolysis, post-reduction neurological damage, avascular necrosis, intra-articular loose bodies and hip instability. Late complications are pain and post-traumatic arthritis.

EXAMINER: What other injuries are associated with this injury pattern?

CANDIDATE: This is determined by the direction of forces and may include patella fracture, PCL rupture, femoral fracture, femoral neck and head fractures.

[Note: The candidate is smiling as the examiner has run out of questions on his crib sheet!]

Structured oral examination question 7

A 78-year-old woman fell out of her bed and sustained this injury. She is in reasonably good health and independently mobile, able to care for herself and do her own shopping. (Figure 8.9.)

Minute 1

EXAMINER: What can you see and how you going to manage her?

CANDIDATE: This is an AP radiograph of the right hip showing a reverse-obliquity inter-trochanteric fracture with subtrochanteric extension. The lesser trochanter is proximally displaced with loss of the medial buttress. I would like to see a lateral radiograph, however, based on just the AP view, it is an unstable fracture pattern.

My management for this patient would start with a thorough assessment and optimization of her general medical condition. We need to exclude the possibility of pathological fracture, although the available radiograph shows no evidence of that. I would obtain full-length radiographs of the femur. Provided she is fit and agrees to surgery, I would aim to manage this fracture operatively and I will do so as early as possible, preferably within

36 hours of admission [new NICE guidelines]. I would use a cephalomedullary device as this has shown better results rather than fixed-angle plating devices in this fracture configuration.[1,2]

Minute 2

EXAMINER: This woman's fracture was managed elsewhere and presents during your on-call week with this complication. Can you explain what has happened? (Figures 8.10 and 8.11.)

CANDIDATE: This lady was treated with a fixed-angled locking plate. Two things are perhaps responsible for this failure: biomechanics and biology.

Looking at the postoperative radiograph, there is a gap at the fracture site especially medially. The fixed-angled device has been used with locking screws with five screws on either side of the fracture, which will make it a very rigid implant. This will prevent any micro-motion necessary for callus formation. In addition, there is a fracture gap and lack of compression that will preclude primary bone union. This has resulted in a delayed union/atrophic non-union at the fracture site.

The implant has been under constant biomechanical load, which has led to the fatigue failure of the implant. In this particular design there is a stress riser at the junction of the last proximal locking hole and the tapered part of the plate, which dictates the failure point in the implant. In addition, the plating device is applied on the lateral aspect of the femur increasing the lever arm for the moment of force as compared with a cephalomedullary device, which further puts the fixed-angle

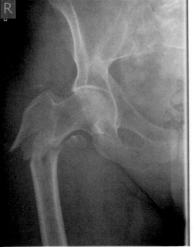

Figure 8.9
Anteroposterior (AP) radiograph right femur demonstrating inter-trochanteric fracture.

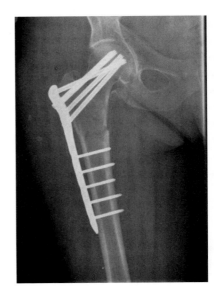

Figure 8.10
Anteroposterior (AP) radiograph right femur with fixed locking plate *in situ*.

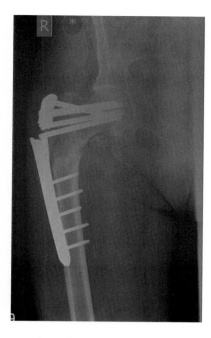

Figure 8.11
Anteroposterior (AP) radiograph right femur demonstrating hardware failure, 4 months postoperative.

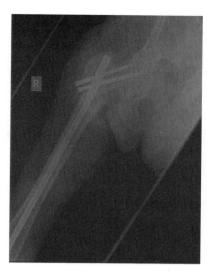

Figure 8.12
Anteroposterior (AP) radiograph demonstrating non-union of the femoral fracture.

plating device in this position at a biomechanical disadvantage. Similar results were reported with the use of compression hip screw and 95° plate.[2] In this type of fracture an intramedullary device has better results and biomechanical stability.

Minute 4

EXAMINER: You fixed it with this recon nail. What do you think about your check X-ray? (Figure 8.12.)

CANDIDATE: As I mentioned earlier the literature reports better results with the use of a cephalomedullary nail. I hope that when the recon nailing was performed bone grafting to the fracture site was performed as well so as to address both biomechanics and biology. The cephalomedullary nail is in slight varus and there is some translation at the fracture site. The screws in the proximal fragment are a bit superior to where I would normally like them. The screws are not absolutely parallel and I would study my lateral radiographs carefully to make sure that the screws have not missed the head.

Minute 5

EXAMINER: How will you follow-up this patient?

CANDIDATE: I would follow-up this patient with clinical reviews and serial radiographs until the fracture heals. I would start her weightbearing as able, stop NSAIDs, counsel against smoking

if she does, keep an eye on her inflammatory markers and do serial radiographs 6 weeks apart. If there is no callus formation at 3–4 months, I would consider revising the intramedullary nail with autologous bone grafting.

1. Sadowski C, Lübbeke A, Saudan M *et al.* Treatment of reverse oblique and transverse intertrochanteric fractures with use of an intramedullary nail or a 95 degrees screw-plate: a prospective, randomized study. *J Bone Joint Surg Am* 2002;**84-A**:372–381.

2. Kregor PJ, Obremskey WT, Kreder HJ, Swiontkowski MF. Evidence-Based Orthopaedic Trauma Working Group. Unstable pertrochanteric femoral fractures (Review). *J Orthop Trauma* 2005;**19**:63–66.

Structured oral examination question 8

A 72-year-old woman, fully independent with good health, was hit by a car when she was walking on a kerb. She was brought to hospital with these injuries. She was assessed following ATLS protocol. She was resuscitated and her injuries were splinted. (Figure 8.13.)

Minute 1

EXAMINER: What your thoughts about this patient's management? Do you have any concerns?

CANDIDATE: This 72-year-old lady has multiple high-energy injuries. This is a serious situation, so although she had good health prior to this accident, I would be concerned about her trauma response and her well-being. Trauma scores show that elderly patients have limited physiological reserves and they tend to do worse than young people. So she needs to be closely

(a) (b) (c)

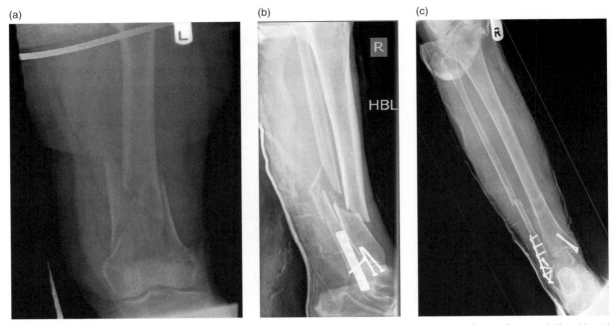

Figures 8.13a, 8.13b and 8.13c Anteroposterior (AP) radiograph left femur demonstrating supracondylar fracture femur and AP and lateral radiographs right lower leg.

observed and kept well hydrated and her condition optimized before undertaking definitive treatment. Fractures of long bone should be stabilized as early as possible for many reasons: for pain relief, to reduce trauma response, to allow for early mobilization and rehabilitation as well as to decrease the complications from bed rest.

Ideally an anaesthetic team and geriatrician should also be involved in planning her treatment, when to take her to theatre.

Minute 2

EXAMINER: What implants are you going to use to fix these fractures?

CANDIDATE: For the left femur fracture, it is a multi-fragment supracondylar unstable fracture, with femur shortening. We need to use a femoral distracter for temporary reduction and then to use either a nail or plate. Personally I would prefer a fixed-angle plate with less invasive technique. Nailing may increase the risk of ARDS and fat embolism.

Regarding the tibia fracture, it is a fracture of the distal third of tibia and there is metalware from a previous ankle fracture fixation. Although an intramedullary nail could be used, we still

have the same argument of fat embolism and ARDS. The fracture could be plated but this means soft tissue stripping and is perhaps not ideal for a 72-year-old woman's leg which is already contused and swollen with the high-impact injury. A circular frame would be a valid option and I would prefer to use it.

Minutes 3 and 4

EXAMINER: Okay, have a look at this radiograph and explain to me the technique the surgeon has used and what the principles are of this technique. (Figure 8.14.)

CANDIDATE: The AP radiograph shows a multifragment distal diaphysis/metaphysis fracture that has been stabilized with a fixed-angle plate, using bridging plating the fracture zone has been bridged. Looking at the skin staples used to close the skin, I can infer that a closed indirect reduction and a less invasive technique was used. This technique was introduced to decrease soft tissue disruption and preserve blood supply. Length, alignment and rotation of bone was restored. Baumgaertel et al. introduced the concept of biological plating and proved that indirect reduction and bridge plating was superior to direct fragment reduction and anatomical fixation in respect to bone healing.[1]

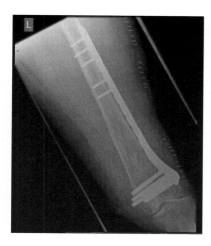

Figure 8.14
Anteroposterior (AP) radiograph left distal femur with locking plate *in situ*.

Minute 5

EXAMINER: Can you tell me the principles of using a circular frame? (Figure 8.15.)

CANDIDATE: It uses tensioned wires for bone fixation and these wires are fixed to rings to form segments proximal and distal to fracture site. Segments of frame can be moved in terms of angulation, rotation, translation and length. The frame can be built to fit all bones and can be temporary or definitive fixation. It can be fitted using a less invasive technique and can be adjusted when needed.

1. Baumgaertel F, Buhl M, Rahn BA. Fracture healing in biological plate osteosynthesis. *Injury* 1998;**29** (Suppl. 3):C3–C6.

Structured oral examination question 9

A 29-year-old female horse rider fell off her horse; she has been fully assessed in A&E and has an isolated closed injury of the foot. (Figure 8.16.)

Minute 1

EXAMINER: What are your views?

CANDIDATE: The radiographs of the left foot, AP and oblique show a displaced fracture of the body of navicular bone with comminution. There is overlap of mid-tarsal bones and I can't exclude fractures of other tarsal bones. The alignment of the foot is still maintained and there is no varus or valgus deformity.

This is a serious injury, probably high energy. I need to assess the patient as a whole: relevant history, clinical examination in general and in particular of the foot ruling out compartment syndrome, any neurovascular damage and assessing the soft tissue envelope of the foot. I would then request further imaging, the modality of choice being CT scan.

I would initially treat the injured foot in a backslab, with strict elevation and intermittent cryotherapy, adequate analgesia and close monitoring for evolving compartment syndrome.

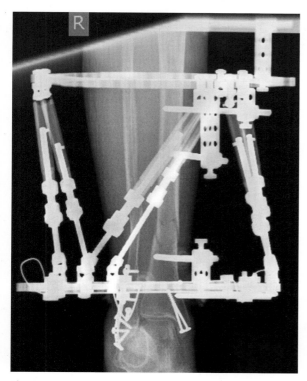

Figure 8.15 Anteroposterior (AP) radiograph right distal tibia with circular frame in situ.

EXAMINER: Can you explain why the surgeon put screws on either ends of the plate and missed the middle?

CANDIDATE: The surgeon intended to increase the working length of the implant (the distance between two points on either side of the fracture where the bone is fixed to plate or nail). This produces an even distribution of forces over a long segment and decreases stress at fracture and implant.

Minute 2

EXAMINER: This is the scan you requested. What do you see, and how would you manage it? (Figure 8.17.)

CANDIDATE: These coronal and sagittal sections of the CT scan confirm X-ray findings of a displaced fracture of the body of navicular bone with comminution. It is an unstable displaced

123

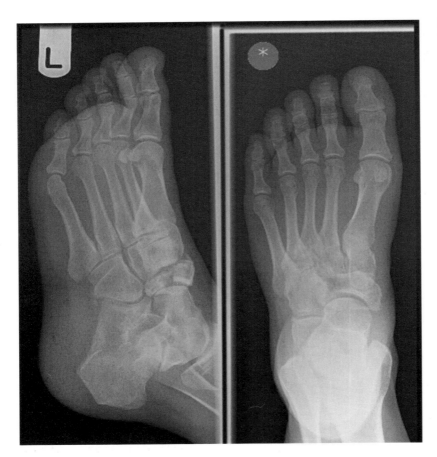

Figure 8.16 Anteroposterior (AP) and lateral radiographs left foot.

(a)

(b)

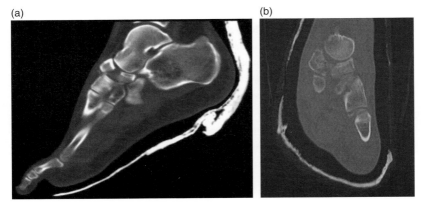

Figures 8.17a and 8.17b CT scan coronal and sagittal sections of left foot.

intra-articular fracture and I would favour operative intervention rather than non-operative. The principles of management are to restore the articular surface, stabilize and hold the fracture to allow early mobilization. The aim of the treatment is to have a mobile, pain-free and functional joint. However, sometimes that is not possible due to severe comminution of the articular surface, in which case I may consider primary fusion of the talonavicular joint.

I would discuss findings, management options, aims of the treatment as well as potential complications with the patient and seek informed consent before proceeding.

Minute 3

EXAMINER: Can you tell us about possible complications associated with this case?

CANDIDATE: These are immediate, early and late complications. Immediate complications are in the perioperative period and include iatrogenic injury to structures, compartment syndrome and anaesthetic problems. Early complications include infection, nerve injury (branches of superficial and deep peroneal nerves) and vascular injury (dorsalis pedis). Late complications include non-union and loss of medial longitudinal arch support, painful talonavicular joint, post-traumatic osteoarthritis, as well as avascular necrosis and collapse.

Minute 4

EXAMINER: Why do non-union and avascular necrosis occur in this fracture?

CANDIDATE: The navicular bone, similar to talus, has a large articular surface area and for the blood supply it relies on the radial arcade of vessels arising from the dorsalis pedis and medial planter arteries and this could be injured either at the time of fracture or during surgery, which could lead to AVN, non-union and/or collapse of the bone resulting in a painful mid-foot.

EXAMINER: What surgical approach are you going to use?

CANDIDATE: I would use a medial approach, between the tibialis anterior and tibialis posterior tendons, preserving the remaining blood supply as much as possible, reduce the articular surface and stabilize with cannulated screws from lateral to medial. The eventual configuration of screws will depend on the fracture pattern.

Minute 5

EXAMINER: Take me through your consent process, in general.

CANDIDATE: I follow GMC guidelines: 'Consent: patients and doctors making decisions together'. I work in partnership with the patient to ensure high quality of care.

(a) I listen to patients and respect their views about their health;

(b) discuss with patients what their views about diagnosis, prognosis, treatment and care involve;

(c) share with patients the information they want or need in order to make decisions;

(d) maximize patients' opportunities, and their ability to make decisions for themselves;

(e) respect patients' decisions.

Remember what the golfer Gary Player said: 'The more I practise the luckier I get'. That is exactly what you need to pass FRCS Orth. Exam, practice and luck!

Chapter

9

Upper limb trauma

Gunasekaran Kumar

Structured oral examination question 1

EXAMINER: A 38-year-old left-hand dominant lady fell onto her right arm when out drinking and attended the casualty department the next day at 16:00 when pain in the right shoulder did not settle down. These are the X-rays of right shoulder. What is your diagnosis? (Figure 9.1.)

CANDIDATE: Fracture dislocation of the right shoulder. It is an anterior dislocation as the humerus is in an abducted position and the greater tuberosity is fractured.

EXAMINER: How will you manage this condition?

CANDIDATE: After assessing the patient for other associated injuries and neurovascular status I will try to reduce the right shoulder dislocation under sedation in casualty.

EXAMINER: What are the risks and complications you anticipate?

CANDIDATE: Since the greater tuberosity is fractured, there is a risk that there may be an undisplaced fracture of the humeral neck not seen on X-ray. Further, during manipulation of the shoulder there is a risk of propagating the fracture through the humeral neck. Other risks are injury to neurovascular structures including axillary nerve and artery or the brachial plexus.

EXAMINER: Attempted closed reduction in casualty failed and it is 19:00 now. What will you do next?

CANDIDATE: I will check with emergency theatres whether there is theatre space available and check with the on-call consultant whether it is okay to get the patient onto the emergency list for closed reduction. In case the humeral neck fractures during manipulation, it will require open reduction and stabilization. I am not experienced with this procedure. Hence, I would prefer the consultant to be around or perform the reduction next day first in the trauma list.

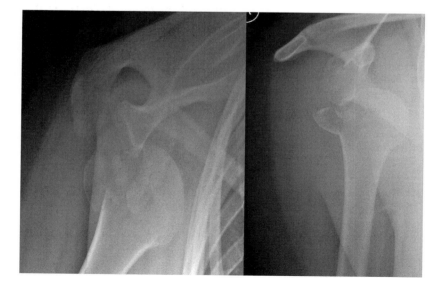

Figure 9.1 Anteroposterior (AP) radiograph right shoulder demonstrating fracture/dislocation.

Postgraduate Orthopaedics: Viva Guide for the FRCS (Tr & Orth) Examination, ed. Paul A. Banaszkiewicz and Deiary F. Kader. Published by Cambridge University Press. © Cambridge University Press 2012.

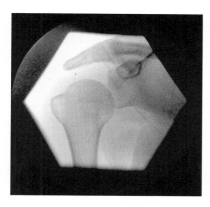

Figure 9.2 II films relocated right shoulder.

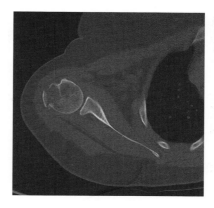

Figure 9.4 CT images right shoulder.

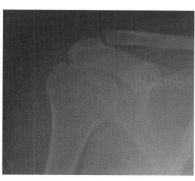

Figure 9.3 Anteroposterior (AP) radiograph right shoulder with greater tuberosity fracture.

EXAMINER: CT scan of the right shoulder shows no humeral neck fracture and axial views of the greater tuberosity are shown in this scan. What will be your management strategy? (Figure 9.4.)

CANDIDATE: The greater tuberosity fragment is displaced. Hence, I would offer her the options of surgical management in the form of open reduction and fixation with screws.

EXAMINER: What are the risks of non-operative management of a displaced greater tuberosity fracture?

CANDIDATE: Non-union, malunion leading to subacromial impingement.

Structured oral examination question 2

EXAMINER: A 24-year-old man fell down the last few steps of a flight of stairs and sustained injury to his left wrist. These are his X-rays. What is this injury? (Figure 9.5.)

CANDIDATE: This is a fracture of the radial styloid that is displaced.

EXAMINER: Is this injury more than just a displaced radial styloid fracture?

CANDIDATE: Yes, it involves dorsal subluxation of the radiocarpal joint also.

EXAMINER: What injuries have occurred other than the radial styloid fracture?

CANDIDATE: Rupture of volar capsular and ligamentous structures.

EXAMINER: How will you manage this injury?

CANDIDATE: I will assess the patient's general condition, look for other injuries, check whether it is a closed or an open fracture

EXAMINER: What manoeuvre would you perform to achieve shoulder reduction?

CANDIDATE: Under complete muscle relaxation, I will manipulate the shoulder with gentle traction, external rotation and adduction with internal rotation.

EXAMINER: Next day in theatre, closed reduction is achieved. What will you do next? (Figure 9.2.)

CANDIDATE: I will assess greater tuberosity fracture reduction. If it is well reduced as the X-ray shows, I will treat it non-operatively with a poly sling for 3 weeks with serial X-rays on a weekly basis and if there is no fracture displacement, I will start shoulder mobilization under physiotherapy care.

EXAMINER: Here is the X-ray of the right shoulder 1 week later. What will you do? (Figure 9.3.)

CANDIDATE: I will reassess the patient clinically including assessing neurovascular status and organize a CT scan of the right shoulder to check for amount of displacement of greater tuberosity fragment and also to check for humeral neck fracture.

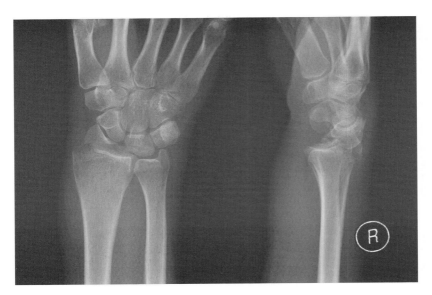

Figure 9.5 Anteroposterior (AP) and lateral radiographs left wrist.

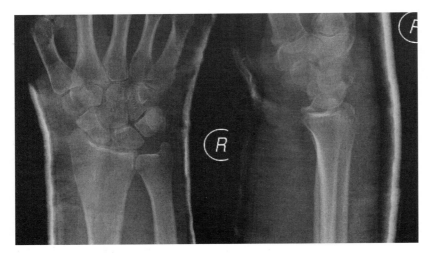

Figure 9.6 Anteroposterior (AP) and lateral post-reduction film left wrist.

and distal neurovascular status. If it is an isolated closed injury, I will attempt closed reduction under sedation in casualty, apply a below-elbow moulded dorsal plaster slab, check distal neurovascular status and get a repeat X-ray of the wrist.

EXAMINER: This is the post-reduction X-ray. How will you manage this injury? (Figure 9.6.)

CANDIDATE: Post-reduction X-rays show that the fracture is well reduced and the radiocarpal alignment is satisfactory. It is a potentially unstable injury due to damage to volar capsular and ligamentous structures. I would offer an examination under anaesthesia of the wrist and if it is unstable I will stabilize the fracture with open reduction and stabilization with screws to achieve compression at the fracture site. I will again examine the wrist for stability; if it is still unstable, I will apply a spanning external fixator with radiocarpal joint well reduced. The external fixator will be removed at 4 weeks post-surgery and I will start mobilization of the wrist with physiotherapy.

Structured oral examination question 3

EXAMINER: A motorcyclist came off his bike at around 80 miles/hour and has sustained an isolated injury to his right elbow. These are his X-rays in casualty. (Figure 9.7.)

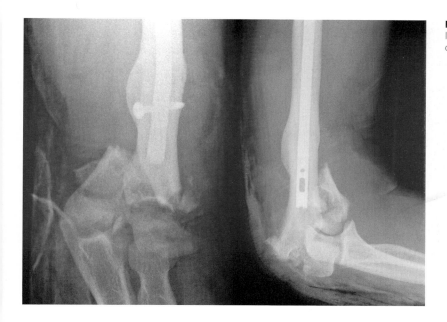

Figure 9.7 Anteroposterior (AP) and lateral radiographs right elbow demonstrating comminuted fracture.

CANDIDATE: These X-rays of the right elbow and distal humerus show a comminuted fracture of the distal humerus. It is difficult to identify the fracture fragments but it is a bicondylar fracture with some intercondylar articular fragments too. There is a retrograde humeral nail in situ. I can see some dressing around the elbow. I will assess the patient according to ATLS protocols and assess to see whether it is an isolated injury with no distal neurovascular deficits. I will also check if it is an open fracture.

EXAMINER: It is an open fracture. How will you deal with the wound in casualty?

CANDIDATE: I will assess the open wound including size, location, any skin loss, active bleeding or any exposed bone. I will remove any gross contamination, clean with normal saline, cover the wound with sterile dressing gauze and OpSite after taking photographs of the wound. I will check the patient's tetanus status and give a booster dose if required and analgesia. I will start the patient on intravenous cefuroxime which will continue until the wound is closed.

EXAMINER: What will be the definitive management and its timing?

CANDIDATE: The timing of debridement is dependent on when a thorough debridement and stabilization of fracture can be performed. It is not essential to perform debridement within 6 hours, as per BOA standards of trauma guidelines.

Principles of management will include a CT scan if possible before surgery to provide a better understanding of the fracture pattern. Wound edges will be excised and extended as appropriate, fracture ends will be debrided including removal of any devitalized soft tissue and bone fragments with no soft tissue attachments. Thorough lavage of the wound with at least 6 litres of gravity-assisted normal saline is then performed. After the debridement is completed, I will assess whether wound and fracture are suitable for definitive stabilization.

EXAMINER: If the wound is satisfactory and definitive stabilization is planned, how will you go about it?

CANDIDATE: I will not remove the retrograde humeral nail but plan stabilization around it. I will perform a posterior approach, incorporating the wound if it is posteriorly. I will perform a chevron olecranon osteotomy after pre-drilling the olecranon. This will allow me to accurately reduce the intra-articular fractures and stabilize them with lag screws. Following this I will stabilize the metaphyseal part of the fracture with medial and lateral pre-contoured plates and try to bypass the nail; if not possible, I will use locking screws in the diaphyseal segment.

EXAMINER: How will you stabilize the olecranon osteotomy?

CANDIDATE: I will use a 6.5 mm partially threaded cannulated screw or a pre-contoured plate fixation, dependent on the bone quality.

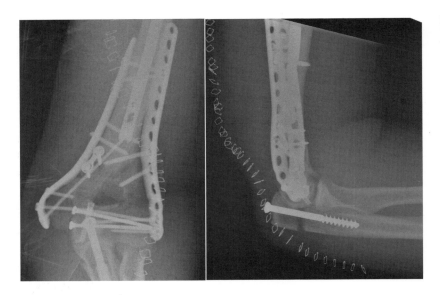

Figure 9.8 Anteroposterior (AP) and lateral radiographs right elbow post fixation.

EXAMINER: This is the postoperative X-ray. What will be your postoperative management? (Figure 9.8.)

CANDIDATE: There appears to be good intra-articular and extra-articular fracture reduction and stabilization. The olecranon osteotomy has been stabilized with a screw but there is a gap in the osteotomy.

I would still proceed with early mobilization of the elbow. If the osteotomy opens up further or does not show signs of healing I will revise the olecranon stabilization.

Structured oral examination question 4

EXAMINER: A cyclist was knocked over by a car and he landed on his elbow. This is an isolated injury. These are his X-rays. (Figure 9.9.)

CANDIDATE: This is a fracture of the proximal ulna associated with an anterior dislocation of the radial head. There is a small fragment seen next to the radial head and it is possibly from the radial head. I will check for distal neurovascular status and for any wounds around the injury.

EXAMINER: Do you know of any eponymous name and classification of this injury?

CANDIDATE: This is a Monteggia fracture dislocation.

A classification based on the direction of radial head dislocation is Bado classification. Types are anterior, posterior, lateral and associated radial fracture. This is a posterior type injury.

EXAMINER: How will you manage this?

CANDIDATE: Once I have fully assessed the patient, I will reduce the fracture under sedation in casualty and apply an above-elbow backslab. After that I will get a check X-ray to make sure the fracture dislocation is reduced.

EXAMINER: Can this fracture be treated non-operatively?

CANDIDATE: It is an unstable fracture configuration with risk of re-displacement. Hence, I will treat this fracture with surgery in the form of open reduction and plate stabilization of the ulna fracture. Most of the time, the radial dislocation will reduce and be stable.

EXAMINER: What is the cause for a radial head still subluxing after ulna fracture stabilization?

CANDIDATE: Malreduction of ulna fracture, incarceration of annular ligament, large radial head fracture.

EXAMINER: This is the postoperative X-ray. What will be your postoperative management? (Figure 9.10.)

CANDIDATE: I will start physiotherapy to mobilize the elbow as tolerated to prevent stiffness and follow up the patient to make sure the wound and fracture have healed along with good functional outcome.

Structured oral examination question 5

EXAMINER: A 23-year-old while on a night out fell on to his left hand and has come to casualty with pain and deformity. This is an X-ray of the left distal forearm (Figure 9.11).

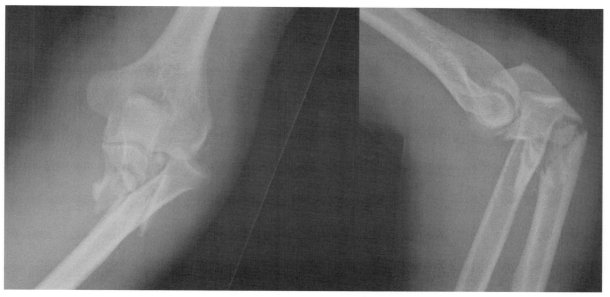

Figure 9.9 Anteroposterior (AP) and lateral radiographs Monteggia fracture/dislocation right elbow.

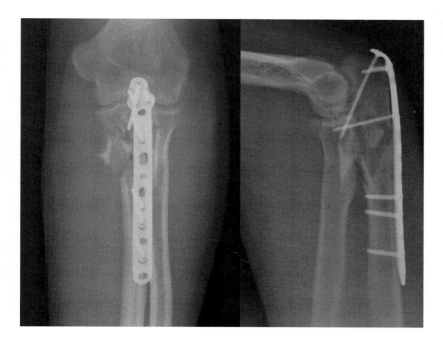

Figure 9.10 Anteroposterior (AP) and lateral radiographs right elbow post-fixation.

CANDIDATE: This is a fracture of radial shaft associated with dislocation of distal radioulnar joint. I will assess the patient with regards to medical conditions, associated injuries, distal neurovascular status and whether it is a closed or open injury.

EXAMINER: This is an isolated closed injury with no distal problems. How will you manage this injury?

CANDIDATE: I will try to reduce the fracture dislocation in casualty under sedation, apply an above-elbow backslab and get an X-ray of the forearm and wrist.

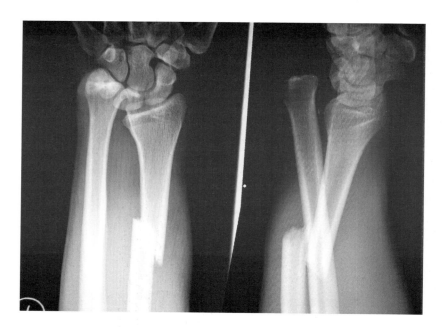

Figure 9.11 Anteroposterior (AP) and lateral radiographs left forearm.

EXAMINER: Check X-ray shows no change in position, the time is now 21:00. What will you do?

CANDIDATE: If there are no signs of any neurovascular deficit, I will prioritize the patient in the next day's trauma list for open reduction and stabilization of radial fracture with stabilization of distal radioulnar joint, if required. Overnight, the arm will be kept elevated and frequent neurovascular assessment will be made.

EXAMINER: During surgery the radius fracture is stabilized but the distal radioulnar joint is still dislocated. What are the causes for this?

CANDIDATE: Malreduction of radius fracture or soft tissue interposition in the distal radioulnar joint or there is significant soft tissue disruption of the joint.

EXAMINER: Radius fracture reduction is satisfactory and there is no interposition but the joint is dislocated. How will you deal with it?

CANDIDATE: I will check if the joint reduces with supination. If the joint reduces, then I will stabilize it with two 2.0 mm K-wires percutaneously.

EXAMINER: What will be your postoperative protocol?

CANDIDATE: I will immobilize the forearm in a below-elbow backslab with wrist in supination. I will convert it to a below-elbow cast with wrist in supination for 4 weeks followed by removal of wires in clinic and start mobilization of wrist under physiotherapy care.

Structured oral examination question 6

EXAMINER: A 58-year-old man sustained an injury to his arm when he fell from standing height. He is right handed, suffers from hypertension and has a sedentary lifestyle. These are his X-rays. (Figure 9.12.)

CANDIDATE: The X-rays show a transverse fracture of the right humerus shaft in the middle third. There is 100% translation and minimal angulation in lateral view and 80% translation in anteroposterior view.

I will check for other injuries, neurovascular status and whether it is a closed or open fracture.

EXAMINER: It is a closed fracture with no associated problems. How will you manage it?

CANDIDATE: In casualty, I will apply a U slab, then check for distal neurovascular status and get a check X-ray.

If there are no further problems and X-ray is satisfactory, then I will bring the patient to the fracture clinic in a few days to convert the U slab to a humeral brace.

EXAMINER: What will you do once the humeral brace is applied?

CANDIDATE: I will get a check X-ray to be sure that the fracture is not displacing. I will also see the patient on a weekly basis for first 3 weeks with X-rays to assess for fracture position.

EXAMINER: This is week 2 X-ray. What will you do?
(Figure 9.13.)

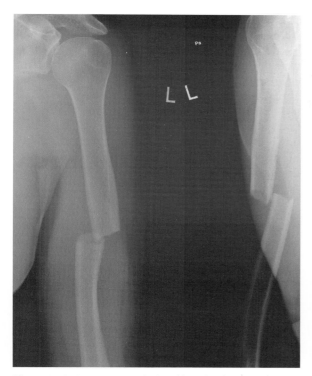

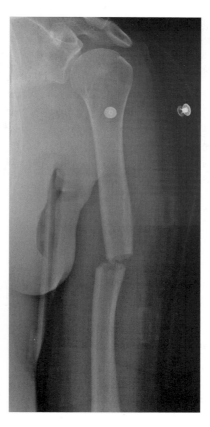

Figure 9.13 Anteroposterior (AP) radiograph distracted right humerus fracture.

Figure 9.12 Anteroposterior (AP) and lateral radiographs transverse fractured right humerus.

CANDIDATE: There is some distraction at the fracture site. This could be an indication of possible non-union in the future. I will discuss this with the patient and continue with non-operative management as planned with adjustment of the humeral brace. However, I will reiterate the possibility of non-union.

EXAMINER: Patient does not want to wait and see. He is keen to have the operation. What will you do?

CANDIDATE: I will discuss with the patient the advantages and risks involved in operative management of humeral fractures, including infection, neurovascular deficit, stiffness, non-union, malunion, implant failure, complex regional pain syndrome.

EXAMINER: What operative intervention will you undertake?

CANDIDATE: The surgical options are intramedullary nail fixation or plate fixation. I prefer plate fixation to avoid the risk of shoulder subacromial symptoms. For this fracture, I will do a plate fixation via an anterior approach.

EXAMINER: This is the X-ray at 3 months. What will you do? (Figure 9.14.)

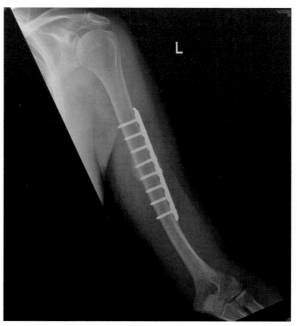

Figure 9.14 Anteroposterior (AP) radiograph non-union right humerus fracture post-plate fixation.

CANDIDATE: My first aim will be to rule out infection. I will check patient for systemic illnesses, like fever, chills, shivering, loss of appetite/weight. I will also perform blood tests – FBC, C-reactive protein.

EXAMINER: Patient has no symptoms and is happy with progress with physiotherapy. Why do you suspect infection?

CANDIDATE: In a plate fixation, absolute stability is the aim. This means that the fracture will heal by primary intention. In the presence of callus formation, I will suspect infection or aseptic implant loosening.

This last question is about primary healing in rigid/stiff fixation. When there is callus formation in these 'rigid fixations' especially of transverse or oblique fractures then the possibility of either early plate loosening or grumbling infection should be kept in mind. Though external callus can occur in plate fixations, in these circumstances the stiffness of the construct is lower and is flexible enough to allow secondary fracture healing as the working length is longer.

A perfectly plated Swiss fracture does not go through endochondral repair.

Chapter

10

Pelvic and spinal trauma

Gunasekaran Kumar and Sherief Elsayed

Pelvic trauma
Structured oral examination question 1

EXAMINER: A 25-year-old professional motor bike racer, at a practice session, came off his bike, at > 100 miles/hour. His only area of pain is left hip. This is an X-ray of his pelvis. What does the X-ray show? (Figure 10.1.)

CANDIDATE: Anteroposterior pelvis X-ray of a skeletally mature adult marking out the ilioinguinal, ilioischial lines, dome, anterior and posterior wall lines show a possible posterior wall injury. Right sacroiliac joint seems wider than the left. There is a small bony avulsion at the pubic symphysis area. Both hip joints appear concentric.

EXAMINER: What will you do next?

CANDIDATE: As per ATLS protocols I will reassess the patient performing primary and secondary surveys to identify any injuries other than left hip. I will assess the range of movements in the left hip joint, distal neurovascular status and examine the left knee and left ankle. I will check the pulse rate, blood pressure and respiratory rate trend.

EXAMINER: Left hip movements are limited to a jog of movements by pain; rest of the examination is unremarkable. What is the next step?

CANDIDATE: I will ensure patient has adequate analgesia and frequent neurovascular assessment of left leg. I will request a CT scan of pelvis and both hips.

EXAMINER: These are axial CT scans of both hips and SI joints. Describe the injury. (Figure 10.2.)

CANDIDATE: The axial section of the left hip shows an intra-articular fragment, marginal impaction of posterior wall, loss of concentricity of hip joint. There is no subluxation of hip or

evidence of femoral head/neck injury. There is also a cystic lesion in the femoral head which looks benign.

Both SI joints appear symmetric and there are no other injuries that I can identify.

EXAMINER: What is the definitive management of this injury?

CANDIDATE: Non-operative management is not recommended due to the intra-articular fragment. Aims of operative management are to remove intra-articular fragment, reduce the marginal impaction, bone graft the bony defect if needed, then buttress plate fixation of the posterior wall.

EXAMINER: When will you operate?

CANDIDATE: The surgery should be performed by an orthopaedic surgeon with interest in pelvic and acetabular fracture fixation. Surgery should be performed ideally within 5 days as per BOAST guidelines.

EXAMINER: What are BOAST guidelines?

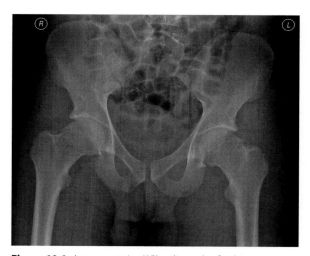

Figure 10.1 Anteroposterior (AP) radiograph of pelvis.

Postgraduate Orthopaedics: Viva Guide for the FRCS (Tr & Orth) Examination, ed. Paul A. Banaszkiewicz and Deiary F. Kader. Published by Cambridge University Press. © Cambridge University Press 2012.

(a)

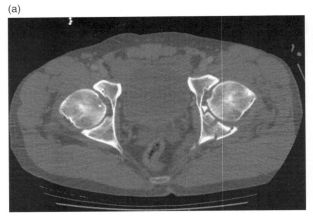

(b)

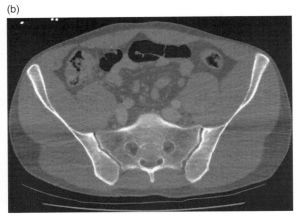

Figure 10.2a and b CT scan of pelvis and SI joints.

CANDIDATE: British Orthopaedic Association Standards of Trauma guidelines.

PELVIC FRACTURES: First line of management is control of haemorrhage – pelvic binder, blood transfusion, pelvic packing or embolization.

Look for genitourinary tract injury and open fractures – wounds in perineum, rectum or vagina.

Surgical treatment of these injuries as soon as possible.

Early CT scan of pelvis.

Transfer images to local referral unit within 24 hours.

Once haemodynamic and skeletal stabilizations are achieved patient should be transferred to specialist unit for surgery within 5 days if possible.

ACETABULAR FRACTURES: Urgent reduction of dislocated hips, skeletal traction should be applied. CT scan within 24 hours and images should be transferred to the specialist unit.

Surgery if needed should be performed within 5 days, ideally.

EXAMINER: What approach will you use? What are the significant risks and complications of the approach?

CANDIDATE: Posterior Kocher–Langenbeck approach.

Important blood supply to femoral head is from the medial femoral circumflex artery that passes close to the insertions of short external rotators of the hip. During surgery the short external rotators should be divided at least 1 cm from their insertions to protect this artery and avoid avascular necrosis of femoral head. Other risks include infection, DVT, PE, loss of fixation, heterotropic ossification, secondary osteoarthritis.

EXAMINER: Does this injury have a good or a bad prognosis, historically?

CANDIDATE: Posterior wall fractures have in general poor prognosis due to the damage to articular surface, impaction and difficulty in achieving anatomic reduction.

EXAMINER: What will be your postoperative rehabilitation protocol?

CANDIDATE: I will start hip range of movement exercises from day 1 and continue with non-weightbearing for 3 months.

Structured oral examination question 2

EXAMINER: A 23-year-old professional dancer is involved in a road traffic accident at 17:00 (motorbike rider versus car). Patient is brought to casualty with GCS of 15, BP 110/70 mmHg, PR 90/min. Patient complained of pain around the right buttock area.

Fifteen minutes after arrival patient's BP dropped to 70 mmHg systolic. What will you do?

CANDIDATE: As per ATLS protocols I will perform primary and secondary surveys making sure two large bore cannulae are introduced and blood taken for FBC, U/E, cross-match 6 units of blood. I will apply a pelvic binder and reassess the chest, abdomen, long bones and look for any open wounds that are bleeding.

EXAMINER: Patient's blood pressure stabilized at 110/70 mmHg and two units of blood were being transfused.

X-ray of pelvis was performed. Describe the injury. (Figure 10.3.)

CANDIDATE: This is a vertical shear type pelvic fracture involving the right hemipelvis with fractures through both superior and inferior pubic rami and through right sacral alae and possibly neural foraminae.

EXAMINER: What are the radiological landmarks/lines you assess for a pelvic fracture? Show them on the normal side.

CANDIDATE: For pelvic fractures I start looking at the pubic symphysis, pubic rami, iliac wing, sacroiliac joints, sacral alae, neural foraminae, sacral bodies, transverse processes of lower lumbar vertebrae, sacral spinous processes. I will also look for associated acetabular fracture by looking at ilioinguinal, ilioischial lines, acetabular dome, anterior and posterior walls, obturator foramen and tear drop.

EXAMINER: How will you manage the patient now?

CANDIDATE: I will assess both lower limbs and distal neurovascular status followed by assessment of both upper limbs. I will also look for any open wounds around perineum, groin, buttocks, vagina, rectum to rule out open fracture. Until spine is assessed patient will have to be log rolled and neck should be triple immobilized.

EXAMINER: Patient has altered sensation in S1 nerve root area in right foot but no motor deficit was noted. What do you do?

CANDIDATE: I will obtain CT scan of cervical spine, chest, abdomen and pelvis to assess for associated injuries and look specifically for evidence of S1 nerve root injury due to the pelvic fracture.

Then, I will perform distal femoral pin traction once I have ruled out any femoral fracture.

EXAMINER: CT scan does not show any other visceral or vascular injuries. No urethral or perineal injuries were identified. What will be the definitive management and the timing?

CANDIDATE: The images and patient details will be sent to the local specialist unit for decision on transfer of patient. Definitive management principles include reduction of vertical shear, usually by skeletal traction, sacral fixation with iliosacral screws, pubic ramus fixation with percutaneous ramus screw fixation or open reduction and plate fixation. If the fixation is still tenuous then external fixation could be used to augment the fixation.

EXAMINER: What are the specific risks involved?

CANDIDATE: Closed reduction of vertical shear may not be possible. If so, then open reduction of the sacral fractures can be performed with patient prone and stabilization with iliosacral screws or posterior rods followed by pubic ramus stabilization.

Other risks include infection, nerve root injury, DVT, PE, failure of fixation, persistent low back pain.

Structured oral examination question 3

EXAMINER: A 75-year-old gentleman who lives in a hostel, independently mobile, not taking any medication, sustained a fall while coming down stairs. Used to smoke 30 cigarettes a day and drink 'a lot'. This is an X-ray of his pelvis. Describe the injury. (Figure 10.4.)

CANDIDATE: This is a right acetabular fracture with medialization of femoral head. Both ilioinguinal and ilioischial lines are broken. Acetabular dome, anterior and posterior wall are also involved.

EXAMINER: How will you manage this patient initially?

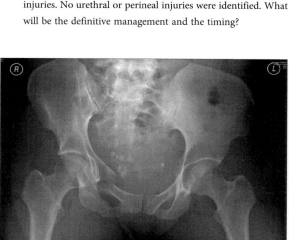

Figure 10.3 Anteroposterior (AP) radiograph of pelvis.

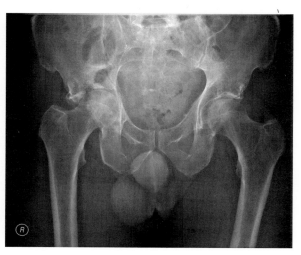

Figure 10.4 Anteroposterior (AP) radiograph of pelvis.

(a)

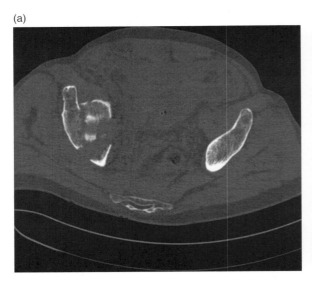

(b)

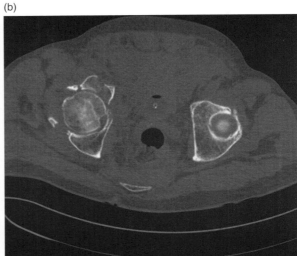

(c)

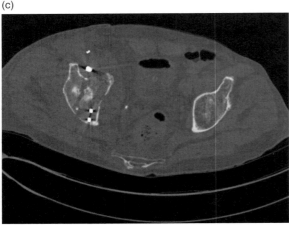

Figure 10.5a, 10.5b and 10.5c CT scan axial views of pelvis.

CANDIDATE: I will examine patient as per ATLS protocols and make sure that there are no other injuries or any distal neurovascular deficits. I will apply distal femoral pin traction after making sure there is no femoral fracture. CT scan of pelvis including both hips will be done as soon as possible. The images will be transferred to the local specialist unit along with patient details for consideration towards surgical management.

EXAMINER: These are the CT scan axial views. What type of fracture is it? Is it common and which group of patients does it occur in? (Figure 10.5.)

CANDIDATE: This fracture involves both anterior and posterior columns. There is an area of intact acetabular dome. Based on the image shown, this fracture looks like anterior wall and column fracture with a posterior hemi transverse fracture.

It is commoner in the older age group due to associated osteoporosis. Hence, these fractures are often due to low-energy injuries, falls from standing height.

EXAMINER: What is your definitive management?

CANDIDATE: Definitive management includes non-operative and operative management. Non-operative management accepts some degree of malunion and if this becomes symptomatic a total hip replacement can be performed. Skeletal traction for 6 weeks followed by a further 6 weeks of non-weightbearing but hip range of movements is started.

Operative management could be either just internal fixation with plate and screws or internal fixation and total hip replacement.

EXAMINER: What are the advantages and disadvantages of just ORIF versus ORIF and THR?

CANDIDATE: ORIF means native hip joint can be salvaged. However, patient has to be non-weightbearing for 3 months. Risk of failure of fixation is higher due to osteoporosis. Even if fixation does not fail, due to increased risk of secondary osteoarthritis, patient could still face a relatively big second operation. Total hip replacement could be performed with relative ease as the fracture should have healed and provides a stable base for the acetabular cup.

ORIF and THR avoids the risks of fixation failure and secondary osteoarthritis. Also the patient could potentially start weightbearing earlier. However, it is a bigger procedure associated with increased risks of dislocation and infection.

Structured oral examination question 4

EXAMINER: A 48-year-old man known to have mental health issues jumped off a bridge from a height of 30 feet landing on concrete pavement. In A&E his injuries identified are all orthopaedic injuries. Lumbar spinal fractures at L2, L3 burst fractures, pelvic and hip injuries as shown in this X-ray, fracture of left radius and ulna, closed intra-articular pilon fracture of left distal tibia. How do you manage this patient? (Figure 10.6.)

CANDIDATE: This patient has sustained multiple significant injuries. As per ATLS protocols I will perform primary and secondary surveys. Closed reduction of left hip as soon as possible and distal femoral pin traction.

Log rolling, neurological assessment, triple immobilization. Soft tissue status of pilon fracture.
Below knee backslab and below-elbow backslab application. Adequate analgesia.
Regular neurological observations, haemodynamic status.
Once haemodynamic stability is achieved CT scan of neck, chest, abdomen and pelvis is performed to rule out other injuries and better identify the fracture patterns.

EXAMINER: What are his injuries on X-ray?

CANDIDATE: Posterior dislocation of left hip with possible fracture, cannot say where the bony fragment has come from. Pubic rami fractures on left side. Both sacroiliac joints, right hip joint, obturator foramen, pubic symphysis appear normal.

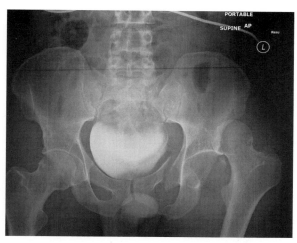

Figure 10.6 Anteroposterior (AP) radiograph of pelvis.

Cystogram has been performed which does not show any extravasation of dye.

EXAMINER: These are axial CT scans of his pelvis. What do they show? (Figure 10.7.)

CANDIDATE: This view shows bilateral sacral alae and neural foraminal fractures. In conjunction with the pubic rami fractures this is an unstable pelvic fracture.

EXAMINER: What other reconstruction view is essential to look at?

CANDIDATE: Sagittal view of sacrum will show whether there are any transverse sacral fractures. If there is also a transverse sacral fracture, then the fracture pattern is 'H' shaped and it is a spinopelvic dissociation.

EXAMINER: How do you classify pelvic fractures?

CANDIDATE: Pelvic fracture can be classified based on the stability of the pelvic ring.

Type A – pelvic ring is intact. Avulsion fractures of ischial tuberosity, iliac wing fractures, etc.
Type B – Incomplete ring injuries. Rotationally unstable. Open-book type fracture, lateral compression fracture.
Type C – complete ring injuries. Rotationally and vertically unstable.

EXAMINER: What is the definitive management plan for this pelvic fracture and its timing?

CANDIDATE: Once patient is stable enough for surgical stabilization, left hip is stressed under fluoroscopy to decide

(a)

(b)

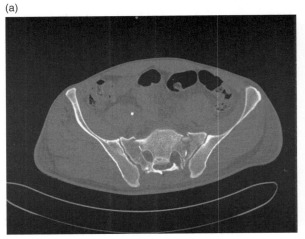
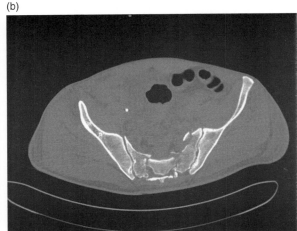

Figure 10.7a and 10.7b CT scan axial views radiograph of pelvis.

whether it is stable. The pelvic fracture fixation is with spinopelvic stabilization with pedicle screws and rod system connecting lumbar fifth vertebra and posterior iliac spines followed by pubic ramus fracture fixation with plate and screws or percutaneous screw fixation.

Structured oral examination question 5

EXAMINER: A 65-year-old lady front-seat passenger of a car involved in a RTA is brought to A&E complaining of pain in her pelvic area and abdomen. GCS is 15, observations are stable. She is obese, suffers from hypertension, NIDDM, has had several laparatomies for diverticulitis, adhesions, total hysterectomy. This is a reconstruction of a CT scan of her pelvis. What is the fracture pattern? (Figure 10.8.)

CANDIDATE: There are pubic rami fractures in the left hemipelvis along with comminuted fracture of left sacral foraminae and alae. There is also vertical displacement along with fractures of left transverse process of fourth and fifth lumbar vertebrae. This is a vertically unstable fracture.

EXAMINER: What are you looking for in examination of this patient?

CANDIDATE: As per ATLS protocols, I will perform primary and secondary surveys. I will look for any associated chest and abdominal injuries, distal neurovascular status.

EXAMINER: This is a CT scan axial view. Describe the injury. (Figure 10.9.)

CANDIDATE: There is a fracture of the left half of the sacrum along the neural foraminae that is displaced.

EXAMINER: Do you know of any classification for sacral fractures?

CANDIDATE: Yes, Denis classification.

Type I – sacral ala fracture.
Type II – fracture through neural foraminae.
Type III – fracture medial to neural foraminae.

This fracture is Type II.

EXAMINER: What is your management plan?

CANDIDATE: Adequate analgesia.
Left distal femoral pin traction.
Regular assessment of left leg neurological status.
Transfer of images and patient information to specialist unit.

EXAMINER: What are the options for managing the pelvic injury?

CANDIDATE: Iliosacral fixation with percutaneous screws after closed reduction with traction or posterior transiliac rods. Anterior stabilization with plate and screws via Pfannenstiel approach.

EXAMINER: What per-operative difficulties do you anticipate?

CANDIDATE: If posterior transiliac rods fixation is planned, then positioning the patient may be difficult.
Intraoperative fluoroscopic images will be suboptimal due to obesity.
Poor bone quality with poor bone purchase of screws.

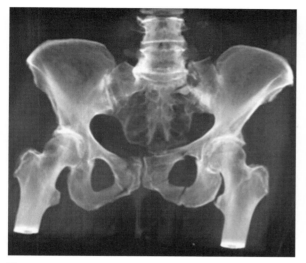

Figure 10.8 Anteroposterior (AP) radiograph of pelvis.

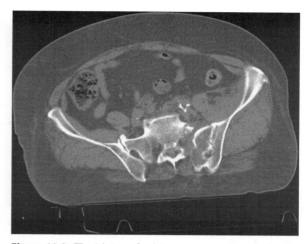

Figure 10.9 CT axial view of pelvis.

Due to previous abdominal procedures, exposing pubic ramus and symphysis may be difficult due to adhesions of bowel and urinary bladder.

Structured oral examination question 6

EXAMINER: A 16-year-old male pedestrian was hit by a car at about 40 miles/hour. GCS at scene was 5–6. Hence, he was intubated at scene. Systolic blood pressure is around 90 mmHg, PR 100/min and peripheral pulses are well felt. Trauma series show no chest or neck injury but a pelvic X-ray has been taken. Describe the injury. (Figure 10.10.)

CANDIDATE: There is a posterior dislocation of left hip with associated acetabular fracture and anterior dislocation of right hip with associated acetabular fracture. Iliac apophysis is still open.

EXAMINER: CT scans of head, neck, chest, abdomen, pelvis were done. These showed cerebral oedema, fluid in abdomen and the injury to both hips as seen here. (Figure 10.11.)

EXAMINER: How will you manage the orthopaedic injuries?

CANDIDATE: Both hip dislocations require urgent reduction and regular check of distal vascular status.

EXAMINER: What are you worried about?

CANDIDATE: The right femoral head is probably very close to the external iliac artery and could compress it along with compressing or stretching the femoral nerve.

EXAMINER: After closed reduction of both hips what will you do?

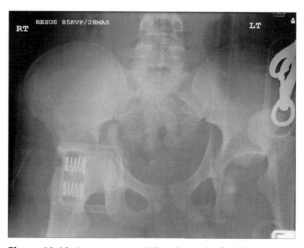

Figure 10.10 Anteroposterior (AP) radiograph of pelvis.

CANDIDATE: I will assess distal vascular status. I will perform distal femoral pin traction for both lower limbs, organize a CT angiogram to confirm the patency of the external iliac artery even if there are good pulsations distally. There is collateral circulation possible that will provide distal blood supply even if there is external iliac artery blockage.

EXAMINER: What will be your definitive management?

CANDIDATE: I will transfer the images to the local specialist unit. When the patient is safe for transfer, he will undergo open reduction and internal fixation of both acetabular fractures either in the same sitting or as a staged procedure.

(a)

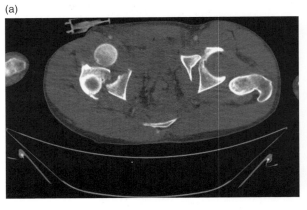

(b)

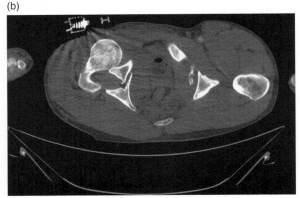

(c)

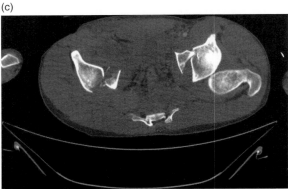

Figure 10.11a, 10.11b and 10.11c CT scan axial views of pelvis.

Spinal trauma
Structured oral examination question 1: Facet dislocation

EXAMINER: What does this X-ray show? (Figure 10.12.)

CANDIDATE: There is anterior translation of the C4 vertebra on C5. This translation is greater than 50% and is highly suggestive of a bifacetal dislocation. The C7/T1 border is not clearly seen and therefore this is an inadequate radiograph.

EXAMINER: How will you manage this patient?

CANDIDATE: I will manage this patient according to ATLS guidelines. I am mindful that a further spinal injury may co-exist, and so until a full neurological examination and full imaging of the spine is obtained, full spinal precautions will prevail. Further management centres on reduction of the dislocation without causing any further neurological damage.

EXAMINER: How will you reduce the dislocation?

CANDIDATE: I would obtain an MRI scan prior to reduction to exclude a disc prolapse (some controversy). Assuming that there is no disc prolapse, and assuming that the patient is lucid and cooperative, I would attempt a closed reduction with the patient awake.

The patient should be in a supine position and should be reverse Trendelenburg. Gardner–Wells tongs are applied to the skull 1 cm above the pinna (below the equator of the skull) in line with the external auditory meatus.

Too anterior placement risks injury to the superficial temporal artery and vein and produces an extension moment to the spine. Too posterior and a flexion moment is applied.

Sequential weights are added to a traction cord. Serial neurological examination is undertaken after the application of progressive weights. An initial weight of 5 kg is applied, with 2 kg weights added sequentially (every 10 minutes). Once the facets have been unlocked, a controlled manoeuvre is undertaken to reduce the facets and the traction is removed.

EXAMINER: What would you do next?

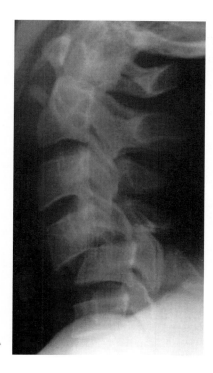

Figure 10.12
Lateral radiograph demonstrating C4 on C5 facet dislocation.

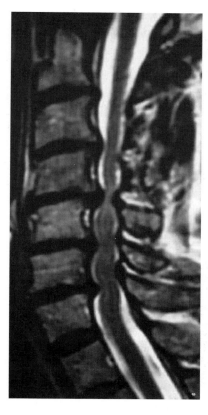

Figure 10.13
T2 sagittal MRI scan cervical spine.

CANDIDATE: A bilateral facet dislocation is typically easier to reduce than a unilateral facet dislocation due to the extensive ligamentous injury, in particular to the PLL. This also suggests gross instability once the initial reduction is undertaken, and so surgical stabilization by way of anterior cervical discectomy and fusion (ACDF) is necessary.

Structured oral examination question 2: Incomplete cord injury

EXAMINER: A 75-year-old female presents with abnormal neurological findings having fallen onto her face; what does the MRI scan show? (Figure 10.13.)

CANDIDATE: The MRI scan demonstrates a hyperintense signal within the parenchyma of the spinal cord at at C4 to C7. In addition, disc bulges of the C5/6 and C6/6 intervertebral discs can be seen (+/− haematoma).

EXAMINER: What pattern of injury do you expect?

CANDIDATE: It is likely that the pattern of injury is one of central cord syndrome, which is the most common incomplete cord injury. The history is characteristic, often an elderly person with an extension injury. The pathophysiology is one of

anterior osteophytes and posterior infolded ligamentum flavum compressing the cord. There is often a background of pre-existing cervical spondylosis which may well have been asymptomatic.

EXAMINER: What do you think the clinical features will be?

CANDIDATE: There will be upper motor neurone weakness affecting the upper and lower limbs. The upper limbs are affected to a greater extent, with the motor deficit especially prevalent in the hand. Sensory loss is variable though sacral sensation is usually present.

EXAMINER: How will you manage this person?

CANDIDATE: Central cord syndrome has a good prognosis though full functional recovery is not likely. It is not unusual to see significant early neurological recovery, and in the absence of spinal instability, I would manage this condition non-operatively. The typical recovery sequence begins with the lower limbs, followed by bladder and bowel function, the proximal muscles of the upper extremity and finally the hands. Typically the patient is ambulatory at final follow-up.

If there is a plateau in recovery with MRI-proven cord compression, or if there are signs of instability, surgical decompression and stabilization should be considered.

EXAMINER: Are you aware of any other incomplete cord syndromes?

CANDIDATE: Anterior cord syndrome, typically caused by a flexion/compression injury, affects the anterior two-thirds of the spinal cord via anterior spinal artery lesions. In this case the lower extremity is affected to a greater extent than the upper extremity but it is useful to note that proprioception and vibratory sense (both carried in the dorsal, unaffected, columns) are preserved. This condition has the worst prognosis.

Brown–Séquard syndrome is a hemitransection of the spinal cord, seen with a penetrating trauma. There is ipsilateral loss of motor function, proprioception and vibratory sense; there is contralateral loss of pain and temperature sensation. This has the best prognosis of the incomplete injuries with 99% of patients ambulatory at final follow up.

Finally a rare syndrome, characterized by a loss of proprioception, is the posterior cord syndrome. Motor, light touch and pain and temperature are all preserved.

Structured oral examination question 3: Thoracolumbar burst fractures

EXAMINER: What does this X-ray show? (Figure 10.14.)

CANDIDATE: There is a fracture of the T12 vertebral body with greater than 50% loss of the vertebral body height. The posterior margin is poorly defined. On the AP view there is widening of the interpedicular distance.

EXAMINER: Is this a stable or unstable injury?

CANDIDATE: This is an unstable injury. Two of Denis' three columns have failed, and there is greater than 50% loss of vertebral body height.

EXAMINER: What is your management?

CANDIDATE: I would manage the patient according to ATLS guidelines and ensure that the spine is kept in alignment at all times. My aims are to exclude any other spinal trauma, concurrent abdominal trauma, and to prevent secondary injury.

A full neurological examination is undertaken and the presence of sacral sparing documented (which is suggestive of a better prognosis). The neurological examination is repeated

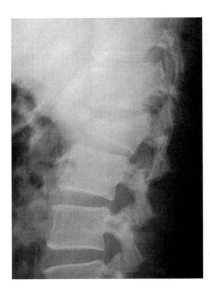

Figure 10.14
Lateral radiograph burst thoracolumbar fracture.

frequently in order to ascertain whether or not there is a progressive neurological deficit.

I would assess the patient for signs of spinal shock, which is a temporary loss of spinal cord function and reflex activity below the level of the injury. It is typically characterized by diaphragmatic breathing (if level appropriate), paralysis, absent reflexes, erection, urinary retention and an absent bulbocavernosus reflex.

EXAMINER: What is the importance of spinal shock and how do you know when it's over?

CANDIDATE: The importance of spinal shock is that one cannot evaluate the neurological deficit until the spinal shock phase has resolved. Resolution is determined by the return of the bulbocavernosus reflex – squeezing the glans penis (or clitoris in the female) or gently pulling on an indwelling urinary catheter elicits an anal sphincter contraction.

EXAMINER: What is neurogenic shock?

CANDIDATE: Neurogenic shock can be thought of as a temporary generalized sympathectomy. Typically the patient will be hypotensive but bradycardic. It is important to exclude other causes of hypotension however (10–15% of patients with spinal injuries have visceral injuries) before attributing hypotension to neurogenic shock.

EXAMINER: The patient is no longer in spinal shock, and has some flickers of movement in his left lower limb only. What is your management now?

CANDIDATE: The patient has an incomplete injury. Given the fact that he also has an unstable spine, as determined by the loss of greater than 50% of vertebral body height (and a kyphosis angle greater than 30°), surgical decompression and stabilization is indicated.

EXAMINER: What if they were to have a complete injury? Is there a role for surgery then?

CANDIDATE: The role of surgery in a complete spinal cord injury is to facilitate rehabilitation by providing a stable and pain-free spine.

EXAMINER: What complications do you expect in the next few days?

CANDIDATE: There are many potential complications, all of which may be anticipated. Proper bedding will avoid any pressure sores as will regular turning (once the spine has been stabilized). Prophylaxis for thromboembolic disease must be provided and strict hygiene undertaken to prevent urosepsis. Paralytic ileus may require the patient to be kept nil-by-mouth and they may require a nasogastric tube to decompress. Prophylaxis should also be provided for stress ulceration (Curling's ulcer).

EXAMINER: What about the bowel?

CANDIDATE: With an upper motor neurone lesion (typically T12 and above), reflex activity is maintained and the bowel will contract and empty. A lower motor neurone lesion (typically at L1 or below) will have return of peristalsis but without the support of the spinal reflex. This leads to faecal retention. I would manage these patients with daily glycerine suppositories, and when bowel sounds return I would prescribe senna and lactulose.

British Orthopaedic Association. *The Initial Care and Transfer of Patients with Spinal Cord Injuries.* London: British Orthopaedic Association, 2006.

Structured oral examination question 4: Odontoid peg fractures

EXAMINER: What does this X-ray show? (Figure 10.15.)

CANDIDATE: This is a lateral radiograph of the cervical spine. The most obvious abnormality is a fracture through the base of the odontoid peg of C2.

EXAMINER: Yes, are you aware of any classification systems for this type of injury?

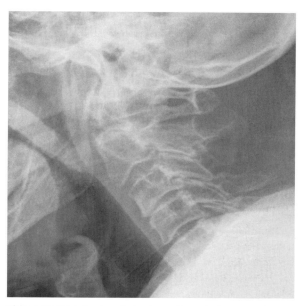

Figure 10.15 Lateral cervical spine radiograph demonstrating an odontoid peg fracture.

CANDIDATE: I am familiar with the Anderson and D'Alonzo classification. This classifies fractures according to their location within the peg. Type I fractures affect the tip of the odontoid and are caused by avulsion of the alar ligaments proximal to the transverse ligament and are usually stable injuries. Type II injuries run through the base of the odontoid peg just below the transverse ligament making them unstable injuries. They have a high ratio of cortical to cancellous bone and so have a higher rate of non-union than other fractures. Type III injuries are seen distal to the base of the peg running through the metaphyseal bone of the vertebral body. As these fractures have a higher proportion of cancellous to cortical bone and a greater surface area they are more likely to heal than Type II injuries.

EXAMINER: So how does this classification guide your management?

CANDIDATE: Type I injuries are stable and so I would treat them in a hard collar such as an Aspen collar. Type III injuries are likely to heal and so I would immobilize them in a halo jacket or possibly in a hard collar in elderly frail individuals due to the risks of halo jackets in the elderly. These injuries would then require follow-up in clinic. Type II injuries are more likely to go on to non-union and so they are the injuries that I would consider fixation as an option as opposed to a halo jacket.

EXAMINER: Are there any factors with Type II injuries that would make it more likely that they would go on to non-union to guide your decision?

CANDIDATE: Yes. If there is more than 4 mm displacement on the initial X-ray, if there is posterior displacement, if there is angulation more than 10°, significant comminution at the base or if there was delayed presentation or failure to reduce or keep the fracture reduced in a halo,[1] these all make it more likely that there will be a non-union and guide the decision towards surgery.

EXAMINER: What are the surgical options for treatment of a Type II fracture?

CANDIDATE: The two options are posterior C1/C2 fusion or screw osteosynthesis of the dens of C2. The benefit of C1/2 fusion is that it is a reliable operation that is not dependent on the fracture configuration but results in a large loss of movement. C2 osteosynthesis gives the benefit of retaining the rotational movement that occurs at the atlantoaxial joint but is technically difficult and is dependent on fracture configuration.

EXAMINER: What factors would guide your choice of surgery?

CANDIDATE: If there is an oblique fracture of the peg in the same orientation as your lag screw then this will lead to poor fixation with a tendency to displacement. In this circumstance I would choose to perform a C1/2 fusion instead. However, if there was an associated fracture of the C1 arch, then it would be preferable to perform screw osteosynthesis.

EXAMINER: Yes, let's move on.

1. Schatzker J, Rorabeck CH, Waddell JP. Non union of the odontoid process: an experimental investigation. *Clin Orthop Rel Res* 1975;**108**:127–137.

Structured oral examination question 5: Hangman's fracture

EXAMINER: What does this X-ray show? (Figure 10.16.)

CANDIDATE: It is a lateral radiograph of the cervical spine. The most obvious abnormality is an anterior subluxation of C2 on C3.

EXAMINER: Do you know what we call this fracture?

CANDIDATE: It is a traumatic spondylolisthesis of C2, also known as a hangman's fracture.

EXAMINER: Do you know any classification systems for this injury?

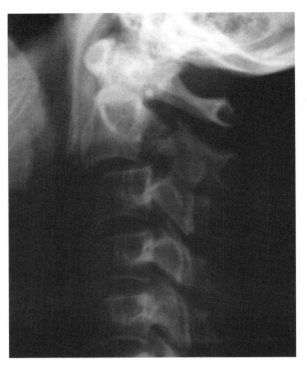

Figure 10.16 Lateral cervical spine radiograph demonstrating hangman's fracture.

CANDIDATE: Yes, I am aware of the Levine classification. It grades the injury as Type I with bilateral pars inter-articularis fractures with less than 3 mm of displacement, in IA one of the fracture lines extends into the foramen transversarium endangering the vertebral artery. Type II injuries involve displacement of more than 3 mm with IIA having more angulation and widening of the disc space posteriorly indicating an intervertebral disc injury. Type III injuries involve fractures or dislocations of the facet joints bilaterally as well as the fractures mentioned previously.

EXAMINER: How would you manage a patient with a hangman's fracture?

CANDIDATE: If the patient is neurologically intact with a hangman's fracture then it is common practice to allow it to heal in situ to reduce the risk of causing a neurological injury on reduction. Therefore, Type I and II fractures are usually treated with halo jackets to allow stability until healing occurs. Type III fractures usually require fixation as they are more unstable due to loss of facet joint stability and are not as easily controlled in a halo jacket.[1]

1. Vieweg U, Schultheiss R. A review of halo vest treatment of upper cervical spine injuries. *Arch Orthop Trauma Surg* 2001;**121**(1–2):50–55.

Structured oral examination question 6: Chance fractures

EXAMINER: What does this picture show? (Figure 10.17.)

CANDIDATE: This is a clinical photograph of a man's abdomen. There is gross bruising across the anterior abdominal wall.

EXAMINER: What do you think has happened to him?

CANDIDATE: I would imagine that he has been involved in a road traffic accident restrained by a seat belt.

EXAMINER: Yes, that's right. So how would you assess this man in the emergency department?

CANDIDATE: I would follow ATLS principles and identify and treat any life- or limb-threatening injuries.

EXAMINER: [interrupting] Yes alright, but what injuries would you expect to find?

CANDIDATE: I would expect this man to have intra-abdominal visceral injuries due to the blunt trauma. With this mechanism I would suspect a chance-type injury which has a 50–60% association with intra-abdominal injuries.[1] I also would want to exclude cervical spine injuries with any flexion–distraction type of injury.

EXAMINER: Tell us about chance-type injuries. (Figure 10.18.)

CANDIDATE: These are flexion–distraction injuries affecting the thoracolumbar spine. It involves an injury to both the anterior and posterior columns (B type injury according to the AO classification system), or all three columns (according to the Denis classification system) making it an unstable injury. It can be purely bony, purely ligamentous or mixed. Typically, the anterior column fails in compression whereas the posterior columns fail in tension.

EXAMINER: So how would you investigate this person in the emergency department?

CANDIDATE: I would request a CT scan of the whole spine to look for any bony injuries.

EXAMINER: What would you expect to see?

CANDIDATE: If there was a bony injury then you could see the pattern of the fracture running through the vertebral body and the posterior elements. If it was a ligamentous injury then there may be some translation of the vertebral bodies at that level and there may be a widening of the interspinous space.

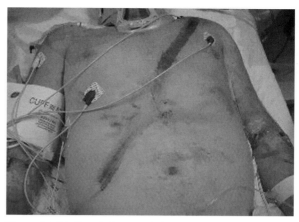

Figure 10.17 Clinical photograph demonstrating gross abdominal bruising. See colour plate section.

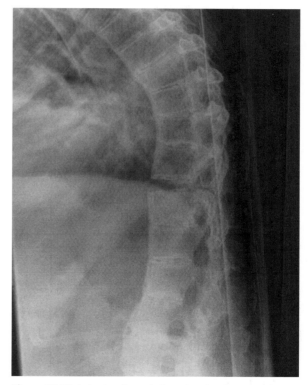

Figure 10.18 Lateral radiograph thoracic spine demonstrating Chance fracture.

EXAMINER: Would you do any further investigations?

CANDIDATE: If there was no bony injury and I suspected a chance-type injury then I would also request an MRI scan to assess the soft tissues.

EXAMINER: How would you manage these injuries?

CANDIDATE: If the patient was neurologically intact and there was minimal displacement of a bony injury it could potentially be managed in a hyperextension brace. This would require very close monitoring to ensure that there is no displacement. If there was any loss of position with this regime then it should be treated operatively. If it is a ligamentous injury then it will require fixation as it will not heal as effectively as a bony injury and will remain unstable. If there is a very displaced fracture that cannot be reduced or held effectively in a brace then they should have surgical stabilization.

EXAMINER: Yes, let's move on.

1. Anderson PA, Rivara FP, Maier RV, Drake C. The epidemiology of seatbelt-associated injuries. *J Trauma* 1991;**31**:60–67.

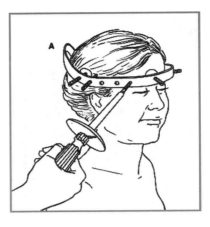

Figure 10.19
Halo traction.

Structured oral examination question 7: Application of a halo

EXAMINER: How do you apply a halo? (Figure 10.19.)

CANDIDATE: I would first explain to the patient what I am going to do and why.

I would match the skull to the appropriate halo ring prior to application. Typically, three people are required to apply a halo with one person maintaining alignment and the remaining two applying the halo.[1]

Using local anaesthetic and antiseptic, four pins are applied to the adult skull (eight in the paediatric population) and tightened with a torque-limiter (8 inch-pounds; 2–4 inch-pounds in the paediatric skull). The pins are placed equidistant and symmetrically in order to allow for stability of the construct.

CARE SHOULD BE TAKEN TO PREVENT DAMAGE TO IMPORTANT STRUCTURES: the superficial temporal artery and vein, the supraorbital nerves and the sinuses.

The anterior pins are placed 1 cm above the lateral one-third of the eyebrow *with the eyes tightly closed*. This is lateral to the supraorbital nerve.

The posterior pins are placed behind the earlobe, just above the mastoid.

An appropriately sized jacket is then applied (or traction as may be necessary).

A radiograph is obtained to ensure correct reduction.

The patient should be instructed to return at 24–48 hours to have the pins retightened, and should be educated on pin hygiene.

EXAMINER: What are the potential complications?

CANDIDATE: Loss of position or reduction, pin site infection and loosening, pain, nerve or vessel injury. One-fifth of patients also complain of pain which can be managed by loosening. Rarely there is a complication of dural puncture (1%).[2,3]

1. Bono CM. The halo fixator. *J Am Acad Orthop Surg* 2007;**15**:728–737.

2. Botte MJ, Byrne TP, Abrams RA *et al*. Halo skeletal fixation: techniques of application and prevention of complications. *J Am Acad Orthop Surg* 1996;**4**:44–53.

3. Garfin SR, Botte MJ, Waters RL *et al*. Complications in the use of the halo fixation device. *J Bone Joint Surg Am* 1986;**68-A**:320–325.

Chapter

11

Hand and upper limb

John Harrison and Santosh Venkatachalam

Structured oral examination question 1: EPL tendon rupture

EXAMINER: What does the photograph show? (Figure 11.1a.)

CANDIDATE: This is a clinical photograph of the hand with the thumb in an abnormally flexed posture at the IP joint.

EXAMINER: The patient has recently come out of plaster for a distal radius fracture. What is a likely pathology?

CANDIDATE: This is usually caused by an ischaemic rupture of the extensor pollicis longus tendon (EPL) in the third dorsal extensor compartment at 4–6 weeks following an undisplaced distal radius fracture.

EXAMINER: How do you manage this?

CANDIDATE: This is surgically reconstructed using a transfer of extensor indicis (EI) tendon.

EXAMINER: How many incisions would you use?

CANDIDATE: Three incisions are needed – a 1 cm transverse incision over the index finger metacarpal head (EI lies ulnar to the EDC index finger), a 3 cm midline dorsal incision proximal to the wrist to bring the divided EI tendon proximal to extensor retinaculum, a zigzag incision over the thumb

metacarpal to identify EPL tendon distal to the rupture. (Figure 11.1b.)

EXAMINER: How do you test for extensor indicis preoperatively?

CANDIDATE: Point the index finger with the middle to little fingers flexed fully (this prevents EDC acting).

Structured oral examination question 2: Enchondroma

An 11 year old reports an injured hand in a fall.

EXAMINER: What do you see in this photograph? (Figure 11.2a.)

CANDIDATE: This is a clinical photograph of a hand showing a swelling at the base of the middle finger with widening of the interspace between the index and middle fingers. No bruising is seen.

EXAMINER: The child has a full range of movements in the hand. Any investigations you would do?

CANDIDATE: I would order a radiograph. The radiograph shows a cystic lesion affecting the proximal phalanx of the middle finger. The proximal radial cortex is markedly thinned and expanded to the radial side causing widening between the middle and index fingers. (Figure 11.2b.)

(a)

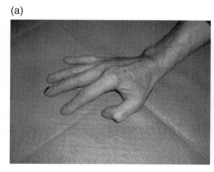

(b)

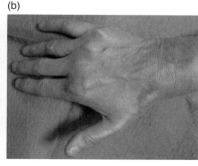

Figure 11.1a Clinical picture of a hand. **11.1b** Showing thumb retropulsion at 6 weeks postoperatively. The three incisions can be seen.

Postgraduate Orthopaedics: Viva Guide for the FRCS (Tr & Orth) Examination, ed. Paul A. Banaszkiewicz and Deiary F. Kader. Published by Cambridge University Press. © Cambridge University Press 2012.

(a)

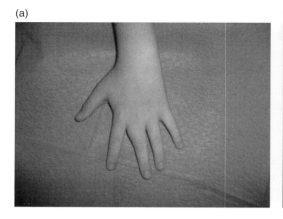

(b)

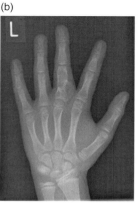

Figure 11.2a Clinical picture of an 11-year-old's hand. **11.2b** Radiograph of the child's hand.

EXAMINER: What is the likely diagnosis?

CANDIDATE: An enchondroma. This is a cartilage tumour of bone.

EXAMINER: How would you manage this lesion?

CANDIDATE: I would take a further history asking about any pain or rapid change in size of the finger. I would look for any bony swellings elsewhere (Ollier's disease – multiple enchondromatosis) or haemangiomas (Mafucci's syndrome). I would explain the tumour has been present prior to the injury and is benign. I would review the patient at 6 weeks and then annually. If it continued to increase in size, I would refer to a hand surgeon for partial excision and bone grafting.

EXAMINER: What is the risk of malignant change?

CANDIDATE: It is very rare for single tumours. The risk is 20–30% for Ollier's disease and near 100% for Mafucci's syndrome.

Structured oral examination question 3: Trans-scaphoid perilunate fracture dislocation

EXAMINER: Tell me what you see here. (Figure 11.3a.)

CANDIDATE: The radiograph demonstrates a trans-scaphoid perilunate fracture dislocation. I would like to see a lateral view.

EXAMINER: This is the lateral view. (Figure 11.3b.) What is the mechanism of injury?

CANDIDATE: Forced wrist dorsiflexion, ulnar deviation, and intercarpal supination. The injury begins at radial side and progresses towards ulnar side through the midcarpal space.

EXAMINER: What classification system do you know of for such an injury?

CANDIDATE: Mayfield has divided it into four sequential stages.

I. Rupture of SL ligament or fracture of the scaphoid.
II. Midcarpal dislocation (dorsal).
III. Lunotriquetral ligament injury.
IV. Lunate dislocation (usually volar).

A greater arc injury goes through the radial styloid, scaphoid and capitate.

EXAMINER: What is the 'spilled tea-cup' sign?

CANDIDATE: Stage IV Mayfield wherein the lunate is dislocated and faces the palm on X-rays. (Figure 11.3c.)

EXAMINER: What is the normal scapholunate angle?

CANDIDATE: Average is 45° (abnormal if < 30° or > 60°).

EXAMINER: How will you manage this patient?

CANDIDATE: I will assess the patient clinically and look for neurovascular impairment particularly median nerve. This will need to be reduced as an emergency procedure in theatre under image intensifier and anaesthesia. The scaphoid needs to be fixed and the dorsal ligaments – scapholunate and lunotriquetral – need to be repaired through a dorsal approach. This can be done at a later stage by a hand surgeon. (Figure 11.3d.)

Structured oral examination question 4: Wrist ganglion

EXAMINER: What do you see? (Figure 11.4a.)

CANDIDATE: There is a swelling over the dorsoradial aspect of the wrist. This is typical site for a dorsal wrist ganglion.

EXAMINER: How would you confirm this?

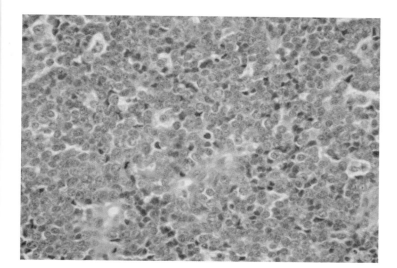

Figure 7.8 Ewing's sarcoma.

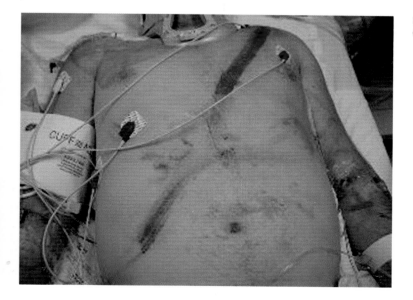

Figure 10.17 Clinical photograph demonstrating gross abdominal bruising.

	Secondary bony epiphysis	
	Reserve zone	Diastrophic dwarfism (Type II collagen synthesis defect) Kneist syndrome (Proteoglycans processing defect) Pseudoachondroplasia (Proteoglycans processing and transport defect)
	Proliferative zone	Gigantism (GH) – Increased profileration Achondroplasia, excessive steriod, malnutrition, radiation injury – decreased proliferation
Hypertrophic zone	Maturation zone	Mucopolysaccharidosis (genetic enzyme defect)
Hypertrophic zone	Degenerative zone	
Hypertrophic zone	Provisional zone	Rickets and osteomalacia
Metaphysis	Primary spongiosa	Metaphyseal chondroplasia (Jansen and Schmid types) – extension of hypertrophic cell into metaphysis. Acute haematogenous osteomyelitis – sluggish blood flow
Metaphysis	Secondary spongiosa	Osteoporosis Osteogenesis imperfecta Scurvy Metaphyseal dysplasia

Figure 12.54 Physeal layers and abnormalities.

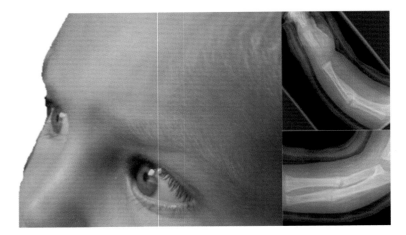

Figure 12.58 A clinical photograph and right forearm X-rays of a child.

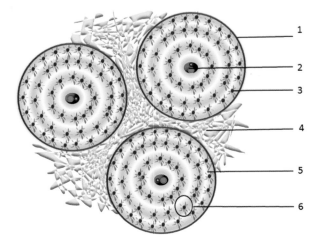

Figure 19.3 Bone architecture.

1
2
3
4
5
6

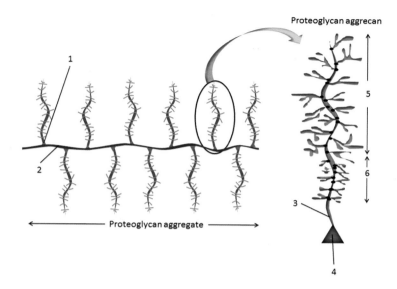

Proteoglycan aggrecan
1
2
3
4
5
6
Proteoglycan aggregate

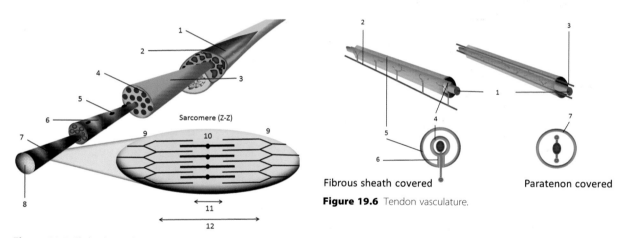

Figure 19.4 Proteoglycan.

1
2
3
4
5
6
7
Sarcomere (Z-Z)
9
10
9
8
11
12

Figure 19.5 Skeletal muscle.

2
3
1
4
5
6
7
Fibrous sheath covered
Paratenon covered

Figure 19.6 Tendon vasculature.

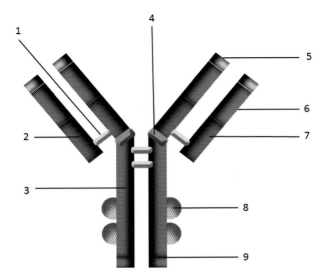

Figure 19.7 Immunoglobulin.

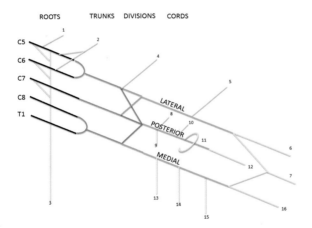

Figure 19.8 Brachial plexus.

ROOTS   TRUNKS   DIVISIONS   CORDS

C5
C6
C7
C8
T1

LATERAL

POSTERIOR

MEDIAL

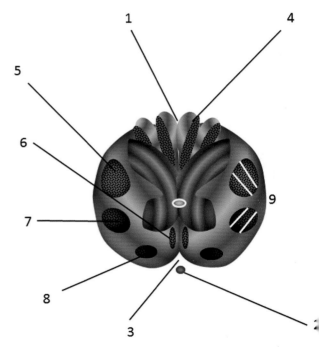

Figure 19.13 Spinal cord anatomy.

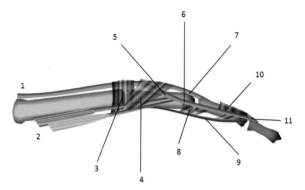

Figure 19.21 Finger extensor tendon.

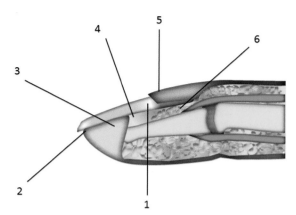

Figure 19.22 Nail anatomy.

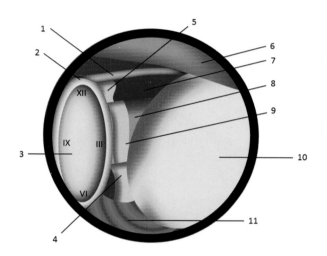

Figure 19.24 Glenohumeral joint arthroscopic view.

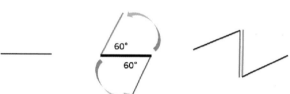

Figure 19.27 Z plasty.

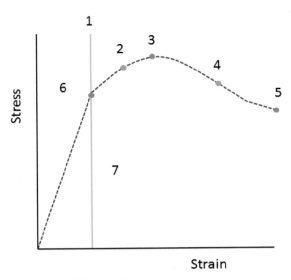

Figure 19.28 Stress–strain curve.

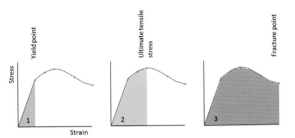

Figure 19.29 Stress–strain curve.

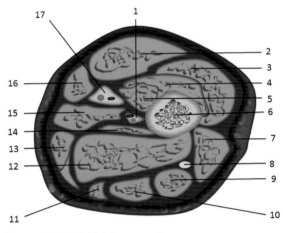

Figure 19.33 Mid thigh cross-section.

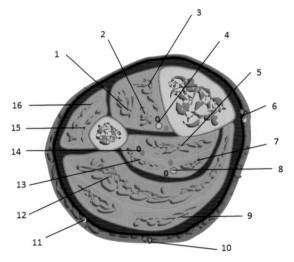

Figure 19.34 Mid leg cross-section.

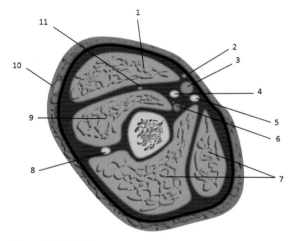

Figure 19.35 Mid arm cross-section.

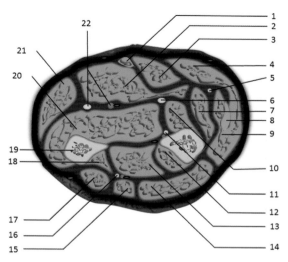

Figure 19.36 Mid forearm cross-section.

Figure 19.37 Distal forearm cross-section.

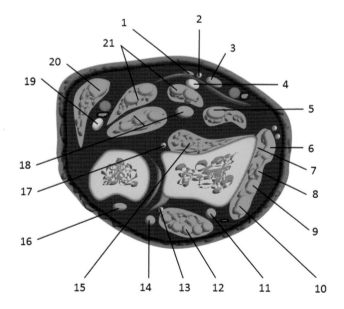

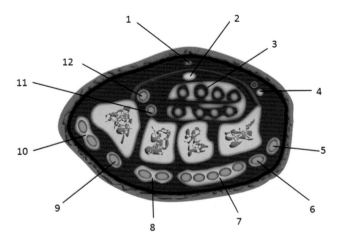

Figure 19.38 Carpal tunnel cross-section.

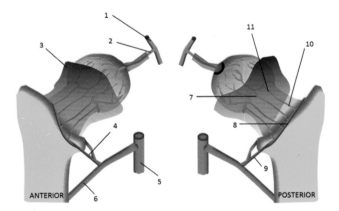

Figure 19.40 Femoral head vascular supply.

ANTERIOR

POSTERIOR

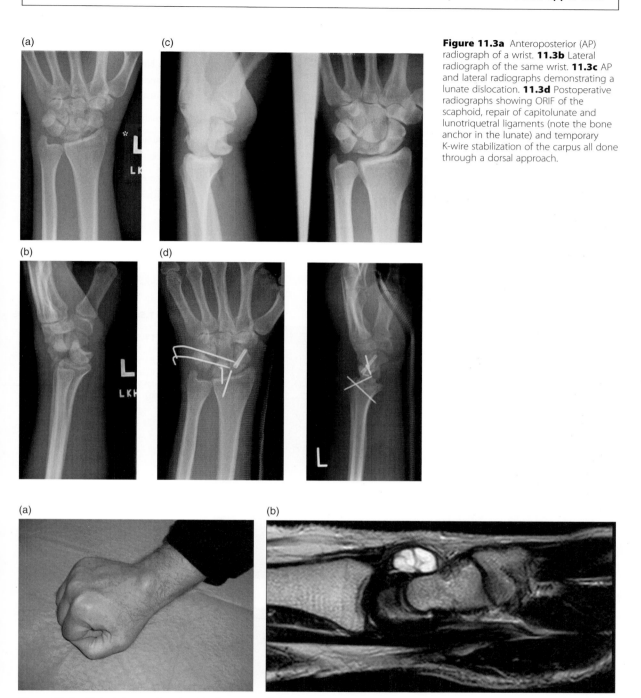

Figure 11.3a Anteroposterior (AP) radiograph of a wrist. **11.3b** Lateral radiograph of the same wrist. **11.3c** AP and lateral radiographs demonstrating a lunate dislocation. **11.3d** Postoperative radiographs showing ORIF of the scaphoid, repair of capitolunate and lunotriquetral ligaments (note the bone anchor in the lunate) and temporary K-wire stabilization of the carpus all done through a dorsal approach.

Figure 11.4a Clinical picture of a wrist. **11.4b** Imaging of the same wrist.

CANDIDATE: Take a history specifically asking about any fluctuation in size. Clinically this is a firm, smooth swelling attached to deep structures which classically transilluminates.

EXAMINER: What does this show? (Figure 11.4b.)

CANDIDATE: This is a T2-weighted MR scan showing a well-circumscribed, focal, multiloculated lesion overlying the lunate and capitate dorsally. The ganglion is likely to have arisen from the scapholunate ligament.

EXAMINER: How would you manage this?

CANDIDATE: Counsel the patient this is a benign condition. As long as there is no history of increasing size or pain this may be the only treatment necessary. If there is pain affecting function especially with forced wrist extension then surgical excision may be offered. The recurrence rate is 5%.

Structured oral examination question 5: Scaphoid fracture (proximal pole)

EXAMINER: An apprentice joiner has fallen on his hand at work. What does this show? (Figure 11.5a.) What is the diagnosis?

CANDIDATE: Proximal pole scaphoid fracture. The fracture is undisplaced.

EXAMINER: What is the relevant anatomy?

CANDIDATE: The proximal pole blood supply is from distal to proximal. A proximal 1/5 fracture has a non-union rate of 80–100% when treated non-operatively.

EXAMINER: How do you manage this injury?

CANDIDATE: Open reduction and internal fixation with a screw placed from a proximal entry point and through a dorsal incision.

EXAMINER: In this case, the fracture was treated non-operatively. This is an X-ray at 4 weeks after immobilization in a plaster cast. (Figure 11.5b.)

CANDIDATE: The fracture ends appear sclerosed with some cyst formation around the edges suggesting this is progressing to a non-union. At this stage, the proximal segment appears to be normal density suggesting no loss of vascularity.

(a)

(b)

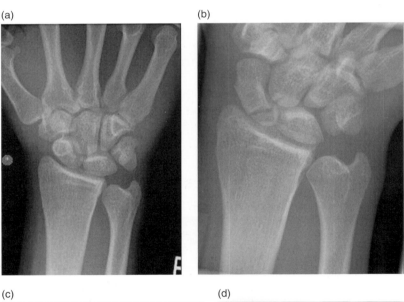

Figure 11.5a AP radiograph of a wrist. **11.5b** AP radiograph of the same wrist at 4 weeks. **11.5c** and **11.5d** Anteroposterior (AP) and oblique radiographs showing union at 8 weeks postoperatively (note the lucency in the distal radius where the graft has been taken from).

(c)

(d)

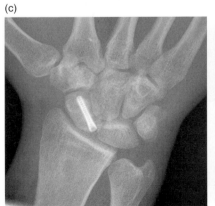 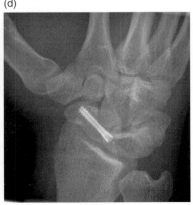

EXAMINER: How would you manage this now?

CANDIDATE: Open reduction through a dorsal approach and internal fixation with a vascularized bone graft using a 1,2-intercompartmental supraretinacular artery (1,2-ICSRA) pedicle.[1] (Figure 11.5c, d.)

EXAMINER: What is the natural history of a scaphoid non-union?

CANDIDATE: This will progress to a scaphoid non-union advanced collapse (SNAC) wrist.

I.   Arthritis between radial styloid and distal scaphoid.
II.   Radioscaphoid fossa involvement.
III. Capitolunate arthritis.
IV.   Generalized wrist arthritis.

EXAMINER: Why does the arthritis affect the radial styloid and distal scaphoid initially?

CANDIDATE: With a non-union, the distal scaphoid typically flexes leading to incongruity between the distal scaphoid and radial styloid, whereas the proximal pole of the scaphoid behaves as a ball and socket joint and is not affected by the scaphoid being flexed.

1. Zaidemberg C, Siebert JW, Angrigiani C. A new vascularized bone graft for scaphoid nonunion. *J Hand Surg Am* 1991;**16**(3):474–478.

Structured oral examination question 6: Base of thumb arthritis

EXAMINER: Describe what this radiograph shows. (Figure 11.6a.)

CANDIDATE: This is a radiograph of the hand. The most obvious abnormality is complete loss of joint space of the thumb carpometacarpal (CMC) joint and subchondral sclerosis.

EXAMINER: Do you know any X-ray view which may better show the thumb CMC joint?

CANDIDATE: A Robert's view – this is a true AP view of the thumb CMC joint, and is taken with the elbow extended, the forearm fully pronated and the thumb abducted. (Figure 11.6b.)

EXAMINER: Do you know any classification system for this?

CANDIDATE: Eaton classification of thumb CMC joint OA. This is a radiological classification.

I.   Widening of the joint.
II.   Joint space narrowing.
III. Complete loss of CMC joint space.
IV.   Pantrapezial arthritis.

EXAMINER: This is a 56-year-old plaster technician with night pain. How would you treat?

CANDIDATE: I would take a detailed history asking specifically for pain and loss of function. I would examine to see if his pain is localized to the thumb CMC joint by looking for squaring-off of the thumb metacarpal base and performing a grind test.

EXAMINER: Show on my hand how you would do the test.

CANDIDATE: I would stabilize your wrist with my left hand then hold your thumb metacarpal with my right hand and compress and rotate the metacarpal base at the CMC joint. The test is positive if this causes pain and then the pain goes with rotation and distraction. Treatment options include painkillers, activity modification, splints and surgery.

EXAMINER: But what would you do?

CANDIDATE: I would offer him a trapeziectomy. There are no randomized controlled studies to show benefit of this procedure over a ligament reconstruction, fusion or joint replacement.[1] I would explain preoperatively that he is likely to have some loss of grip strength on a permanent basis. (Figure 11.6c.)

1. Davis TR, Brady O, Barton NJ, Lunn PG, Burke FD. Trapeziectomy alone, with tendon interposition or with ligament reconstruction? *J Hand Surg Br* 1997;**22**(6): 689–694.

Structured oral examination question 7: Kienböck's disease

EXAMINER: A 30-year-old electrician presents with wrist pain. What does this show? (Figure 11.7a.)

CANDIDATE: Radiograph shows increased density of the lunate with some cyst formation and partial collapse. There are no obvious arthritic changes in the surrounding joints.

EXAMINER: What is the diagnosis?

CANDIDATE: Kienböck's disease – avascular necrosis of the lunate.

EXAMINER: How do you classify Kienböck's disease?

CANDIDATE: Lichtman classification (radiological).[1]
    I. Normal X-rays (changes seen on MRI). II. Lunate sclerosis. IIIA. Fragmentation and collapse of lunate without fixed scaphoid rotation. IIIB. Fragmentation and collapse of lunate with fixed scaphoid rotation. IV. Radiocarpal and midcarpal arthritis.

(a)

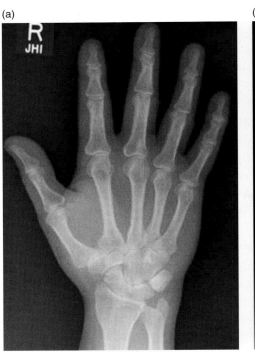

(b)

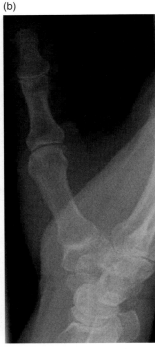

Figure 11.6a Anteroposterior (AP) radiograph of a hand. **11.6b** Robert's view (true AP view of the thumb CMC joint). **11.6c** In this case a fusion was done as this possibly allows improved grip strength in a manual worker but has a higher incidence of complications such as non-union.

(c)

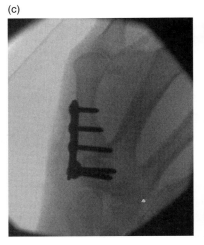

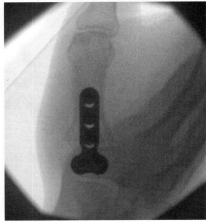

EXAMINER: Any predisposing factors?

CANDIDATE: These include ulnar minus variant – this is thought to lead to increased loading on the lunate, poor intraosseous anastomosis and a single extraosseous nutrient vessel.

EXAMINER: What are patterns of intraosseous blood supply?

CANDIDATE: These were described by Gelberman who described a Y pattern (60%), I pattern (30%) and an X pattern (10%).

EXAMINER: What are the treatment options for this condition?

CANDIDATE: This depends on the patient's symptoms and functional demands. Conservative treatment with a period of time in splintage can be discussed. For symptomatic patients with Stage I/II/IIIA disease and if ulnar minus, I would offer a joint levelling procedure, either a radial shortening or an ulnar lengthening. I would prefer a shortening osteotomy since the incidence of non/delayed union is less. If ulnar neutral or plus, consider a procedure aiming to reduce loading on the lunate – either a partial carpal arthrodesis (STT or scapho-capitate) or a

(a)
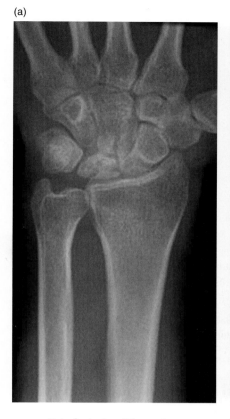

(b)
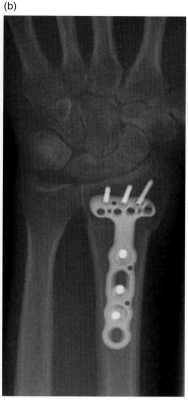

Figure 11.7a Anteroposterior (AP) radiograph of a wrist. **11.7b** Radiograph demonstrating a joint levelling procedure (radial shortening).

capitate shortening. Other options are a vascularized bone graft with 4,5-ICSRA or a distal radial osteotomy.

For Stage IIIB/IV disease, surgical options include a neurectomy, or salvage procedures such as a proximal row carpectomy or a wrist arthrodesis.

EXAMINER: How would you manage this case?

CANDIDATE: I would confirm these were length films for ulna variance, i.e. a wrist PA view with the shoulder flexed 90°, elbow 90° and forearm midprone. If these were, the wrist appears to be ulnar minus and I would offer a joint levelling procedure with a radial shortening. (Figure 11.7b.)

1. Allan CH, Joshi A, Lichtman DM. Kienbock's disease: diagnosis and treatment. *J Am Acad Orthop Surg* 2001; **9**(2):128–136.

Structured oral examination question 8: Dupuytren's disease

EXAMINER: What do you see? (Figure 11.8a.)

CANDIDATE: This is a clinical photograph of a hand showing a cord across the first web space causing a contracture. There is

also a cord affecting the index finger causing fixed flexion of the MCP and PIP joints.

EXAMINER: What is the most likely diagnosis?

CANDIDATE: Dupuytren's contracture.

EXAMINER: What is the primary cell involved?

CANDIDATE: Myofibroblasts. They contain smooth muscle actin and lead to contracture of the cord.

EXAMINER: What is Dupuytren's diathesis?

CANDIDATE: This is an aggressive form of the disease with a high recurrence rate. It includes bilateral disease, onset < 40 years, radial side hand involvement, involvement of feet/genitalia, and presence of Garrod's pads.

EXAMINER: What are the predisposing factors?

CANDIDATE: Family history, male, diabetes, epilepsy, alcoholism, smoking, COPD.

EXAMINER: What structures make up a spiral cord and how does it affect the neurovascular bundle?

(a)

(b)

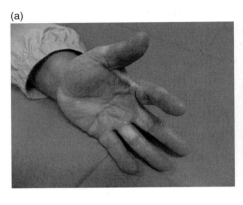

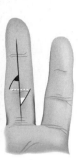

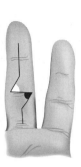

Figure 11.8a Clinical picture of a hand. **11.8b** Illustration of a Z plasty. Mark a perpendicular (white dotted line) to main incision. Mark skin flaps with 60° angles. Make incisions and cross over skin flaps.

CANDIDATE: The pretendinous, lateral and spiral bands, and Grayson's ligament. A spiral cord pulls the neurovascular bundle midline.

EXAMINER: What is a thumb web space contracture called?

CANDIDATE: Commissural cord.

EXAMINER: What are the surgical options for treatment?

CANDIDATE: These are fasciotomy (division of the cord), fasciectomy (excision of the cord) and dermofasciectomy (cord and overlying skin excised).

EXAMINER: What is a Z-plasty? Can you draw it?

CANDIDATE: Technique to manage skin deficiency. Angles should be made at 60° to the incision to achieve a 75% increase in length. (Figure 11.8b.)

EXAMINER: How would you consent me for a fasciectomy?

CANDIDATE: The operation will be carried out under general anaesthetic (you will be put off to sleep) and as a day-case procedure. The aim is to restore lost movement. You will wake up with your hand in a heavy bandage and let home once you are comfortable. You will be seen at 10 days for removal of your sutures. You will then have physiotherapy to help with scar management and regaining finger movement and may need a splint. Complications include the following: early – infection, bleeding and haematoma formation, arterial or nerve injury, amputation and delayed wound healing, or late – recurrence (50% recur but most do not require further surgery) and complex regional pain syndrome.

EXAMINER: Do you know any new treatments for a Dupuytren's contracture?

CANDIDATE: Collagenase (Xiapex*) injections are now licensed in Europe for a Dupuytren's contracture. Two

randomized controlled studies of 374 patients comparing Xiapex* to placebo have shown benefit with 60% showing correction to 5° of full extension.[1] The patient has an injection at three points along the cord and returns the next day for a finger-extension procedure.

1. Hurst LC, Badalamente MA, Hentz VR *et al*. Injectable collagenase from *Clostridium histolyticum* for Dupuytren's contracture. *New Engl J Med* 2009; **361**(10):968–979.

Structured oral examination question 9: Ulnar collateral ligament injury thumb

EXAMINER: What is being tested? (Figure 11.9a.)

CANDIDATE: Clinical photograph showing stressing of the ulnar collateral ligament of the thumb. This shows opening of > 20° but should be compared with the opposite side.

EXAMINER: What is shown in this intraoperative photograph? (Figure 11.9b.)

CANDIDATE: This is an intraoperative photograph showing an approach to the medial side of the thumb MCP joint possibly for an ulnar collateral ligament repair.

EXAMINER: What structure has been divided to give this view?

CANDIDATE: The adductor pollicis tendon attachment to the EPL tendon.

EXAMINER: What lesion is shown in the photograph?

CANDIDATE: A Stener lesion. The torn proximal end of the ligament is retracted proximal to the adductor pollicis tendon and prevents the ligament from healing.

(a)

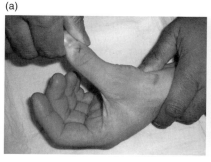

(b)

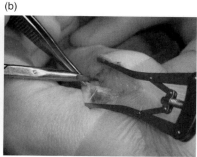

Figure 11.9a Clinical picture of a thumb. **11.9b** Intraoperative picture of a thumb during a UCL repair. The scissor tips are pointing at the bare insertion of the ligament to the base of the proximal phalanx. This is a chronic case and the scarred proximal ligament is lying bunched up over the metacarpal head.

(a)

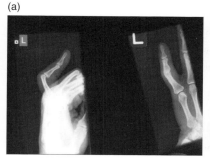

(b)

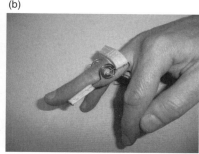

Figure 11.10a Anteroposterior (AP) and lateral radiographs of a little finger. **11.10b** Picture of a splint used to manage a Boutonnière deformity.

Structured oral examination question 10: Boutonnière deformity

EXAMINER: A rugby player has injured his finger during a game. He has pain and swelling and attends casualty where X-rays are taken. Describe what you see and the likely diagnosis. (Figure 11.10a.)

CANDIDATE: The radiographs show flexion at the PIP joint of the little finger and hyperextension at the DIP joint.

EXAMINER: How would you manage this?

CANDIDATE: I would test the central slip of the extensor mechanism by Elson's test – the PIP joint is flexed to 90° over the edge of a table, and the patient is asked to extend the finger against resistance (the examiner presses on the middle phalanx). A positive test shows weakness of extension of the PIP joint with hyperextension of the DIP joint due to recruitment of the lateral bands.

CANDIDATE: A closed central slip rupture if left may lead to a Boutonnière deformity. I would offer a dynamic splint – a Capener – to keep the PIP joint passively extended but allow active flexion. (Figure 11.10b.) This needs to be worn for 6 weeks. I would explain a mild flexion deformity is likely even with treatment.

Structured oral examination question 11: Rheumatoid arthritis

EXAMINER: What does this picture show? (Figure 11.11a.)

CANDIDATE: Clinical photograph of a hand with swelling of the MCP joints and ulnar drift of the digits. These are features of rheumatoid arthritis.

EXAMINER: How would you treat this patient?

CANDIDATE: I would ask about pain and any functional loss asking specifically about ADLs such as doing up buttons, writing, handling coins, etc. The patient may also be concerned about cosmesis. If the patient is struggling with pain I would offer her MCP joint replacements using silastic implants. I would explain surgery aims to correct the deviation of the fingers and would improve any pain from those joints, the appearance of the hand and the ability to pinch (the range of movement and grip strength are unlikely to improve).

EXAMINER: Any medications you would ask about pre-operatively?

CANDIDATE: I would ask about any steroid medication which would need covering perioperatively. Newer anti-TNF alpha treatments such as Infliximab and Etanercept should not be given within a couple of weeks of surgery and until after the

(a)

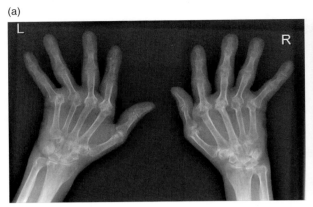

(b)

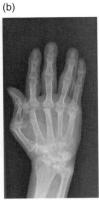

Figure 11.11a Radiographs of a patient's hands. **11.11b** Postoperative anteroposterior (AP) radiograph of a hand.

wound has healed. Methotrexate can be continued as there is no evidence to suggest it increases the risk of infection.

EXAMINER: What are the possible complications of MCP joint replacements? (Figure 11.11b.)

CANDIDATE: Early – infection, dislocation prosthetic stem. Late – recurrence ulnar drift, prosthesis wear/breakage, silicone synovitis.

EXAMINER: What are the three most common rheumatoid hand operations?

CANDIDATE: Wrist fusion, MCP joint replacement and thumb MCP joint fusion.

Other potential cases

- Distal radius fracture.
- Infection.
- Flexor tendon injury.

Chapter

12

Children's orthopaedics

Sattar Alshryda and Akinwande Adedapo

Introduction

The aims of the FRCS exam are to see if you have enough knowledge to practise as a consultant orthopaedic surgeon safely; not to test you as a paediatric orthopaedic consultant. Hence, the depth of knowledge required is not huge. Nevertheless, a substantial number of candidates fail this section.

This is partly because this section is not well covered by most exam books. Reading paediatric orthopaedic textbooks for the exam is not practical and can be confusing for the inexperienced. Most candidates, particularly those who could not have a paediatric placement, rely on a few good courses to consolidate this area of knowledge.

With this in mind, we used a different approach to cover this section in which we married actual exam questions gathered over the past few years with comprehensive and expanded answers. This keeps the theme of a viva book, provides comprehension of the topics and extra knowledge that may help high fliers to score high marks. Hence, you may find candidate answers with diagrams, X-rays and graphs; these are for your benefit rather than expected answers.

We stuck to the exam principle, where a simple question is asked concerning a clinical picture, X-ray or video clip, followed by increasingly difficult questions to explore the candidate depth and breadth of knowledge. Some of the questions are deliberately difficult and beyond average candidate level, some are easy and the majority are average.

We wish you the best of luck.

Station 1: Paediatric hip

Q 1: You have been referred a 12-year-old boy who presented with left knee pain for the last 3 weeks. No history of trauma. How would you approach this child?

My approach is to take a detailed history, perform thorough examination and order the appropriate investigations guided by my examination and provisional diagnosis.

Q 2: What goes through your mind when you face such a scenario?

Although my aim is to reach the correct diagnosis, I do not want to miss or delay diagnosing conditions that require immediate attention.

Am I dealing with septic arthritis, or juvenile arthritis?

Is it the knee or the hip? Could it be a slipped upper femoral epiphysis (SUFE)?

Q 3: How does a SUFE patient present?

The classic presentation is an overweight child presenting with groin, thigh and/or knee pain (referred pain, obturator nerve) and limping. There may be a history of minor trauma. The age is usually between 11 and 14 years old. It is more common in boys (boys 3 : 1. Boys age 12–14, girls age 11–13). The child may be able to weight bear and ambulate (stable slip) or may not be able to do so even with crutches (unstable). If he can walk, there is an external rotation of the involved limb and he cannot sit comfortably without keeping his leg straight (as he cannot bend the hip). There is usually restriction in the flexion, abduction and internal rotation of the affected hip.

Q 4: How can you confirm your diagnosis?

By radiological test; pelvis AP and cross-table lateral views of both hips. I do not prefer frog lateral as it may worsen the severity of the slip.

Postgraduate Orthopaedics: Viva Guide for the FRCS (Tr & Orth) Examination, ed. Paul A. Banaszkiewicz and Deiary F. Kader. Published by Cambridge University Press. © Cambridge University Press 2012.

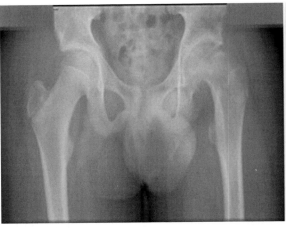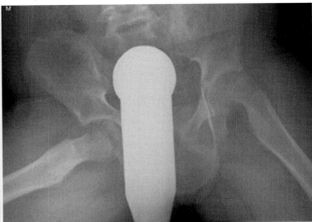

Figure 12.1 Pelvis X-ray of 12-year-old child with knee pain.

Q 5: These are his pelvis X-rays. What can you see? (Figure 12.1.)

These are AP and lateral X-rays of both hips. The most obvious abnormality is the slipped upper femoral capital epiphysis on the left side:

- Trethowan's sign is positive; a line (often referred to as Klein's line) drawn on the superior border of the femoral neck on the AP view should pass through the femoral head. In SUFE, the line passes over the head rather than through the head (compare left and right hip).
- Decreased epiphyseal height as the head is slipped posteriorly behind the neck.
- Remodelling changes of the neck with sclerotic, smooth superior part of the neck and callus formation on the inferior border. This may not be seen in acute slip.
- Increased distance between the tear drop and the femoral neck metaphysis.
- There are other radiological signs of SUFE which are not present on this radiograph such as widening and irregularity of the physeal line (early sign) and Steel's blanch sign which is a crescent-shape dense area in the metaphysis due to superimposition of the neck and the head.

Q 6: Can you grade the severity?

There are two radiological grading systems:

a. Severity of the slip by Wilson.
b. Grading using the lateral epiphyseal–shaft angle of Southwick.

I consider this grade II or moderate slip, although the AP gives a false impression of mild slip. (Figures 12.2, 12.3.)

Q 7: Are you aware of any other grading or classifications system?

Randall Loder[1] in his classic paper evaluated the presenting symptoms and radiographs of 54 patients (55 hips) and reclassified the slipped epiphyses as unstable or stable, rather than acute, chronic or acute-on-chronic.

I. Stable slip: child is able to weight bear and ambulate with or without crutches.
II. Unstable slip: child is not able to weight bear and ambulate.

Thirty of these were unstable and 25 were stable. All slips were treated with internal fixation. Avascular necrosis developed in 14 (47%) of the unstable hips and in none of the stable hips. Fourteen (47%) of the 30 unstable hips and 24 (96%) of 25 hips had a satisfactory result.

It is important to notice that a reduction occurred in 26 unstable hips and in only two of the stable hips. He was not able to demonstrate an association between early reduction and the development of AVN.

Q 8: Why does it happen?

There are several theories to explain the aetiology of SUFE. Some are more convincing than others; but none is perfect. These can be summarized as follows:

- The biomechanical theory: There are several anatomical features that lead to increase the shear forces across the physis and lead to slip:

1. Increased weight (> 80th centile).
2. Femoral retroversion (> 10°).
3. Increased physis height due to widened hypertrophic zone.

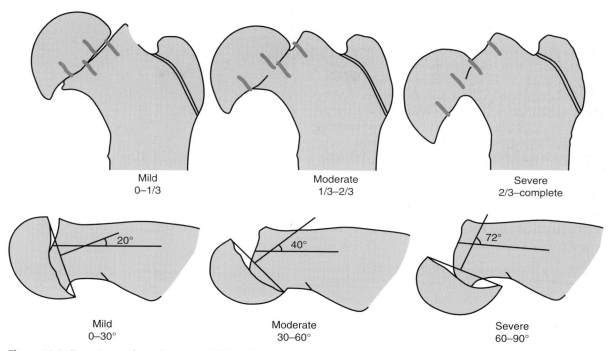

Figure 12.2 Slipped upper femoral epiphysis (SUFE) radiological grading.

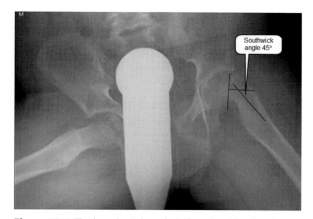

Figure 12.3 The lateral epiphyseal–shaft angle of Southwick.

4. More vertical slope of the physis.
5. Trauma.
- Structural defect of the physis theory:
    1. Hormonal theory: several endocrine disorders have been implicated with causation of SUFE. Bilateral slip is more common with endocrine diseases.
        i. Hypothyroidism.
        ii. Growth hormone deficiency.

    iii. Sex hormone (more common in boys 3:1. Boys age 12–14, girls age 11–13).

    iv. Renal osteodystrophy. It is associated with the highest risk (90%) of bilaterality. By contrast, idiopathic SUFE has a 20% risk of bilaterality initially and a further 10% to 20% risk until maturity. It is also associated with the highest risk (43%) of progressing to grade III slip. The slip goes through the metaphysis rather than the hypertrophic zone of the physis.

2. Radiotherapy.
3. Racial/ethnic (more common in blacks).
4. Idiopathic.
- Combined: increased sheer forces on abnormal physis.

Q 9: How would you treat this child?

This child has a grade II slip and I would treat him with pinning in situ (PIS). The primary aim of the treatment is to stabilize the slip and prevent further progression until physis closure. There is almost a universal agreement that grade I and grade II slips can be treated with PIS using a single cannulated screw. Some advise multiple smooth pins in a younger age group (< 8 years) to allow some growth.

However, there is controversy on the best treatment for grade III. Some advocate pinning in situ and a re-alignment procedure later if the remodelling is not optimum. There are several re-alignment procedures recommended such as subtrochanteric, intertrochanteric and neck osteotomies. Others recommend acute open reduction and fixation using Dunn or Fish osteotomy and more recently using flip osteotomy and surgical dislocation (Ganz technique).

Q 10: I agree, PIS is a reasonable option here. How soon do you want to do it?

The timing of operation is still controversial. Given the rarity of the condition (incidence 3/100 000), most studies that looked at the timing of surgery and outcome are suboptimum. Peterson *et al.*[2] showed early stabilization within 24 hours was associated with less AVN (3/42 = 7%) in comparison with those stabilized after 24 hours (10/49 = 20%). Kalogrianitis and colleagues[3] showed that AVN developed in 50% (8/16) of the unstable SUFE in their series. All but one were treated between 24 and 72 hours after symptom onset. They recommend immediate stabilization of unstable slips presenting within 24 hours; if this is not possible, delaying the operation until at least a week has elapsed.

Q 11: Would you pin the other non-slipped, asymptomatic side?

This is also controversial. The quoted risk of contralateral slip varies from 18 to 60%. Prophylactic PIS is not free of risk and it should be weighed against the benefit. The proponents and opponents have some evidence to support their views.[4] The following factors play a role in decision making:

1. Age of the child (< 10 years is associated with a higher risk of bilaterality).
2. The aetiology of the slip (renal osteodystrophy and endocrine disorders have a high incidence of bilaterality).
3. The ability and the compliance of the child and family.
4. The nature of current slip (very bad slip occurring over a very short period of time may justify pinning the other side).

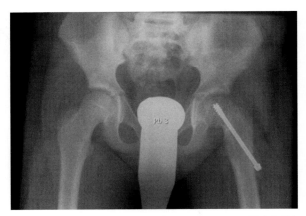

Figure 12.4 Postoperative X-ray after pinning in situ of left SUFE.

Q 12: This is the postoperative X-ray of the child. Any comments? (Figure 12.4.)

This is an AP pelvis plain X-ray with a single cannulated screw in situ. It is centred in the neck and epiphysis. There are about three threads in the epiphysis. Ideally, I would like to see five threads, but without seeing the lateral view, I cannot criticize this.

Q 13: A few months later, your secretary received a phone call from his general practitioner (GP) because he develops pain in the other hip. The GP asks if you could see him in your next available clinic.

Contralateral slip is not uncommon and I always warn my patients to seek urgent medical advice if they develop pain in the other hip. I would bring this child to hospital for urgent X-ray rather than waiting to see him in the routine clinic. Some of these slips progress rapidly to severe slip.

Q 14: This is the X-ray you requested. What do you see? (Figure 12.5.)

As I expected, there is a contralateral slip (probably mild) and I would consider pinning in situ.

Q 15: I agree. What do you think of the other side?

I think he is outgrowing the screw. There is a single thread of the screw left in the epiphysis and the physis is still open. I will exchange this for a longer screw. It should be relatively easy. I will pass the guide wire through the cannulated screw and exchange it for a longer screw.

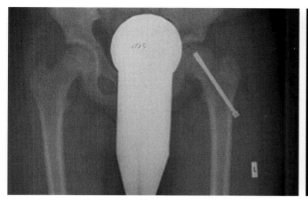
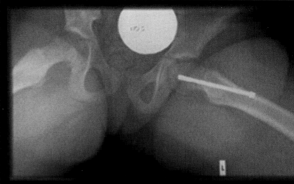

Figure 12.5 Pelvis X-ray (AP and lateral) of a child with right hip pain.

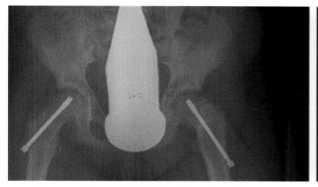
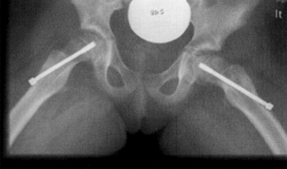

Figure 12.6 Postoperative plain X-ray of the pelvis after the second operation.

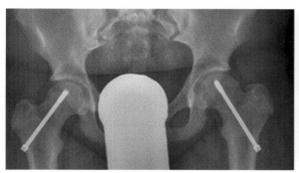
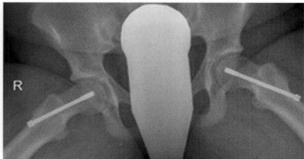

Figure 12.7 Pelvis X-rays 7 years after pinning in situ.

Q 16: This is exactly what was done. (Figure 12.6.) A few years later, the patient asks whether you would leave the screws or remove them. He is asymptomatic. His X-ray is shown in **Figure 12.7.**

The X-rays shows the physes have been closed, hence the screws become redundant. Interestingly there is a reasonable remodelling of the neck and the joints are not arthritic. I usually offer my patients removal of the screws and my justification is that this would make future hip replacement (if it is needed) more difficult; particularly if the screw heads are fully covered with bone. Of course, removing the screws is associated with risk and the patient has to be informed.

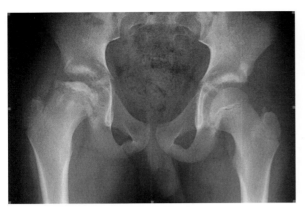

Figure 12.8 Pelvis X-ray of a child with right hip pain and limping.

Table 12.1 Blood supply of the femoral head.

Age	Birth–4 years	4 years–adult	Adult
Source	Medial and lateral circumflex arteries from profunda femoris artery Ligamentum teres with posterior division of obturator artery	Posterosuperior and posteroinferior retinacular from medial femoral circumflex artery Negligible lateral circumflex artery Minimum ligamentum teres	Medial femoral circumflex to lateral epiphyseal artery

Q 17: This is a pelvic X-ray of a 9-year-old boy who has been limping over the last 3 months. What can you see? (Figure 12.8.)

This is an AP view of the pelvis in a skeletally immature patient. The most obvious feature is the collapse of the right femoral head with increased bone density. There is a widening of the joint space on the right side. At the top of my list is Legg–Calvé–Perthes disease (LCPD), but other diagnoses such as infection need to be excluded.

Q 18: What is Perthes' disease?

It is a non-inflammatory AVN of the femoral head in a growing child caused by interruption of blood supply. The condition was first described by Waldenstorm, but he attributed it to tuberculosis; it was then described more accurately by Arthur Legg (1874–1939), Jacques Calvé (1875–1854) and George Perthes (1869–1927) almost at the same time; hence the name Legg–Calvé–Perthes disease (LCPD).

It is not common (1\10 000), affecting children between 4–9 years old of low socioeconomic class. Child is often small with delayed bone age by usually 2 years. It is bilateral in 15% of cases but involvement is usually asymmetrical and never simultaneous (in contrast to multiple epiphyseal dysplasia). There may be a family history.

Q 19: What does it happen?

The aetiology is unknown; however, several theories have been put forward to explain it:

1. The anatomical theory.
The blood supply to the femoral head changes as the child grows (Table 12.1). The change over to adult pattern may be affected comprising the blood supply to the femoral head leading to ischaemic necrosis.

2. Hydrostatic pressure theory.
This theory attributes the reduction in blood supply to the femoral head to the increase in the intraosseous venous pressure which has been noticed in several cases.

3. Thrombophillic theory.
There is evidence of association of LCPD with various forms of thrombophilia. In one study, 72 patients with LCPD were compared with 197 matched healthy controls.[5] The factor-V Leiden mutation was more common in LCPD (8/72) than in the controls (7/197) (chi-square = 5.7, p = 0.017). A high level of anticardiolipin antibodies was found in 19 of the 72 LCPD compared with 22 of the 197 controls (chi-square = 9.5, p = 0.002). Other studies showed association of LCPD with protein S and C abnormalities.[6,7] It is important to remember that association does not always mean causation.

Q 20: What is your differential diagnosis?

In this scenario where the right side only is involved, my differential diagnoses are:

1. Septic arthritis (usually the child is unwell, fever with high inflammatory markers).
2. Sickle cell (history, sickling test, Hb electrophoresis).
3. Eosinophilic granuloma (other lesions particularly in skull, radiological features, biopsy).
4. Transient synovitis.

Bilateral LCPD is not common and requires skeletal survey and blood tests to exclude:

1. Hypothyroidism.
2. Multiple epiphyseal dysplasia.
3. Spondyloepiphyseal dysplasia.
4. Meyer's dysplasia.
5. Sickle cell.
6. Gaucher's disease.

Q 21: Do you know any grading or classification system?

There are several classifications to address different aspects of LCPD. These include the following.

Classification addressing chronological radiographic stages (Waldenstrom)

I. Initial (sclerotic/necrotic) stage

It lasts 6–12 months. Ischaemia leads to subchondral bone death and necrosis (dead bone looks dense on plain radiograph). There is joint space widening due to continuous cartilage growth (nutrient from synovial fluid). This can be subdivided into early (no loss in epiphysis height) or late where there is some loss of epiphyseal height but the epiphysis is still in one piece.

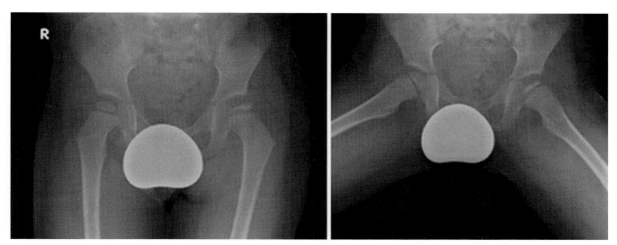

Figure 12.9 Legg–Calvé–Perthes disease (LCPD): initial (sclerotic/necrotic) stage.

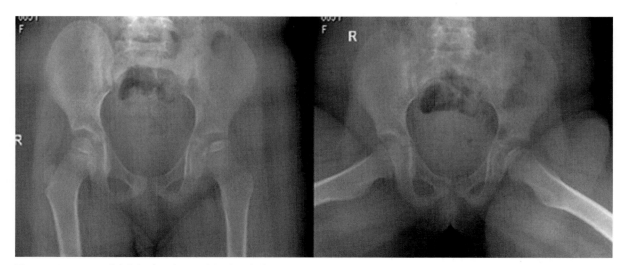

Figure 12.10 Legg–Calvé–Perthes disease (LCPD): early fragmentation stage.

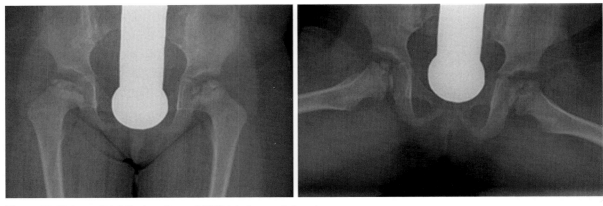

Figure 12.11 Legg–Calvé–Perthes disease (LCPD): late fragmentation stage.

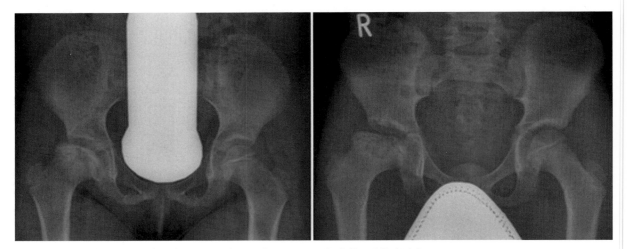

Figure 12.12 Legg–Calvé–Perthes disease (LCPD): reossification stage; IIIa (left) and IIIb (right).

II. Fragmentation (resorption) stage

In this stage, revascularization has started bringing osteoblasts and osteoclasts. The latter remove dead and necrotic bone causing radiolucent fissures among dead fragments. This usually lasts from 12–24 months. This stage can be further divided into early (1–2 fissures only) or late when the head is in several fragments.

III. Reossification (healing) stage

Osteoblasts form new bone which is soft and pliable. It starts peripherally and progresses centrally. This usually appears as a small and expanding fragment on the lateral part of the epiphysis marking the beginning of this stage IIIa. This soft bone matures and covers more than a third of the epiphysis in stage IIIb. This stage usually lasts 6–24 months.

It is critical to keep the soft head within acetabulum for natural moulding in order to maintain its sphericity. If uncontained the soft head will be extruded, collapse and lose its sphericity leading to early OA of head and acetabulum. This is the basis of containment treatment.

IV. Remodelling (residual) stage

The head is considered to have healed when there is no avascular bone visible on the radiographs; however it continues to remodel until skeletal maturity. The head becomes large (coxa magna) and hard with residual deformity of head according to the shape at the end of the fragmentation phase.

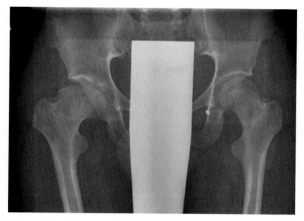

Figure 12.13 Legg–Calvé–Perthes disease (LCPD): remodelling (residual) stage.

Classification addressing severity of head involvement

Catterall 1971 (Figure 12.14)

Based on extent of head involvement at fragmentation phase. Catterall advised four stages:

Catterall I

- 0–25% head involvement.
- Only anterior epiphysis (therefore seen only on the frog lateral film).

Catterall II

- 25–50% head involvement.
- Anterior and central segment – fragmentation (sequestrum).
- Lateral part/rim is intact (protects the central involved area).
- Junction – clear.
- Metaphyseal reaction present – anterior.
- Subchondral fracture – anterior.

Catterall III

- 50–75% head involvement.
- Anterior segment involved. Lateral head – also fragmented.
- Only the medial portion is spared.
- Loss of lateral part/support worsens the prognosis.
- Junction – sclerotic.
- Metaphyseal reaction present – anterior and lateral.

Catterall IV

- > 75% head involvement.

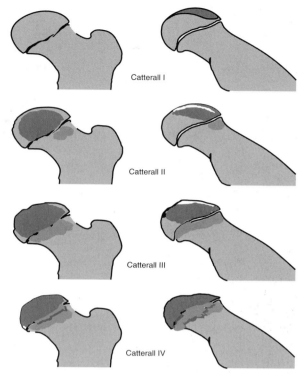

Catterall I

Catterall II

Catterall III

Catterall IV

Figure 12.14 Legg–Calvé–Perthes disease (LCPD): Catterall classification.

Salter and Thompson 1984

Salter and Thompson recognized that Catterall's first two groups and second two groups were distinct and therefore proposed a two-part classification; this is often referred to as modified Catterall's classification.

Salter and Thompson Group A: Less than 50% of the head is involved.

Salter and Thompson Group B: More than 50% of the head is involved.

Again the main difference between these two groups is the integrity of the lateral pillar.

(Herring) lateral pillar 1992

This is based specifically on the integrity of the lateral pillar on the AP film only, at the beginning of the fragmentation phase.

Group A

- Normal height of the lateral one-third of the head is maintained.
- Fragmentation occurs in the central segment of the head.

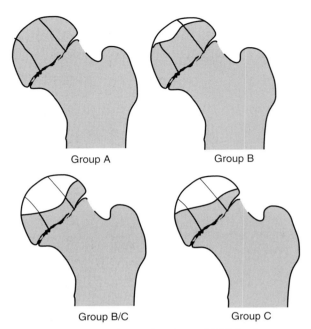

Group A   Group B

Group B/C   Group C

Figure 12.15 Legg–Calvé–Perthes disease (LCPD): Herring classification.

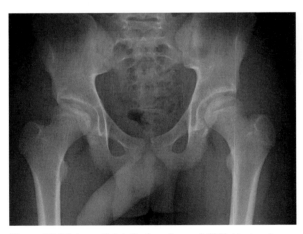

Figure 12.16 Legg–Calvé–Perthes disease (LCPD): Herring A.

Group B
- More than 50% of the original lateral pillar height is maintained.
- There may be some lateral extrusion of the head.

Group C
- Less than 50% of the original lateral pillar height is maintained.
- The lateral pillar is lower than the central segment early on.

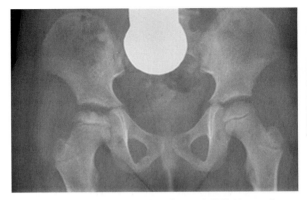

Figure 12.17 Legg–Calvé–Perthes disease (LCPD): Herring B.

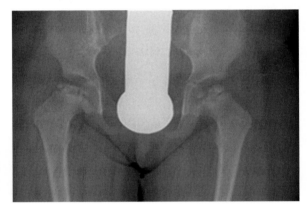

Figure 12.18 Legg–Calvé–Perthes disease (LCPD): Herring C (right) and Herring B/C left.

Group B/C
- Less than 50% of the original lateral pillar height is maintained.
- The lateral pillar is higher than the central segment.

Classification addressing outcome
Mose classification
Using the concentric circle technique to compare and classify the final outcome in PD at the end of growth. The final shape of the head may be compared with a perfect circle using the Mose template and both AP and lateral images.

Given that a congruous but aspherical head can perform well suggests that the Mose criteria are too strict and impractical.

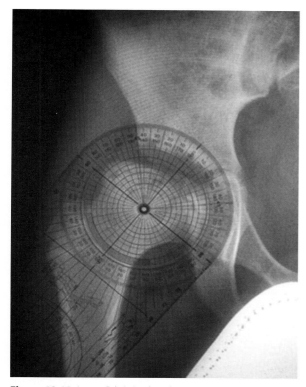

Figure 12.19 Legg–Calvé–Perthes disease (LCPD): Mose grading.

Table 12.2 Mose grading.

Outcomes	Description
Good outcome	Aspherical head contour is within 1 mm of a given circle on both views
Fair outcome	Aspherical head contour is between 1–2 mm
Poor outcome	Aspherical head contour is > 2 mm

Stulberg classification

Stulberg showed that a lack of sphericity and congruency were both predictors for poor outcome.[8] Table 12.3 summarizes Stulberg's classification. A modified version of the Stulberg classification is becoming more popular. It consists of three groups: group A hips (Stulberg I and II) have a spherical femoral head; group B (Stulberg III) have an ovoid femoral head; and group C (Stulberg IV and V) have a flat femoral head.

Table 12.3 Stulberg grading.

Congruency	Class	Description
Spherical congruency	I	Normal spherical head
	II	Spherical head, coxa magna/breva, steep acetabulum
Aspherical congruency	III	Ovoid or mushroom-shaped head
	IV	Flat head on flat acetabulum (may hinge on abduction)
Aspherical incongruency	V	Flat head but normal acetabulum

Table 12.4 Legg–Calve–Perthes disease: poor prognostic signs.

Poor clinical prognostic signs (FOOBS)	Poor radiological prognostic signs
Male	Gage's sign (V-shape lucency at lateral epiphysis; Figure 12.20)
Older age	Horizontal growth plate – implies a growth arrest phenomenon and deformity
Obesity	Lateral calcification (lateral to the epiphysis – implies loss of lateral support and head extrusion)
Bilateral	Lateral subluxation – implies loss of lateral support. Uncovering of the femoral head > 3 mm in excess of opposite side (measured as the horizontal distance between a vertical line through the outer lip of acetabulum and lateral edge of femoral head physis)
Stiffness	Metaphyseal rarefaction/cyst

Q 22: What do you think about this child's prognosis?

Unfortunately, this child already has three poor prognostic signs. He is a boy, 9 years old and the plain X-ray showed Herring C. There are other clinical and radiological prognostic signs which I would look for in my assessment (Table 12.4).

Q 23: How would you treat this patient?

I would start treating this child symptomatically with rest, analgesia, anti-inflammatory medication, temporary

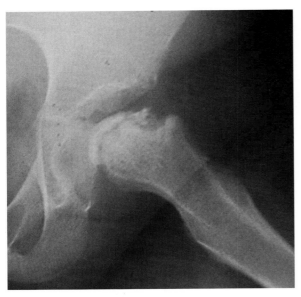

Figure 12.20 Legg-Calvé-Perthes disease (LCPD): Gage sign.

non-weightbearing with crutches and I may consider admitting for a short period of gentle traction. Physiotherapy plays an important role in improving range of motion. Several types of braces have been advocated but their values have been heavily questioned and compliance is a real issue in this age group.

Q 24: Would you consider surgery?

It depends which surgery you are referring to. I would not recommend containment surgery (femoral varus osteotomy or Salter osteotomy) for this boy. There is evidence that containment surgery is beneficial in certain subgroups of LCPD. Patients with lateral pillar B and B/C involvement and aged 8 years or older are likely to benefit from surgery.[9,10]

Unfortunately, studies have not shown benefit of containment surgery for lateral pillar C hips patients. However, one study suggests that early distraction with hinged external fixation may be of value in such patients.[11]

Q 25: Which studies are you referring to?

Herring *et al.* report on the results of the Legg–Perthes Study Group.[9] Thirty-nine surgeons from 28 centres took part in a prospective study. Each surgeon agreed to apply a single treatment method to each patient who met the study criteria. All patients were between 6 and 12 years of age at the onset of the

disease, and none had had prior treatment. The treatment groups were no treatment, range of motion treatment in which the patient did exercises once a day, Atlanta brace treatment, femoral varus osteotomy, and Salter osteotomy.

The study showed that age, lateral pillar grading and treatment methods were significantly related to outcome.

In group B hips with an age at onset of more than 8 years, 73% of the operated hips had a Stulberg I or II result compared with 44% of the non-operated hips (p = 0.02). For the group B hips with onset at 8 years or younger, there was no advantage demonstrated for the surgical group. The group C hips were not shown to benefit from surgical or non surgical treatments.

Wiig *et al.* reported on a nationwide prospective study.[10] Twenty-eight hospitals in Norway were instructed to report all new cases of LCPD over a period of 5 years.

A total of 368 with unilateral disease were included in the study. For patients over 6 years of age at diagnosis with more than 50% necrosis of the femoral head (152 patients), the surgeons at the different hospitals had chosen one of three methods of treatment: physiotherapy (55 patients), the Scottish Rite abduction orthosis (26) and proximal femoral varus osteotomy (71). The study showed that the strongest predictor of poor outcome was femoral head involvement of more than 50% (modified Catterall classification) followed by age at diagnosis, then lateral pillar grades. In children over 6 years at diagnosis with more than 50% of femoral head necrosis, proximal femoral varus osteotomy gave a significantly better outcome than orthosis or physiotherapy. There was no difference in outcome after any of the treatments in children under 6 years.

Other small studies showed the benefit of shelf acetabuloplasty as a salvage operation for extruded head;[12,13] valgus osteotomy in hinged abduction;[14] and trochanteric growth arrest or advancement when there is overgrowth.

Q 26: This becomes confusing. Can you simplify it?

I agree it is confusing and this reflects the current state. However, for the sake of simplicity:

< 6 years old
- Prognosis is good for the majority.
- Bed rest, traction, pain-relieving anti-inflammatory medication and rest.

- No evidence that abduction splints or surgical intervention is warranted in the majority of these younger patients.

> 8 years old (think of this as a range rather than absolute number)

- Herring lateral pillar classification A may do well and do not need surgery.
- Herring lateral pillar classification B and B/C; containment of the head within the acetabulum seems to be warranted.
- Herring lateral pillar classification C is associated with poor outcome and containment surgery does not improve outcome. However, shelf acetabuloplasty may be useful in the early stage of the disease. Valgus osteotomy if patient develops hinged abduction late in the disease.

For the best result, surgery should be performed in the earliest stage of the disease; maybe even before being able to classify the severity. If all children older than 8 were to be offered surgical treatment, the group A and C hips would not likely benefit. These groups combined represent only 13% of hips presenting at age older than 8, and this approach may be justified.[15]

Q 27: What do these three clinical photographs demonstrate in this 6-month-old child? (Figure 12.21.)

The top left photo shows that the left thigh is shorter than the right (Galleazzi test is positive). The other two pictures show an abnormal skin crease (top right) and limitation of the left hip abduction (bottom). My suspicion is that this child has a dislocated left hip.

Q 28: How would you manage this child?

I always take a detailed history and perform a thorough examination. In the history, risk factors for developmental dysplasia of the hip (DDH) are important. These include (6 Fs):

1. First baby (the uterus is tighter and less elastic).
2. Female (lax ligament due to maternal hormones).
3. Family history (may be genetic predisposition).
4. Fetal malposition (breech presentation).
5. Fetal packaging disorders (oligohydramnios, twins, feet and neck torticollis).
6. LeFt side (60% left hip, 20% right and 20% both). May be related to the fetal position.

There are other risk factors of less importance and even the above risk factors vary in their importance.

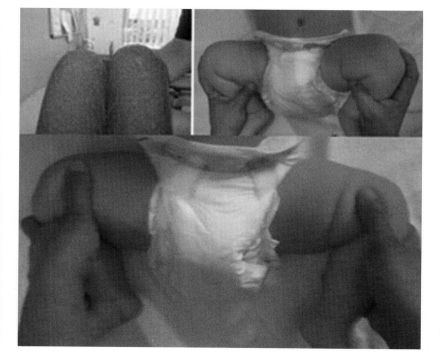

Figure 12.21 Clinical photographs of a 6-month-old child.

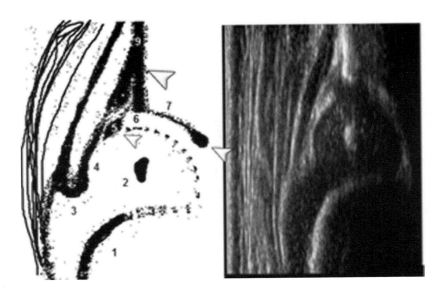

Figure 12.22 Infant hip ultrasound.

Family history and breech presentation are probably the most important.

Usually a child of this age is asymptomatic with no discomfort or pain. There may be asymmetrical skin fold (not very specific) or leg asymmetry as in Figure 12.21.

Ortolani and Barlow tests are very important in the early weeks of life but their value becomes less as the child gets older. Ortolani test identifies a dislocated hip that can be reduced. By flexing the infant's hip and knee to 90°, the thigh is then gently abducted with the middle finger over the greater trochanter to feel for the reduction of the dislocated head as it comes from the dislocated position to the socket. With time, it becomes more difficult to reduce the femoral head into the acetabulum, and the Ortolani test becomes negative. Barlow test is rarely positive after 10 weeks.

Q 29: How accurate are these tests?

Unfortunately, all these tests have limitations and the examiner should be aware of these. Bilateral limitation of abduction, asymmetrical skin crease and LLD are inaccurate in neonates. However, unilateral limited abduction has 70% sensitivity and 90% specificity for DDH in infants > 3 months.[16]

Ortolani and Barlow tests have a 60% sensitivity and 100% specificity in expert hands in comparison with ultrasound which has 90% sensitivity and specificity.[17]

Q 30: How does ultrasound help your diagnosis?

The role of ultrasound is well established in diagnosing and grading the DDH. There are two different techniques in use:

1. Graf: Static alpha and beta angles.[18]
2. Harcke: Dynamic provocation test.[19]

With a bit of experience, it is easy to identify the anatomical structures of infant hips and decide whether they are normal or not, and the severity of the dysplasia and dislocation.

The anatomical landmarks of normal infant hips in ultrasound include (Figure 12.22–12.27):

1. Chondro-osseous junction.
2. Femoral head.
3. Synovial fold.
4. Joint capsule.
5. Labrum.
6. Cartilage part of the roof. This is pliable and can be deformed with dislocation. Labrum and the cartilage part of the roof are sometimes collectively called limbus.
7. Bony part of the roof.
8. Bony rim (or the turning point between concavity and convexity of the roof).
9. Ilium.

These landmarks should be identified in the same sequence every time to enhance reproducibility.

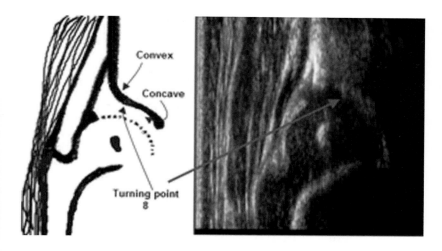

Figure 12.23 Infant hip ultrasound: turning point.

The acetabular roof line, starts from the lower limb, runs tangentially to the acetabular roof to the lowest end of bony acetabulum

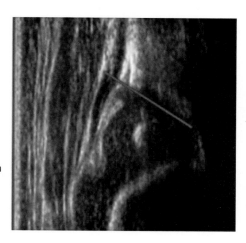

Figure 12.24 Infant hip ultrasound: The bony roof line.

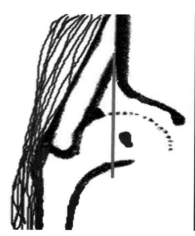

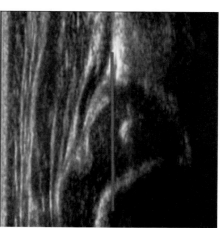

Figure 12.25 Infant hip ultrasound: The baseline.

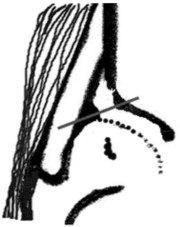

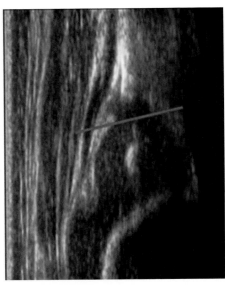

Cartilaginous roof line connects the turning point and the middle of labrum

Figure 12.26 Infant hip ultrasound: The cartilage roof line.

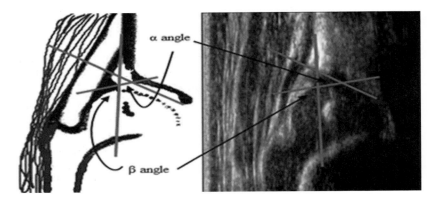

α angle

β angle

Figure 12.27 Infant hip ultrasound: alpha and beta angles.

Three of these landmarks are essential to establish the standard plane (marked with arrow heads): the lower limb of the acetabular roof (usually it is the brightest and largest lower end of the bony roof); the midportion of the ilium and the labrum. If any of these points is missing or not clearly shown, the sonogram is worthless and should not be used. The only exception is when the joint is fully dislocated (Graf III and IV).[20]

Three important lines are to be identified:

1. The bony roof line which runs tangentially from the lower limb to the bony roof touching the turning point as in Figure 12.24.
2. The baseline runs tangential to the outer surface of the ilium where the cartilaginous roof meets the ilium. (Figure 12.25.)
3. The cartilage roof line (or the inclination line) is drawn from the turning point (the bony rim) to the centre of the labrum. (Figure 12.26.)

The angle between the bony roof line and the baseline is the alpha angle (α) whereas the angle between the cartilage roof line and the baseline is the beta angle (β) (Figure 12.27). Importantly, notice that the bigger the alpha angle and the smaller the beta angle the better the hip is (within limits).

Based on the above, Graf classified infant hips into several types (this has been updated on several occasions – Table 12.5 shows the most up to date). It has been simplified for ease recall.

Table 12.5 Graf sonographic grading for developmental dysplasia of the hip.

Type	Alpha angle (α)			Beta angle (β)		Descriptions
I	> 60°			< 55°	Ia	Normal hip (at any age). This grade is further divided into Ia (β < 55°) and Ib (β > 55°). The significance of this subdivision is not yet established
				> 55°	Ib	
II	50–59°	IIa		< 77°		If the child is < 3 months. This may be physiological and does not need treatment
		IIb		< 77°		>3 months, delayed ossification
	43–49°	IIc	Stable Unstable	< 77°		Critical zone, labrum not everted. This is further divided into stable and unstable by provocation test
D	43–49°			> 77°		This is the first stage where the hip becomes decentred (subluxed). It used to be called IId, but for the above reason, it is a stage on its own
III	< 43°	IIIa IIIb				Dislocated femoral head with the cartilaginous acetabular roof pushed **upwards**. This is further divided into IIIa and IIIb depending on the echogenicity of the hyaline cartilage of the acetabular roof (usually compared with the femoral head) which reflects the degenerative changes
IV	< 43°					Dislocated femoral head with the cartilaginous acetabular roof pushed **downwards**

Q 31: How would you treat a child with DDH?

The principles of treating DDH are:

1. Achieve a concentric reduction.
2. Maintain stability in the concentric reduction.
3. Promote the normal growth and development of the hip.
4. Minimize complications.

There are different methods to achieve the above principles depending on the child's age, reducibility of the dislocation and the availability of resources and expertise. There are accepted guidelines on managing children with DDH, who are grouped into the following age ranges:

1. Children from birth up to 6 months. (Figure 12.28.)
2. Children from 6 months to 18 months. (Figure 12.29.)
3. Children from 18 months to 30 months. (Figure 12.30.)
4. Children above 30 months. (Figure 12.31.)

The charts in Figures 12.28–12.31 summarize the treatment of DDH in different age groups.

Q 32: This is the sonogram of a 7-week-old child's hip? What can you see? (Figure 12.32.)

This is a sonogram of a newborn's hip. I can easily identify the chondro-osseous border and the femoral head and less easily the synovial fold. The capsule, labrum and the cartilaginous roof seem to be pushed down by the decentred femoral head (hence it is Graf IV). The bony roof is steep and shallow. In the picture on the right, the sonographers tried to quantify the dislocation by measuring α and β angles but I have a reservation on doing so for several reasons. The picture is not in the standard plane, and the cartilage roof line was not drawn correctly as it should pass through the labrum.

Q 33: What are your treatment options?

The options are:

1. Splinting the hip.

   i. Rigid such as Craig splint (Although user-friendly, it is out of favour. It may be useful in certain situations such as respiratory compromise.)

   ii. Dynamic splint such as Pavlik harness. (Table 12.6, Figure 12.33.)

   iii. Hip spica.

A Pavlik harness is my preferred option. It is sized by measuring the chest circumference. There are five sizes (premie, small, medium, large and extra-large). The harness has shoulder and leg straps. The anterior leg straps are to keep the hip flexion more than 90°

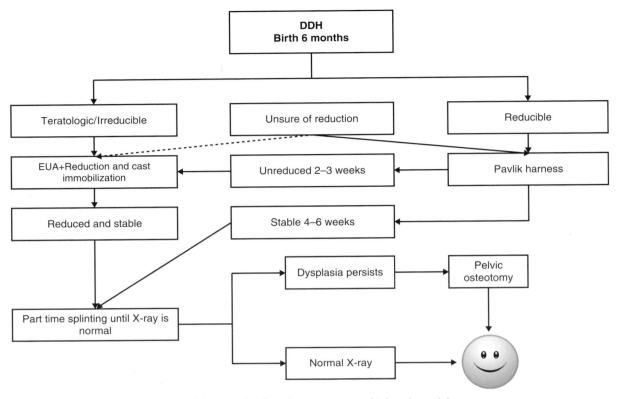

Figure 12.28 Developmental dysplasia of the hip (DDH) flow chart management (birth to 6 months).

while the posterior leg straps are to keep hip abduction in the safe zone. It allows motion within the range of stability. This motion is essential for stimulating the growth of the acetabulum. It is essential to do frequent checking of the child with a Pavlik harness (2–4 weeks) for the reduction, ultrasound progression, fitness (as the child may outgrow the harness) and to document active knee extension (functioning femoral nerve).

Q 34: Apart from DDH, are you aware of any other indication for a Pavlik harness?

Yes, femoral shaft fracture in infants. A retrospective study of 40 patients by Podeszwa et al. compared application of the Pavlik harness versus spica casting for the treatment of infant femoral shaft fracture.[21] No difference was found in radiographic outcomes, but approximately one-third of all spica patients experienced development of a skin complication. The authors conclude that all children younger than 1 year with a femoral shaft fracture should be considered for treatment with a Pavlik harness.

Q 35: This is a plain pelvis X-ray of a 7-month-old child. Her mother noted stiffness of the right leg when she applies a nappy. Can you tell me what might be wrong? (Figure 12.34.)

This plain radiograph of the pelvis shows the right acetabulum is shallow and there may be a false acetabulum a bit higher. Both femoral heads are not visible. They normally start ossifying by 8 weeks; however, there is normal variation. I would like to draw Hilgenreiner's line and Perkins' lines. I suspect the right femoral head (which is at the top of the femoral neck) lies in the upper lateral quadrant consistent with right hip dislocation.

Q 36: I agree, he has a dislocated right hip. How would you treat this child?

Provided there is no contraindication, I would take this child to theatre for EUA and try to reduce closed. If I am successful and the hip reduces satisfactorily, I would immobilize the hip in a hip spica. However, if I am not certain about the reduction, I will perform a hip arthrogram.

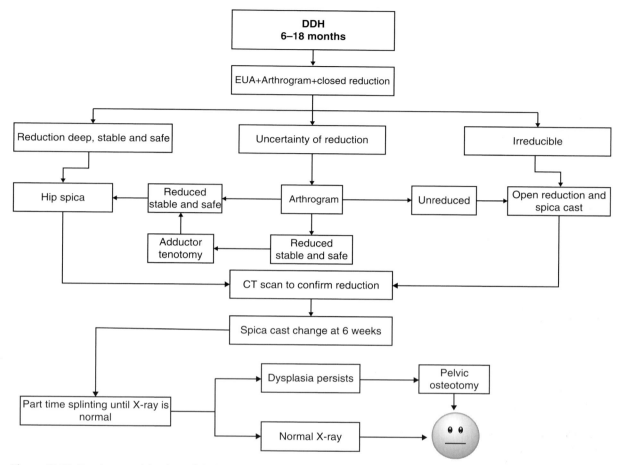

Figure 12.29 Developmental dysplasia of the hip (DDH) flow chart management (6–18 months).

Q 37: These are the intraoperative hip arthrogram pictures. Do you want to comment on the findings? (Figure 12.35.)

This arthrogram nicely shows the outline of the cartilaginous part of the femoral head. The capsule is distended. Pictures 2 and 3 show the hour-glass shape caused by the iliopsoas tendon (not visible) compressing the capsule in the middle. The top four pictures confirm hip dislocation where the head is not sitting in the acetabulum and there is significant medial dye pooling (>7 mm). The ligamentum teres is thickened and elongated (best seen in picture 3). The surgeon seems to evaluate the hip reductions in different positions; I think the hip is shown to be reduced in pictures 6 and 7. Pictures 6 and 7 show the effect of rotation on reduction, where external rotation led to dislocation. If a satisfactory reduction (as shown in pictures 6 and 7) has been achieved within the safe zone and without extreme abduction or flexion, then the hip can be immobilized in a hip spica.

Q 38: What would you have done if you could not have reduced the above hip closed?

This will be an indication for open reduction (OR). Open reduction is indicated:

1. If the reduction is not possible.
2. If the reduction is not concentric.
3. If the hip reduced but remains unstable (narrow safe zone).
4. If stability can only be achieved by holding the hip in extreme abduction or internal rotation (high risk of AVN).

There is controversy on the best time to do the OR. Some delay it until the ossification nucleus of the

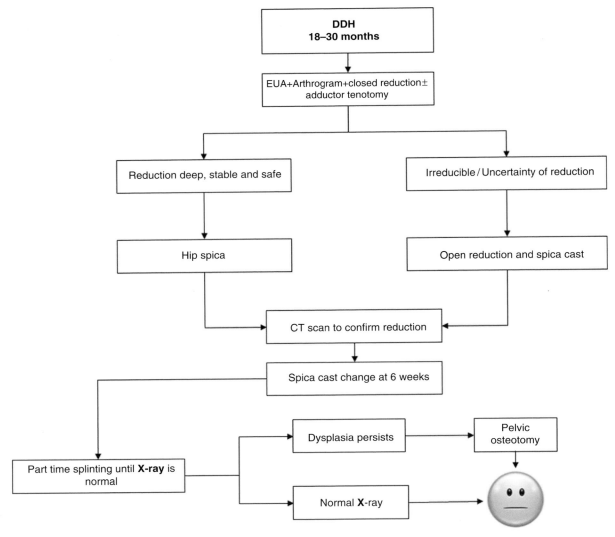

Figure 12.30 Developmental dysplasia of the hip (DDH) flow chart management (18–30 months).

head is visible on the X-rays. They claim there is less risk of AVN and the child is bigger and easier to operate on. Others do it when the closed reduction fails regardless of the age of the child.

Q 39: This is a plain pelvis X-ray of the hip belonging to a 19-month-child. Grandparents noticed that she walks oddly. What can you say about the X-ray? (Figure 12.36.)

The obvious feature is the high dislocation of the left hip. The femoral nucleus is small and is not sitting in

the acetabulum (compare with the other side). There is a false acetabulum and if I draw Hilgenreiner's and Perkins' lines, the head will be sitting in the upper lateral quadrants. There is a break in the inferior and lateral Shenton's lines.

Q 40: How would you treat this child?

She is 19 months old. I will be surprised if this hip can be reduced closed. So I would take this child to theatre for EUA and trial of CR, but I will consent parent for OR ± pelvic osteotomy ± femoral shortening.

Table 12.6 Pavlik harness (complications and contraindications).

Complications	Contraindication
Failure of reduction	Major muscle imbalance such as myelomeningocoele
Damage to the posterior acetabular wall (persistent posterior dislocation)	Major stiffness as in arthrogryposis
Avascular necrosis of the head of the femur (AVN) 2.4%	Ligamentous laxity such as in Ehlers–Danlos syndrome
Skin damage	Severe respiratory compromise (Craig splint may be useful)
Femoral nerve palsy	Irreducible hip >6 months
Brachial plexus injury	
Knee dislocation	

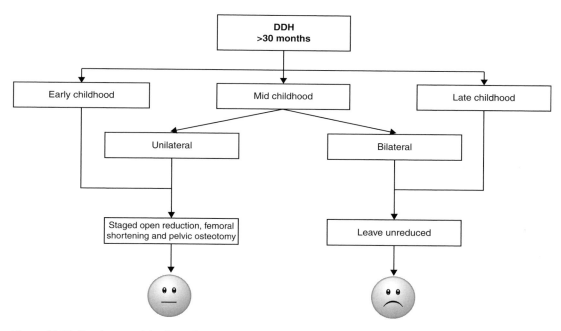

Figure 12.31 Developmental dysplasia of the hip (DDH) flow chart management (> 30 months).

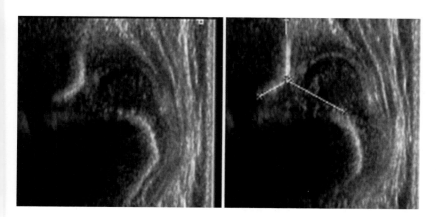

Figure 12.32 Infant hip ultrasound: 7-week-old child.

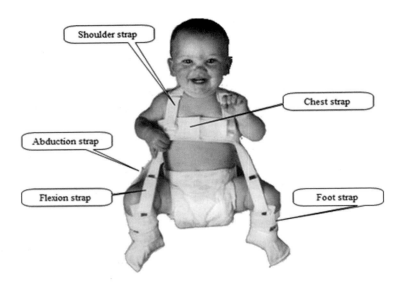

Figure 12.33 Pavlik harness (picture courtesy of Wheaton Brace Company).

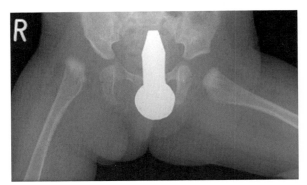

Figure 12.34 Plain pelvis X-ray of 7-month-old child.

Q 41: This is the child's hip arthrogram. Do you want to comment on the findings? (Figure 12.38.)

The arthrogram shows the femoral head is dislocated from the normal socket and articulating with a false acetabulum on the ileum. The capsule is distended and displays the classic hour-glass shape (visible in pictures 2 and 6). The ligamentum teres is thickened and elongated (pictures 2–6). None of the pictures demonstrates a reduced hip and there is significant medial dye pool. So I believe this hip is not reducible.

Q 42: What prevents reduction?

There are several anatomical structures that can prevent reduction. These can be summarized as:

1. Inverted limbus.
2. Thickened and elongated ligamentum teres.

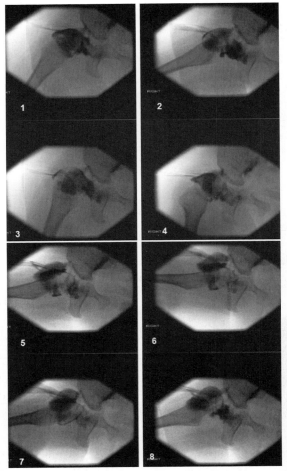

Figure 12.35 Hip arthrogram of 7-month-old child.

3. Interposed iliopsoas tendon.
4. Pulvinar (fibro-fatty tissues filling the acetabulum).
5. Capsule constriction.
6. Contracted transverse ligament giving the acetabular cartilage classic horseshoe shape.

Q 43: What is the limbus?

There is not a normal anatomical structure called limbus, but it is the name given to the labrum with the attached cartilaginous roof of the acetabulum moulded and pushed into the acetabulum preventing the femoral head reduction.

Q 44: So what would you do in the above situation?

I would proceed to OR through the anterior hip approach (Smith Petersen).

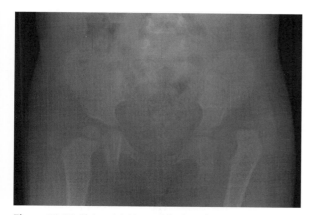

Figure 12.36 Plain pelvis X-ray of the hip of a 19-month-old child.

Q 45: This is a pelvis X-ray of a child with cerebral palsy. Can you describe the main problem and how you would treat it? (Figure 12.39.)

There is bilateral subluxation of the hips with Reimer's migration index (RIM) of more than 75% (Figure 12.40); bilateral coxa valga and femoral anteversion. Although the acetabuli look reasonable there might be deficient posterior wall which is common in these patients. Ideally, this should have been dealt with before it reached this advanced stage.

Q 46: How would you manage this child?

Patients with cerebral palsy (CP) should be managed by a multidisciplinary team including a paediatrician, physiotherapist, orthotist and paediatric orthopaedic surgeon as well as the family. Thorough history and assessment are essential with particular focus on current symptoms, mobility and other comorbidities that may preclude general anaesthesia.

This child needs substantive tissue release (adductors and iliopsoas muscles) with exploration of the hip joint. If the articular cartilage is healthy and not damaged, the hip should be reduced. Femoral (varus derotation osteotomy; VDRO) and pelvis osteotomy (Dega) are often necessary to achieve concentric stable reduction. Table 12.7 summarizes general recommendations for treating neurogenic hip dislocation. There is some controversy about certain aspects.

Q 47: A 6-year-old boy is referred to you with a painful right hip and limping. No history

Figure 12.37 Pelvis X-ray of the hip of a 19-month-old child.

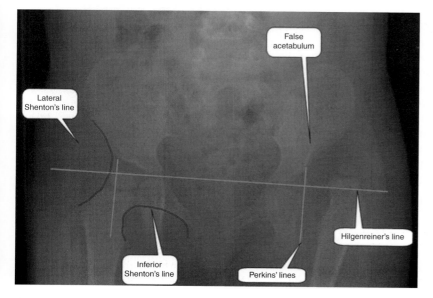

False acetabulum

Lateral Shenton's line

Inferior Shenton's line

Perkins' lines

Hilgenreiner's line

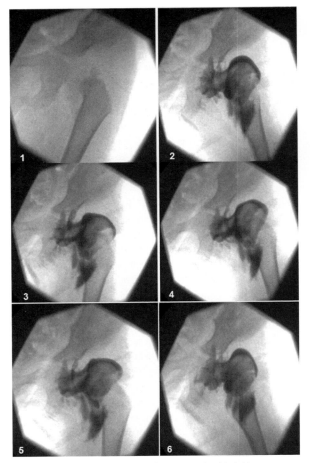

Figure 12.38 Hip arthrogram of a 19-month-old child.

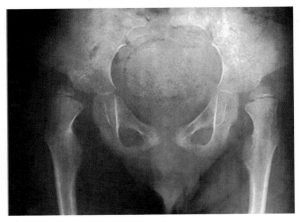

Figure 12.39 Pelvis X-ray of a child with CP.

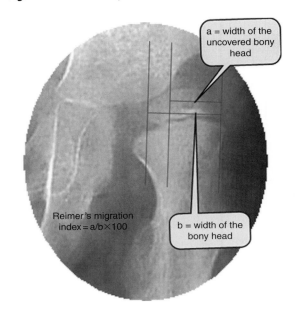

a = width of the uncovered bony head

Reimer's migration index = a/b × 100

b = width of the bony head

Figure 12.40 Reimer's migration index.

of trauma and he was previously fit and healthy. How would you approach such a patient?

I would like to know more (any constitutional symptoms, recent upper respiratory infection, previous similar episodes, involvement of other joints, contact with unwell children, etc.). Then I would perform a thorough examination (temperature, how unwell the child looks, walking, the involved limb and joints and other limbs and joints etc.). I would arrange for appropriate investigations. In such a situation, I usually request blood tests (FBC, CRP, ESR and blood culture if there is fever or the child looks unwell) and pelvis X-ray (AP and lateral).

Q 48: What goes through your mind?

This is quite a common scenario and most of the time, the diagnosis is irritable hip or transient synovitis which is a benign condition; however, I do not want to miss serious conditions such as septic arthritis, osteomyelitis or tumours.

Q 49: The child does not have a temperature, WCC is 10.4, ESR and CRP are 20 and the X-ray did not show anything abnormal. What would you do?

This is reassuring result and fits in with irritable hip. According to Kocher's criteria (Table 12.8), infection is very unlikely (but not impossible). My treatment will be symptomatic with analgesia, anti-inflammatory (not aspirin due to the possible link with Reyes' syndrome), antihistamine but no antibiotic. Depending on few logistic considerations, I may discharge this child home with 48-hour open access to come back to the ward if things deteriorate, otherwise I will review

Table 12.7 Management of neurogenic hip dislocation.

Severity	Passive hip abduction < 30°	Subluxation (RIM 20–40%) No coxa valga No acetabular dysplasia	Subluxation (RIM 40–60%) ± Coxa valga No acetabular dysplasia	Subluxation (RIM 40–60%) ± Coxa valga + Acetabular dysplasia	Subluxation (RIM > 60%) OR Dislocation No pain	Severe painful subluxation or dislocation
Interventions	Adductor release + Physiotherapy	Adductor release + Intramuscular release of psoas at pelvic brim + Physiotherapy	Adductor release + Intramuscular release of psoas at pelvic brim (in ambulant child) OR from lesser trochanter in non-ambulant child + Femoral osteotomy + Physiotherapy	Adductor release + Intramuscular release of psoas at pelvic brim (in ambulant child) OR from lesser trochanter in non-ambulant child + Femoral osteotomy + Acetabular augmentation if acetabulum is small or Dega osteotomy if acetabulum is large + Physiotherapy	Arthrotomy + If articular cartilage is healthy, then open reduction and treat as in column 3 or 4	Excision of the femoral head with valgus subtrochanteric osteotomy and muscle interposition

Table 12.8 Kocher's four criteria.[22]

Kocher's four criteria	Significance
Non-weightbearing ESR > 40 mm/hour (or CRP >20)[23] Fever (> 38.5) WBC > 12 000/mm³	Four criteria met: 99% septic arthritis Three criteria met: 93% septic arthritis Two criteria met: 40% septic arthritis One criterion met: 3% septic arthritis

Table 12.9 Joint fluid analysis.

Conditions	WCC (per mm³)	PML (%)	Other characteristics
Non-inflammatory	200	25	Joint aspirate glucose and protein equal to serum values
Inflammatory	2000–75 000	50	↓ Joint aspirate glucose, low viscosity, yellow–green, friable mucin clot. Synovial complement is low in RA but normal in AS
Infectious	> 80 000	> 75	Thick, cloudy fluid + Gram stain + Cultures ↓ Joint aspirate glucose ↑ joint aspirate protein

him in clinic in 1 week. For example, if the parents are sensible, do not live far away and have a means of transport, this is a practical approach.

Q 50: What is the difference in the synovial fluid analysis between infection and non-infectious conditions?

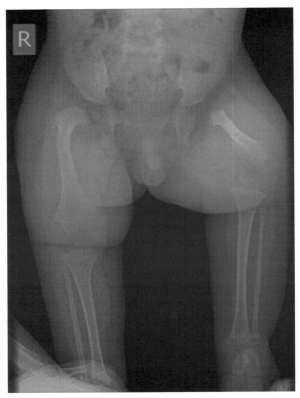

Figure 12.41 A child with short limb.

Q 51: This is an X-ray of a child with a short lower limb. Describe what you see. (Figure 12.41.)

This X-ray shows the left femur is short and dysplastic. The proximal parts (head and trochanter) are not visible; features consistent with proximal focal femoral deficiency (PFFD). There is coxa vara of the right side indicating the right side may be affected as well (bilateral involvement in 15%). The left fibula seems to be shorter than the right side raising the possibility of fibular hemimelia (two-thirds of patients). It is difficult to comment on the state of the hip and knee joints from a single plain film and further assessment is required.

Q 52: How would you approach such a patient?

Treatment of this condition is a challenge and it should be undertaken in specialized centres with interest and experience in its treatment. The National Institute for Health and Clinical Excellence (NICE) has issued guidance to the NHS hospitals on combined bony and soft tissue reconstruction for PFFD

(IPG297 on 22 April 2009). Treatment must be tailored to individual patients based on LLD, hip and knee stability, femoral rotation, proximal musculature, foot condition, availability of the expertise and patient and family motivation. The two broad options are reconstructive surgery or amputation and prosthetic replacement.

A few classifications have been advised to aid assessment and treatment:

1. **Gillespie and Torode**

   a. Group A: congenital short femur by about 20%. The child can weight bear on the affected leg.

   b. Group B: The LLD is around 40% and there is anterior projection of the thigh and flexed knee.

   c. Group C: The thigh is short and bulbous and the leg is externally rotated with the foot at or near the level of the other knee.

2. **Aitken's classification**

Treatment recommendations: Reconstruction and lengthening if femoral length > 50% (usually grade A and B where there is a head). Amputation, fusion, Van Ness rotational arthroplasty if the femoral length < 50%.

3. **Paley classification**

This is the most recent and comprehensive classification, however it is still not widely adopted.

Type I: Intact femur with mobile hip and knee.

   a. Normal ossification proximal femur.

   b. Delayed ossification proximal femur.

Type II: Mobile pseudarthrosis (hip not fully formed, a false joint) with mobile knee.

   a. Femoral head mobile in acetabulum.

   b. Femoral head absent or stiff in acetabulum.

Type III: Diaphyseal deficiency of femur (femur does not reach the acetabulum).

   a. Knee motion > 45°.

   b. Knee motion < 45°.

Type I is further subclassified into:

0. ready for surgery; no factors to correct before lengthening.

1. One factor to correct before lengthening.

2. Two factors to correct before lengthening.

3. Three factors to correct before lengthening.

4+. etc.

Table 12.10 Aitken's classification of proximal focal femoral deficiency (PFFD).

Type	Diagram	Description
A		There is a normal acetabulum and femoral head. The femur is short. Bony connections exist between all components. The cartilaginous neck ossifies later on, although this is often associated with a pseudarthrosis. This may heal, however the X-rays show severe coxa vara with significant shortening of the femur
B		The femoral head is more rudimentary and the deficiency of the proximal femoral shaft is more extensive. Pseudarthrosis between femoral shaft and head is always present
C		The acetabulum is markedly dysplastic and the femoral head never ossifies. The femoral shaft is very short and its upper end tapers sharply to a point. The hip is very unstable
D		Both the femoral head and acetabulum are absent and the deficiency of the femoral shaft is more significant

Table 12.11 Management options for leg length discrepancy.

LLD	Options
0–20 mm LLD	Conservative: nothing, insole or shoe raises
20–50 mm LLD	Consider epiphysiodesis of the opposite side at appropriate age, unless the child is already very short, when you may consider lengthening of the short limb after appropriate consultation. After skeletal maturity, acute shortening of the long limb is an option
Over 50 mm LLD	Offer lengthening of the short limb ± epiphysiodesis of the long limb

Examples of factors requiring correction prior to lengthening of femur are NSA $< 90°$, delayed ossification proximal femur, CEA $< 20°$, subluxing patella and/or dislocating knee.

The strategy of management is staged corrections of the abnormalities to reach stage I0 which is amenable to lengthening. For example, type Ia-3 is converted to Ia-2, then Ia-1, then Ia-0, followed by lengthening.

Pre-existing knee stiffness is the most functionally limiting factor and should be considered a relative indication for amputation versus reconstruction. Hip dysplasia or deficiency is reconstructable and is not a limiting factor. Hip reconstruction should be performed prior to lengthening.

Q 53: What are the principles of LLD management?

It depends on current LLD, the predicted LLD at skeletal maturity and patient's perception of discrepancy.

- Current LLD.
  - Clinical.
  - Radiological.
    - Teleoroentgenography.
    - Orthoroentgenography.
    - Parallel beam scanogram.
    - CT scanogram.
- Predicted LLD at maturity.
  - Menelaus rule of thumbs.
  - Moseley straight line method.
  - Eastwood and Cole method.
  - Paley's multiplier method.

- Patient's perception of discrepancy.
  - How tall is the child? Is the child taller or shorter than average?
  - How tall are the parents or family members?

Station 2: Paediatric knees

Q 1:   This is the clinical photograph of a 2-year-old child who was referred because of bowed legs. How would you approach such a child? (Figure 12.42.)

Bowed legs and knocked knees are common referrals to children's orthopaedics. Most are physiological (i.e. normal for the age of the child), however, this must be differentiated from pathological causes (Table 12.12).

The average child is born with genu varum of 15° which decreases through infancy. The legs are straight at some point in the second year then go into progressive valgus reaching maximum valgus of average 10° at around 3–4 years of age. Valgus then gradually decreases reaching the adult value (5° of valgus) at around age 8 (see Selenius curve; Figure 12.43).

Q 2:   So how can you tell whether the bowing is physiological or pathological?

In most cases, history, examination and appropriate investigations are adequate to differentiate between pathological and physiological bowing. However, sometimes it is not possible to be certain whether it is physiological or pathological and follow-up becomes necessary. It is important to win parent confidence. Reassuring them without adequate explanation and a future plan may not be enough.

Genu varum is more likely to be pathological if it is:

1. Present after 2 years.
2. Unilateral or with asymmetry of more than 5°.
3. Associated with shortening of the limb (or stature).
4. Severe (beyond 2 SD of the mean as per Selenius chart; SD = 8°).
5. In a child with obesity.

And genu valgus is more likely to be pathological if it is:

1. Severe (intermalleolar distance > 10 cm at 10 years or > 15 cm at 5 years).
2. Unilateral.

The following radiological assessment can be very helpful:

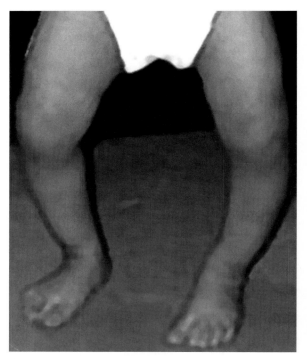

Figure 12.42 A child with bowed legs.

Table 12.12 Causes of genu varum (bow legs) and genu valgus (knocked knees).

Bowed leg	Knocked knees
Physiological	Physiological
Tumours such as osteochondromas	Tumours such as osteochondromas
Skeletal dysplasia	Skeletal dysplasia
Blount's disease	Primary tibia valga
Infection	Infection
Trauma	Trauma
Metabolic (vitamin D deficiency, fluoride poisoning)	Renal osteodystrophy
Osteogenesis imperfecta	Neuromuscular disease (polio) and tight iliotibial band

1. Tibiofemoral angle as per Selenius curve.
2. Metaphyseal–diaphyseal angle of Levine and Drennan (normal < 11°, abnormal > 16°).
3. Metaphyseal–epiphyseal angle (normal < 20°).

Mean tibiofemoral angle according to age (SD = 8°)

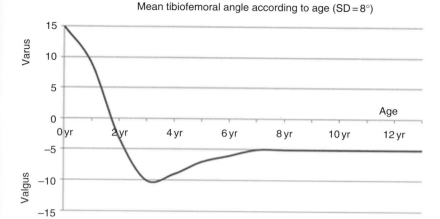

Figure 12.43 Selenius curve.

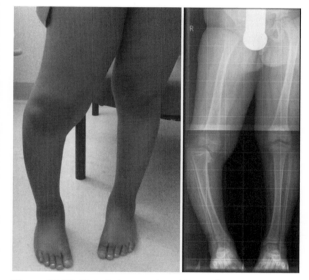

Figure 12.44 Clinical photograph and X-ray of a 7-year-old African child.

Q 3: This is a clinical photograph and X-ray of a 7-year-old African child with right knee deformity. What do you think the diagnosis is? (Figure 12.44.)

There is an obvious deformity of the right leg, specifically around the knee. The child looks big. The X-ray shows classic features of Blount's disease (idiopathic tibia vara) which is medial physeal closure of the proximal tibia with varus (and internal rotation) deformity – Type VI.

Q 4: What is Blount's disease?

Blount's disease is an uncommon growth disorder characterized by disordered ossification of the medial aspect of the proximal tibial physis, epiphysis and metaphysis. This is probably caused by a combination of excessive compressive forces on the proximal medial metaphysis of the tibia and altered enchondral bone formation. There are two recognized types:

1. Infantile (0–4).
2. Adolescent (> 10 years).

In infantile tibia vara, patients generally start to walk early (9–10 months); it is more prevalent in females, blacks, and those with marked obesity. It is bilateral in approximately 80% of cases and associated with a prominent metaphyseal beak, internal tibial torsion, and LLD. The deformity is usually painless.

In the adolescent type, patients complain of pain at the medial aspect of the knee. These patients are overweight and involvement is unilateral in 80% of cases with LLD.

Q 5: Can you draw the following angles? And tell me the significance of these angles?

1. Tibiofemoral angle.
2. Metaphyseal–diaphyseal angle of Levine and Drennan.
3. Metaphyseal–epiphyseal angle.

The tibiofemoral angle is 20° varus. In a 7-year-old child, the tibiofemoral angle approaches the mean adult value which is 5° valgus; hence there is 25° total varus deformity. This is an extreme deformity even after allowing for the quoted standard deviation of 8°. Drennan angle is 21° (normal value is 11° and above

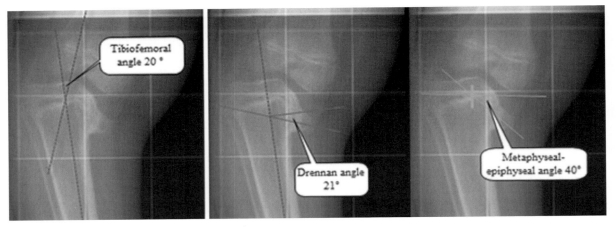

Figure 12.45 Radiological measurement in Blount's disease.

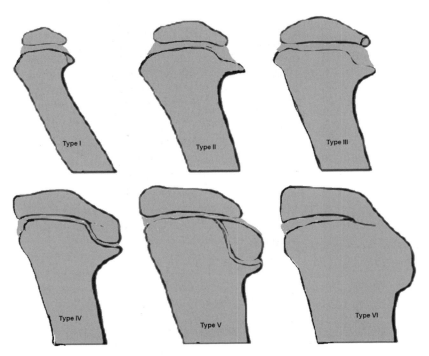

Figure 12.46 Langenskiold classification of Blount's disease.

16° is considered abnormal) which reflects varus deformity of the proximal tibia rather than the knee joint. The same can be said for the metaphyseal–epiphyseal angle.

Q 6: Are you aware of any classification of this condition?

Langenskiold proposed a six-stage radiological classification (Figure 12.46). This classification was not intended for use in determining the prognosis or

the most desirable type of treatment. However, it is generally accepted that surgical treatment commonly is needed for any child with stage 3–6 changes (Table 12.13).

Q 7: So what would you offer this girl?

This girl has stage 6 so surgical treatment is indicated. She has 25° of varus deformity so epiphysiodesis alone will not be adequate (usually correct 1°/month); moreover, the medial physis has been closed so you cannot

Table 12.13 Langenskiold classification of Blount's disease.

Stages	Descriptions	Treatment
Stage 1	Medial beaking, irregular medial ossification with protrusion of the metaphysis	Orthotic for < 3 years
Stage 2	Cartilage fills depression. Progressive depression of medial epiphysis with the epiphysis sloping medially as disease progress	Failure of full correction or progression to type III → surgery
Stage 3	Ossification of the inferomedial corner of the epiphysis	Surgery
Stage 4	Epiphyseal ossification filling the metaphyseal depression	
Stage 5	Double epiphyseal plate (cleft separating two epiphyses)	
Stage 6	Medial physeal closure	

rely on medial growth even after epiphysiolysis. So the only option left is proximal tibial osteotomy and either acute correction using internal fixation or gradual correction using an external fixator.

Station 3: Paediatric feet

Q 1: This is a clinical photograph of a newborn's feet. What can you see? (Figure 12.47.)

This photograph shows the classic feature of bilateral club feet. The deformity is quite complex involving the ankle, subtalar and midtarsal joints. The ankles are usually in equinus. The hind feet are in varus. This is produced by a coupled inversion and adduction deformity at the subtalar joints. The forefeet are adducted and plantar-flexed in relation to the hindfoot.

Q 2: Tell me about the causes of club feet. Why was this child born with club feet?

The cause in the majority of cases is unknown (idiopathic). A few theories have been introduced to explain the aetiology:

1. The neuropathic theory.[25] Biopsies were taken from the posteromedial and peroneal muscle groups in 60 patients mostly under the age of 5 years. Evidence of neurogenic disease was seen in most instances and was more obvious in the older patients.
2. The myopathic theory.[26] A histochemical analysis was made of 103 muscle biopsies taken from 62 patients with idiopathic club feet. The authors noticed the muscles in patients aged under 6 months contained 61% Type 1 fibres in the affected legs, compared with 44.3% in normal legs.
3. Arrest of development of the growing limb bud.

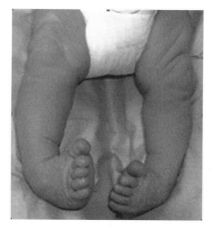

Figure 12.47
A clinical photograph of a newborn's feet (picture courtesy of Dr Lynn Staheli and Global Help Publication).[24]

4. Congenital constriction of the annular band.
5. Viral infection.
6. Mechanical moulding theory.
7. Multifactorial:
   a. Common in Polynesian and rare in the Japanese race.
   b. Not more common in consanguinity.
   c. 10% risk if first-degree relative affected – combination of environmental/genetic factors.[27]
   d. 25% have a family history.

Although less common than idiopathic, there are identifiable causes for club feet which need to be excluded. These include the following:

1. Neurological causes: spina bifida (myelomeningocoele), polio, cerebral palsy.
2. Sacral agenesis.
3. Fetal alcohol syndrome.
4. Congenital myopathy.

5. Down syndrome (may include vertical talus).
6. Arthrogryposis.
7. Hand anomalies (Streeter's dysplasia/constriction band syndrome).
8. Diastrophic dwarfism.
9. Prune belly.
10. Tibial hemimelia.

Q 3: How would you manage this child?

Having established the diagnosis of idiopathic club feet, my management is serial casting by the Ponseti method. The treatment should be started as early as possible; the severity of the deformity is quantified using Pirani score, then serial casting weekly for up to 3 months.

Sequence of deformity corrections (**CAVE**):

1. **C**avus.
2. **A**dduction of the forefeet and **V**arus of the heel. This is achieved concomitantly using the talus head as a fulcrum.
3. **E**quinus of the heel. Tendo-Achilles tenotomy is required in 90% of the patients to correct the heel equinus.

This can be repeated if necessary and can be utilized up to the age of 1 year. Successful correction is

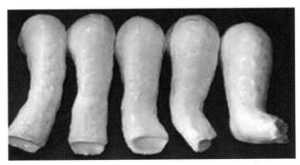

Figure 12.48 Ponseti's weekly serial casting (picture courtesy of Dr Lynn Staheli and Global Help Publication).[24]

followed by a regime of using Denise-Browne boots continuously for 3 months, after which they will be used at nap and night time for 3 years.

Q 4: These are Denise–Browne boots. Can you describe the different parts and their functions? (Figure 12.49.)

The brace consists of open-toe high-top straight-last shoes attached to a bar. The bar should be of sufficient length so that the heels of the shoes are at shoulder width. This can be adjusted using the sliding clamp in the middle. The bar should be bent 5–10° to hold the feet in dorsiflexion.

For unilateral cases, the brace is set at 60–70° of external rotation on the clubfoot side and 30–40° of external rotation on the normal side. In bilateral cases, it is set at 70° of external rotation on each side.

Q 5: Explain the Pirani score for club feet.

The Pirani score is simple and reproducible. It uses six clinical signs to quantify severity of each component of the deformity. Each component is scored as 0 (normal), 0.5 (mildly abnormal) or 1 (severely abnormal) (Table 12.14).

The six clinical signs Pirani used are divided equally between the hindfoot and midfoot and then added for a total score of 0–6:

Hindfoot contracture score (HFCS) 0–3

1. Equinus.
2. Deep posterior crease.
3. Empty heel.

Midfoot contracture score (MFCS) 0–3

1. Curved lateral border.
2. Medial crease.
3. Lateral head of talus.

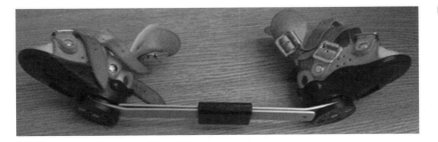

Figure 12.49 Denise–Browne boots.

Table 12.14 Pirani score for club feet. (Pictures courtesy of Dr Lynn Staheli and Global Help Publication.)

Hindfoot contracture score	Equinus	0	0.5	1.0

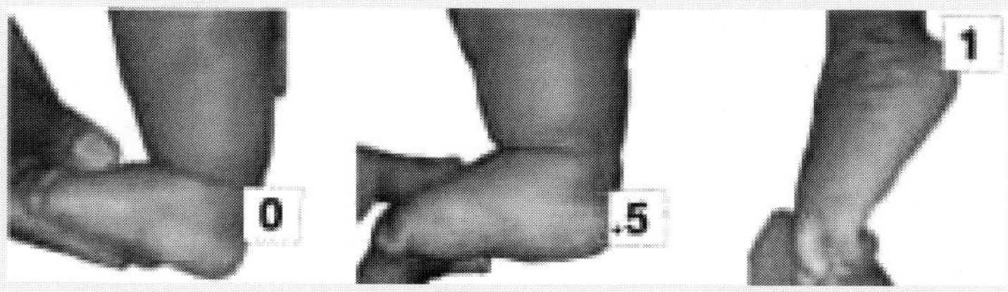

	Deep posterior crease	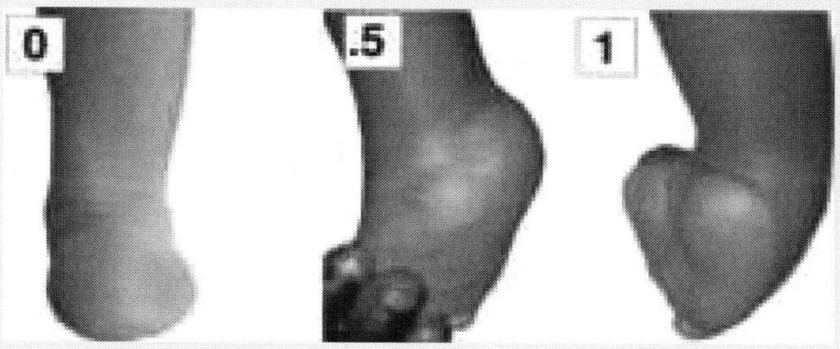		

	Empty heel	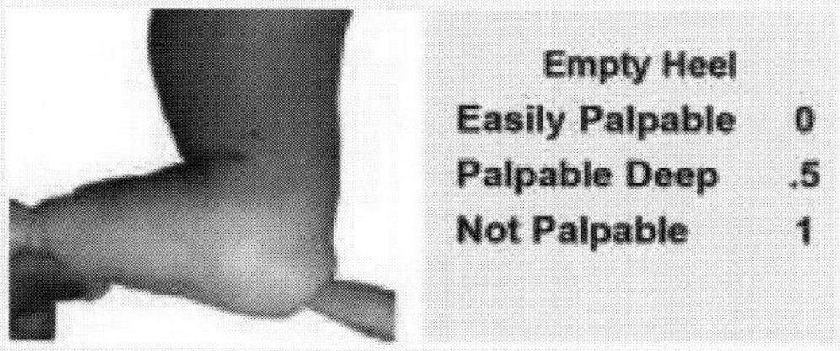		

Empty Heel

Easily Palpable	0
Palpable Deep	.5
Not Palpable	1

Midfoot contracture score	Curved lateral border	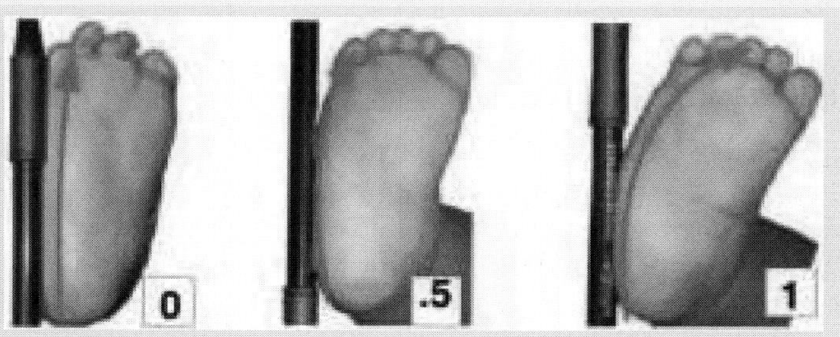		

	Medial crease	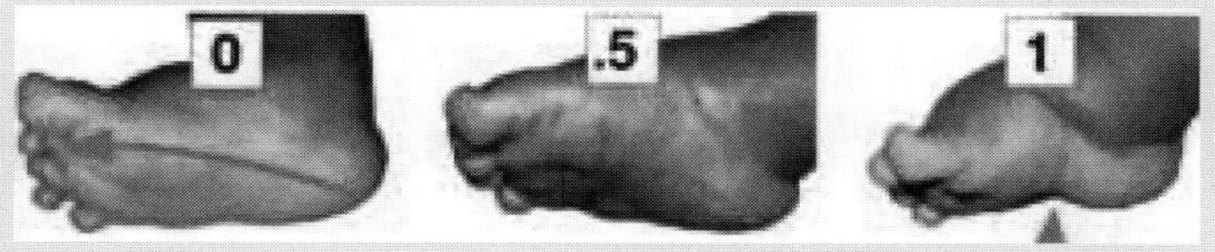		

	Lateral head of talus	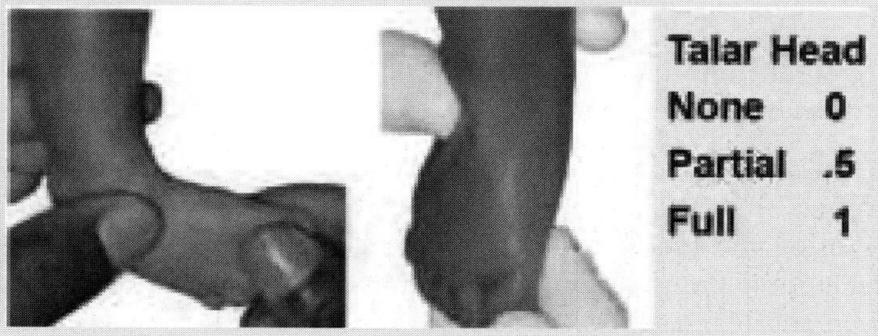		

Talar Head

None	0
Partial	.5
Full	1

Table 12.15 Dimeglio scoring system.

Rating	4	3	2	1	0
1. Equinus	45°–90° Plantar flexion	20°–45° Plantar flexion	20°–0° Plantar flexion	0°–20° Dorsiflexion	>+20° Dorsiflexion
2. Varus	45°–90° Varus	20°–45° Varus	20°–0° Varus	0°–20° Valgus	> 20° Valgus
3. Supination	45°–90° Supination	20°–45° Supination	20°–0° Supination	0°–20° Supination	>20° Supination
4. Adductus	45°–90° Adduction	20°–45° Adduction	20°–0° Adduction	0°>–<20° Adduction	> 20° Abduction
5. Posterior crease				Yes	No
6. Medial crease				Yes	No
7. Cavus				Yes	No
8. Deviant muscle function				Yes	No

Q 6: Do you know any other scoring system for club feet?

Yes, there is the Dimeglio classification which consists of eight items. Scorings for four items range from 0–4 (best to worst). Four items only score 0 or 1. Total score ranges between 20–0 (very severe: 16–20, severe 11–15, moderate 6–10, and postural 0–5). (Table 12.15.)

Q 7: This is another child who was born with bilateral club feet. Have a look at the picture and tell us how you would treat him. (Figure 12.50.)

The striking feature of this child is the lack of skin creases over the joints (hips, knees and elbows) which is very suggestive of arthrogryposis. As far as the club feet are concerned, I would still treat them as idiopathic club feet. Researchers from SickKids hospital in Toronto studied 40 non-idiopathic club feet and compared them with 249 idiopathic club feet and showed the success rate of Ponseti serial casting in the former group is less successful (10% failure rate; 4/40) and recurrence rate is higher (44%; 16/36), and more patients needed additional operations.[28] Nevertheless, correction was achieved and maintained in most patients.

Q 8: What other complications of Ponseti treatment are there?

In contrast to the above example, some patients may develop excessive heel valgus and external tibial torsion while using the brace. In such instances, the external rotation of the shoes on the bar should be reduced from approximately 70° to 40°.

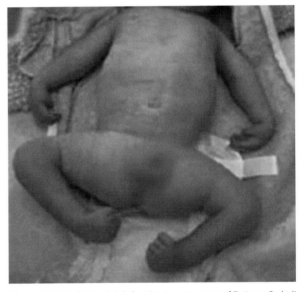

Figure 12.50 Bilateral club feet (picture courtesy of Dr Lynn Staheli and Global Help Publication).[24]

Q 9: These are lateral views of the left and right feet of a child who was brought to your clinic with a right foot deformity. What can you see? (Figure 12.51.)

These are weightbearing views of both feet. There is a vertical orientation (i.e. the talus is plantar flexed) of the talus of the right foot and the long axis of the first metatarsal is not in line with the navicular bone and the long axis of the talus. In comparison, the talus of

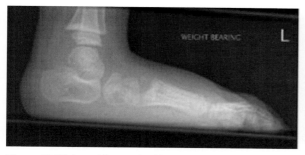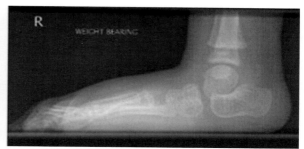

Figure 12.51 Lateral foot and ankle X-rays of a child with foot deformity.

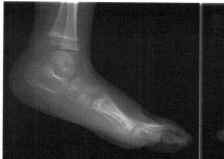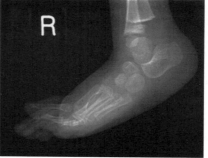

Figure 12.52 Plantar flexion lateral foot and ankle X-rays of a child with foot deformity.

the left foot seems to be pointing to the navicular bone; however, it is not perfectly aligned with the first metatarsal. I suspect there is a congenital vertical talus on the right-hand side. I would like to see lateral views with the ankle joint in hyperextension and hyperflexion.

Q 10: These are what you requested. How can they help? (Figure 12.52.)

These views help me differentiate between the congenital vertical talus and flexible oblique talus. In the former, the hind foot is rigid and the calcaneum and the talus remain in plantar flexion (right foot) and the alignment of the three bones (talus, navicular and first metatarsal) is not restored while it is not the case on the left side. Also, the soft tissue shadow shows a convex contour to the sole (rocker bottom).

Q 11: So, what is a vertical talus?

It is a rare congenital foot deformity characterized by a dislocation of the talonavicular joint. The navicular dislocates dorsally and the head of the talus points towards the plantar. The heel in equinus and valgus and the forefoot in dorsiflexion and abduction produce the classic rocker-bottom appearance. It is usually associated with other conditions such as:

1. Arthrogryposis.
2. Multiple pterygium syndrome.
3. Neuromuscular diseases (poliomyelitis, CP).
4. Spinal muscular dystrophy.
5. Genetics (trisomy 13, 15, 17, 18 and Turner syndrome).
6. Sacral agenesis.
7. Neural tube defects (myelomeningocoele, diastematomyelia).
8. Visceral anomalies.
9. Malformation syndromes (Marfan syndrome, nail patella syndrome, Freeman–Sheldon syndrome).

Q 12: How would you treat this child?

The aims of the treatment are:

1. Reduction of joint dislocation.
2. Maintenance of the joint reduction and restoration of normal foot biomechanics.
3. Identify any associated diseases and treat them (need multidisciplinary input).

There are a few techniques to achieve and maintain reduction depending on the age of presentation, severity of the condition and other associated disorders.

1. Serial casting and percutaneous surgery.[29,30]

This is sometimes called a reversed Ponseti technique. The abducted forefoot is gently plantar flexed and inverted with one hand while the other hand is pushing the talar head upward to correct the plantar-flexed position. This procedure is repeated at weekly intervals. Four or five casts are usually required until the plantar-flexed talus is in line with the first metatarsal.

A K-wire is introduced from the dorsum of the forefoot in line with the first metatarsal, through the navicular bone and talus so that it keeps the talonavicular joint reduced. Percutaneous tendoachilles tenotomy is performed to correct the hind foot equinus and valgus. The foot is then put in cast in 5° dorsiflexion for 4 weeks. The K-wire is removed at 4 weeks; the foot is recast for another 4 weeks in 15° of dorsiflexion. Then a solid AFO to keep the foot in 15° planter flexion and 15° adduction is used until the age of 2 years.

2. Open soft tissue release.

In older children and severe cases, the closed reduction can be unsuccessful by the above method. Hence, open talonavicular joint reduction with soft tissue release is required. It is usually performed around 9–12 months. All contracted tissues are released or lengthened such as tendoachilles, posterior capsule, dorsal tendons (extensor digitorum longus, peroneus tertius). Rarely, excision of the navicular may be necessary.

3. Tibialis anterior transfer to the talar neck to prevent the talus from plantar flexing.

4. Triple fusion as a salvage procedure.

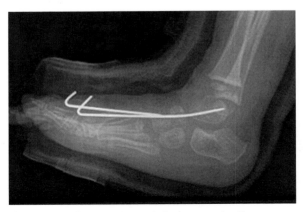

Figure 12.53 Postoperative vertical talus correction X-ray.

Station 4: Miscellaneous

Q 1: Can you draw me the different layers that the growth plate (physis) consists of and give me an example of a disease that affects each layer? (Figure 12.54.)

Q 2: **What classifications do you use for physeal fractures?**

Several classification systems have been developed for physeal fractures. The most widely used system today is the Salter–Harris classification (Figure 12.55).

- Type I injuries involve complete separation of the epiphysis through the physis without fracture through the metaphysis.
- Type II injuries involve separation of a portion of the physis with the fracture progressing out of the metaphysis.
- Type III injuries involve a fracture that runs through a portion of the physis and out through the epiphysis.
- Type IV fractures are longitudinal splits through the epiphysis, physis and metaphysis.
- Type V fractures involve a crush injury of the growth plate and are not evident on radiographs at the time of injury.

This classification has been modified by Peterson, Rang and Ogden. Peterson added another two types: Type VI with metaphyseal fractures extending to the physis and Type VII with loss of the physis (VIIa for central and VIIb for peripheral). (Figure 12.56.)

Ogden from his series of 443 physeal fractures has added another three (Figure 12.57):

Type VII: Epiphyseal fractures not involving physis.
Type VIII: Metaphyseal fractures affecting later growth.
Type IX: Periosteal damage affecting later growth.

Q 3: **What is the significance of this classification?**

This classification predicts the impact of injury on the growth plate function; the higher the grade the worse the prognosis (Table 12.16). The location of the physeal fracture is also an important prognostic factor. Undulant physis or irregular physis (such as distal femur and distal tibia) have the worst prognosis as the fracture is more likely to affect several layers of the physis.

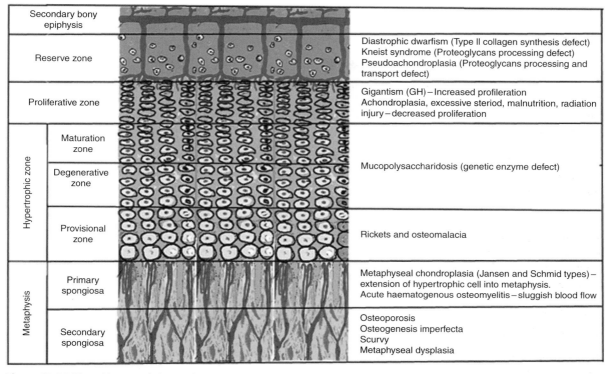

Secondary bony epiphysis		
Reserve zone		Diastrophic dwarfism (Type II collagen synthesis defect) Kneist syndrome (Proteoglycans processing defect) Pseudoachondroplasia (Proteoglycans processing and transport defect)
Proliferative zone		Gigantism (GH) – Increased profileration Achondroplasia, excessive steriod, malnutrition, radiation injury – decreased proliferation
Hypertrophic zone	Maturation zone	Mucopolysaccharidosis (genetic enzyme defect)
	Degenerative zone	
	Provisional zone	Rickets and osteomalacia
Metaphysis	Primary spongiosa	Metaphyseal chondroplasia (Jansen and Schmid types) – extension of hypertrophic cell into metaphysis. Acute haematogenous osteomyelitis – sluggish blood flow
	Secondary spongiosa	Osteoporosis Osteogenesis imperfecta Scurvy Metaphyseal dysplasia

Figure 12.54 Physeal layers and abnormalities. See colour plate section.

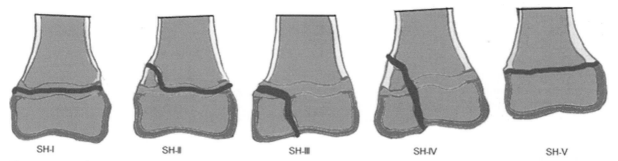

Figure 12.55 Salter–Harris classification.

SH-I   SH-II   SH-III   SH-IV   SH-V

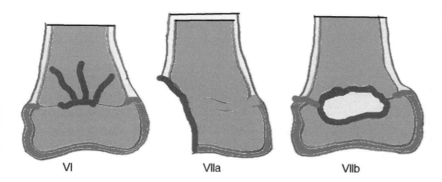

VI   VIIa   VIIb

Figure 12.56 Peterson modification of Salter–Harris classification.

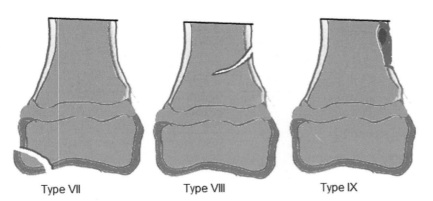

Figure 12.57 Ogden modification of Salter–Harris classification.

Type VII   Type VIII   Type IX

Table 12.16 Risk of growth disturbance after physeal injury.

Location	Risk of growth disturbance
Distal radius	1–6%
Distal femur	20–25%
Proximal tibia	10%
Distal tibia	15%

Type	Risk of growth disturbance
I	7%
II	2–3%
III	14%
IV	18%

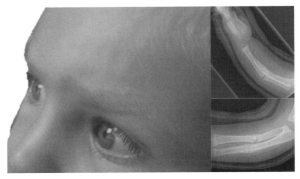

Figure 12.58 A clinical photograph and right forearm X-rays of a child. See colour plate section.

Q 4: This is a clinical photograph and right forearm X-rays of a child who was investigated for non-accidental injury (NAI) after presenting with two fractures with minor trauma. What are your thoughts? (Figure 12.58.)

The clinical photograph focuses on the eyes and the surrounding areas. The sclera has a blue tinge to it with no signs of trauma (such as subconjunctival haemorrhage, hyphema or skin bruises). The X-ray shows a healing forearm fracture with callus formation. There is a slight angulation of the radius of about 20°. The two possible underlying diagnoses are NAI or osteogenesis imperfecta (OI).

Q 5: How would you approach such a scenario?

There is a moral and legal duty of all healthcare providers to initiate child protection procedures if child abuse is suspected. Most hospitals have standard operating procedures to deal with such a situation.

This is best managed as a multidisciplinary team (paediatrician, orthopaedics, radiologist and social services).

Q 6: What is the basic pathology of OI?

Osteogenesis imperfecta (OI) is caused by mutations in the genes that produce type I collagen (COL1A1 and COL1A2). Type I collagen fibres are found in the bones, joint capsules, fascia, cornea, sclera, tendons and skin. Qualitative defects (an abnormal collagen I molecule) and quantitative defects (decreased production of normal collagen I molecules) have been both described in OI and this leads to bone fragility and other features of OI. Sillence described four major classes of OI (Table 12.17);[31] however, syndromes resembling osteogenesis imperfecta have been described in the literature that are not caused by mutations in the type I collagen genes. They present with congenital brittle bones and, often, with other distinctive characteristics (e.g. blindness, congenital contractures, redundant callus formation). In most cases, these are recessive conditions.

Table 12.17 Sillence classification of osteogenesis imperfecta.

Type	Genetics	Inheritance	Sclera	Bone fragility	Comments
I	Decreased production of normal collagen	AD	Blue	Mild to moderate	Most common type, normal height, presenile hearing loss or impairment in 50% of patients. Tooth involvement is rare
II	Abnormal collagen structure	AD or AR	Blue	Extreme	Almost always perinatally lethal Subtype A: Broad crumpled long bones; beaded ribs Subtype B: Broad, crumpled long bones; discontinuous or no beading of ribs Subtype C: Thin, fractured long bones; thin beaded ribs
III	Abnormal collagen structure	AD or AR	Normal, pale blue, or grey at birth; normal by adolescence	Moderate to severe	Significant short stature. Variable hearing impairment. Tooth involvement is common
IV	Abnormal collagen structure	AD	Normal, pale blue, or grey at birth; normal by adolescence	Mild to moderate	Variable short stature. Hearing impairment less common than type I

Q 7: How would you diagnose OI?

History, examination and appropriate investigations are essential. In my centre, this is usually in liaison with a clinical geneticist who reviews the child and the family. Family history and radiological tests usually raise suspicion; however, confirmation is by skin biopsy (biochemical analysis of collagen produced by cultured fibroblast) or genetic testing to detect the culprit mutation.

Q 8: How would you treat a patient with OI?

Osteogenesis imperfecta patients are a heterogeneous group and treatment is best tailored at individual level. Fractures are treated as necessary. Although the bones fracture easily, they take longer than normal to heal. Prevention of fractures is the mainstay of treatment; correct positioning and supporting of the patient, muscle strengthening, bracing or even prophylactic nailing using a growing rod may become necessary in severe forms.

Treatment with bisphosphonates such as pamidronate has been shown to increase bone mass and to decrease bone pain and frequency of fractures.[32,33] However, the long-term effects of bisphosphonate treatment, which may compromise bone quality over time, are not known yet. Use of growth hormone to correct OI-associated short stature is also under investigation.

Q 9: Back to the possibility of non-accidental injury, what might make you suspect a NAI?

Unfortunately, child abuse is more common than most expect. It is estimated that 7% of children suffer serious physical abuse. If diagnosis is not considered and missed, there might be a serious outcome including death. Twenty-five per cent of fatally abused children have been seen recently by a healthcare provider.[34]

The overall pattern or combination of features should raise suspicion:

- The injuries are multiple, frequent or of different ages.
- Injury is not consistent with history stated or the developmental age of child.
- Delayed presentation, reluctance to seek help, fear of medical examination.
- Child is brought to different surgeries/ departments (to avoid detection of repeated injuries).
- Unexplained denial or aggression.
- No explanation for the injuries, a story that changes on repetition, or child's story differs from carer's.

- Bruising in the shape of a hand, ligature, stick, teeth mark, grip, fingertips or an implement. Bruises at sites where accidental bruising is unusual: face, eyes, ears (bruising around the pinna may be subtle), neck and top of shoulder, anterior chest, abdomen.
- Petechiae (tiny red or purple spots) not caused by a medical condition – may be due to shaking or suffocation.
- Although there is no fracture absolutely specific for NAI, some should raise suspicion:

  1. Rib fractures.
  2. Metaphyseal fractures.
  3. Complex or wide (diastatic) skull fractures.
  4. Digital fractures.
  5. Outer end of clavicle.
  6. Any scapular fracture.
  7. Fractures of different ages.
  8. Bilateral or multiple diaphyseal fractures.

Q 10: If you suspect a NAI, how would you investigate it further?

This is best managed as a multidisciplinary team. Standards for radiological investigations of suspected NAI were published by the Royal College of Radiologists and Royal College of Paediatrics and Child Health in March 2008. A full skeletal survey involves a significant amount of radiation (17 exposures) and it should not be taken lightly. A chest X-ray represents an exposure equivalent to 3 days of background radiation while a full skeletal survey may equate to 8 months of background radiation.

Q 11: What does a skeletal survey involve?

A skeletal survey is a radiological screening to discover occult pathologies. In the context of NAI, these are occult bony injuries. In children under 2 years with suspected NAI, a full skeletal survey is indicated (ideally after discussion among senior members of the child medical protection team). This involves the following series of images:

1. Anteroposterior (AP) skull.
2. Lateral skull.
3. AP chest.
4. Oblique left ribs.
5. Oblique right ribs.
6. AP abdomen and pelvis.
7. Lateral spine.
8. Dorsopalmar both hands.
9. Dorsoplantar both feet.
10. AP left humerus.
11. AP right humerus.
12. AP left forearm.
13. AP right forearm.
14. AP left femur.
15. AP right femur.
16. AP left tibia/fibula.
17. AP right tibia/fibula.

In children over 2 years, this should be guided by history and physical examination. This is different from a skeletal survey performed for other conditions such as dysplasia or neoplasia.

1. Loder RT, Hensinger RN, Alburger PD *et al*. Acute slipped capital femoral epiphysis: the importance of physeal stability. *J Bone Joint Surg Am* 1993;**75-A**: 1134–1140.
2. Peterson MD, Weiner DS, Green NE *et al*. Acute slipped capital femoral epiphysis: the value and safety of urgent manipulative reduction. *J Pediatr Orthop* 1997;**17**(5): 648–654.
3. Kalogrianitis S, Tan CK, Kemp GJ, Bass A, Bruce C. Does unstable slipped capital femoral epiphysis require urgent stabilization? *J Pediatr Orthop B* 2007; **16**(1):6–9.
4. Jerre R, Billing L, Hansson G, Wallin J. The contralateral hip in patients primarily treated for unilateral slipped upper femoral epiphysis. Long-term follow-up of 61 hips. *J Bone Joint Surg Br* 1994;**76-B**:563–567.
5. Balasa VV, Gruppo RA, Glueck CJ *et al*. Legg–Calve–Perthes disease and thrombophilia. *J Bone Joint Surg Am* 2004;**86-A**:2642–2647.
6. Thomas DP, Morgan G, Tayton K. Perthes' disease and the relevance of thrombophilia. *J Bone Joint Surg Br* 1999;**81-B**:691–695.
7. Hayek S, Kenet G, Lubetsky A *et al*. Does thrombophilia play an aetiological role in Legg-Calve-Perthes disease? *J Bone Joint Surg Br* 1999;**81-B**:686–690.
8. Stulberg SD, Cooperman DR, Wallensten R. The natural history of Legg–Calve–Perthes disease. *J Bone Joint Surg Am* 1981;**63-A**:1095–1108.
9. Herring JA, Kim HT, Browne R. Legg-Calve-Perthes disease. Part II: Prospective multicenter study of the effect of treatment on outcome. *J Bone Joint Surg Am* 2004;**86-A**:2121–2134.
10. Wiig O, Terjesen T, Svenningsen S. Prognostic factors and outcome of treatment in Perthes' disease: a prospective study of 368 patients with five-year follow-up. *J Bone Joint Surg Br* 2008;**90-B**:1364–1371.

11. Maxwell SL, Lappin KJ, Kealey WD, McDowell BC, Cosgrove AP. Arthrodiastasis in Perthes' disease. Preliminary results. *J Bone Joint Surg Br* 2004;**86-B**: 244–250.

12. Daly K, Bruce C, Catterall A. Lateral shelf acetabuloplasty in Perthes' disease. A review of the end of growth. *J Bone Joint Surg Br* 1999;**81-B**: 380–384.

13. Domzalski ME, Glutting J, Bowen JR *et al.* Lateral acetabular growth stimulation following a labral support procedure in Legg–Calve–Perthes disease. *J Bone Joint Surg Am* 2006;**88-A**:1458–1466.

14. Bankes MJ, Catterall A, Hashemi-Nejad A. Valgus extension osteotomy for 'hinge abduction' in Perthes' disease. Results at maturity and factors influencing the radiological outcome. *J Bone Joint Surg Br* 2000; **82-B**:548–554.

15. Wright JG. (Ed.) *Evidence-Based Orthopaedics. The Best Answers to Clinical Questions.* Philadelphia, PA: WB Saunders, 2009.

16. Jari S, Paton RW, Srinivasan MS. Unilateral limitation of abduction of the hip. A valuable clinical sign for DDH? *J Bone Joint Surg Br* 2002;**84-B**:104–107.

17. Jones, D. Neonatal detection of developmental dysplasia of the hip (DDH). *J Bone Joint Surg Br* 1998;**80-B**: 943–945.

18. Graf, R. The diagnosis of congenital hip-joint dislocation by the ultrasonic Combound treatment. *Arch Orthop Trauma Surg* 1980;**97**:117–133.

19. Harcke HT, Clarke NM, Lee MS, Borns PF, MacEwen GD. Examination of the infant hip with real-time ultrasonography. *J Ultrasound Med* 1984; **3**(3):131–137.

20. Graf R. (Ed.) Hip sonography. In *Diagnosis and Management of Infant Hip Dysplasia.* Berlin: Springer, 2006.

21. Podeszwa DA, Mooney IF III, Cramer KE *et al.* Comparison of Pavlik harness application and immediate spica casting for femur fractures in infants. *J Pediatr Orthop* 2004;**24**(5):460–462.

22. Kocher MS, Mandiga R, Murphy JM *et al.* A clinical practice guideline for treatment of septic arthritis in children: efficacy in improving process of care and effect on outcome of septic arthritis of the hip. *J Bone Joint Surg Am* 2003;**85-A**:994–999.

23. Caird MS, Flynn JM, Leung YL *et al.* Factors distinguishing septic arthritis from transient synovitis of the hip in children. A prospective study. *J Bone Joint Surg Am* 2006;**88-A**:1251–1257.

24. Staheli L, Ponseti I *et al. Clubfoot: Ponseti Management.* Global Help Publications, 2009.

25. Isaacs H, Handelsman JE, Badenhorst M, Pickering A. The muscles in club foot – a histological, histochemical and electron microscopic study. *J Bone Joint Surg Br* 1977;**59-B**:465–472.

26. Gray DH, Katz JM. A histochemical study of muscle in club foot. *J Bone Joint Surg Br* 1981;**63-B**:417–423.

27. Wynne-Davies, R. Genetic and environmental factors in the etiology of talipes equinovarus. *Clin Orthop Relat Res* 1972;**84**:9–13.

28. Janicki JA, Narayanan UG, Harvey BJ *et al.* Treatment of neuromuscular and syndrome-associated (nonidiopathic) clubfeet using the Ponseti method. *J Pediatr Orthop* 2009;**29**:393–397.

29. Alaee F, Boehm S, Dobbs MB. A new approach to the treatment of congenital vertical talus. *J Child Orthop* 2007;**1**(3):165–174.

30. Bhaskar, A. Congenital vertical talus: treatment by reverse Ponseti technique. *Indian J Orthop* 2008;**42**:347–350.

31. Sillence DO. Osteogenesis imperfecta nosology and genetics. *Ann N Y Acad Sci* 1988;**543**:1–15.

32. Letocha AD, Cintas HL, Troendle JF *et al.* Controlled trial of pamidronate in children with types III and IV osteogenesis imperfecta confirms vertebral gains but not short-term functional improvement. *J Bone Mineral Res* 2005;**20**(6):977–986.

33. Zacharin M, Bateman J. Pamidronate treatment of osteogenesis imperfecta – lack of correlation between clinical severity, age at onset of treatment, predicted collagen mutation and treatment response. *J Pediatr Endocrinol Metab* 2002;**15**(2):163–174.

34. Lucas DR, Wezner KC, Milner JS *et al.* Victim, perpetrator, family, and incident characteristics of infant and child homicide in the United States Air Force. *Child Abuse Negl* 2002;**26**(2):167–186.

Chapter

13

Anatomy and surgical approaches

Tom Symes

Structured oral examination question 1: Approach to hip for total hip arthroplasty

Q 1: What approach do you use for THA?
Example answers:

Posterior, lateral (Hardinge/Omega), anterolateral (Watson-Jones).

Probably the most common approach you will be asked to describe. Talk about the approach that you know and use. If you try to describe something that you have only read in a book you will probably forget it and come unstuck. Read up on your favoured approach beforehand especially the neurovascular intervals and potential dangers.

Q 2: Describe the approach from skin, fat, fascia, bursa, muscular interval if relevant to joint

Posterior – Incision centred on posterior aspect of greater trochanter (GT), curve posteriorly, incise fat and fascia in line with the skin incision, sweep fat off short external rotators (ER), divide ER where they attach into the greater trochanter, divide capsule and dislocate the femoral head.

Lateral – Longitudinal incision centred on greater trochanter, incise fat and fascia in line with skin, incision in fibres of gluteus medius/vastus lateralis avoid taking dissection too far proximal (injury to superior gluteal nerve), H- or T-shaped capsulotomy, dislocate femoral head.

Anterolateral – Straight incision centred on tip of greater trochanter, fat and fascia in line with skin distally but in line with fibres proximally towards ASIS, develop interval between tensor fascia lata and gluteus medius, release origin of vastus lateralis. Detach abductor mechanism by either (1) trochanteric trochanteric osteotomy or (2) partial

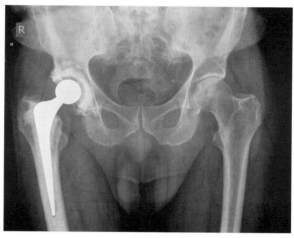

Figure 13.1 Radiograph of total hip arthroplasty (THA).

detachment of abductors. Detach reflected head of rectus femoris from the joint capsule, then an H- or T-shaped capsulotomy, dislocate femoral head with external rotation.

Q 3: What nerve is at risk in each approach and when?

Posterior – Sciatic nerve during the approach, femoral nerve during retraction/exposure of anterior acetabulum, obturator nerve during inferior acetabulum retraction.

Lateral – superior gluteal nerve (3–5 cm above the upper border of greater trochanter) during approach through abductors.

Anterolateral – femoral nerve during retraction.

Q 4: What is the consequence of damage in terms of sensory loss, weakness?

Sciatic – most commonly affects the peroneal branch, therefore foot drop and sensory loss dorsum of the foot.

Postgraduate Orthopaedics: Viva Guide for the FRCS (Tr & Orth) Examination, ed. Paul A. Banaszkiewicz and Deiary F. Kader. Published by Cambridge University Press. © Cambridge University Press 2012.

Femoral – weak knee extension and loss of sensation over the medial border of leg and foot.

Superior gluteal nerve – abductor weakness, Trendelenburg gait.

You must know your peripheral nerve lesions and sensory dermatomes for many different topics e.g. spinal injuries, ATLS assessment, brachial plexus.

Q 5: Which approach is more extensile for revision hip surgery?
Posterior.

If you can justify another approach that is equally acceptable.

Q 6: What manoeuvres can be performed to:

i. Improve exposure of the acetabulum

Release piriformis, anterior capsule, reflected head of rectus femoris, psoas tendon.

ii. Facilitate removal of cement and/or a stem which is difficult to remove.
Extended trochanteric osteotomy.
Trochanteric osteotomy.
Window in femur.

Q 7: Describe how you would perform an ETO.
Pre-op planning, osteotomy length is determined from tip greater trochanter, hip placed in extension, internal rotation with knee flexed, osteotomy extends along posterolateral aspect of the proximal femur slightly anterior to the gluteus maximus insertion. Saw directed posterolateral to anterolateral and should include posterolateral third proximal femur, corners rounded to minimize risk of stress fracture. Multiple osteotomes used to lever osteotomy site from posterior to anterior.

Answering questions 6 and 7 will get you a 7 or 8 depending on your level of detail.

Structured oral examination question 2: Approach to the hip for drainage

A 5-year-old boy presents to A&E with a 2-day history of fevers, off legs, c/o painful hip and knee. This is his X-ray. (Figure 13.2.)

Q 1: After taking a history and examination what tests would you perform? [Likelihood of hip sepsis.]

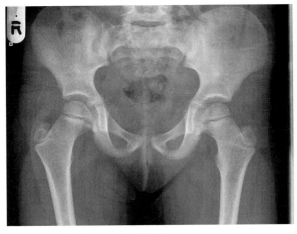

Figure 13.2 Radiograph of child's hip.

FBC, CRP, ESR, USS, ?MRI.

Hip sepsis in children is a common question at several points in the exam and needs to be known well. There are studies that have produced prediction of the likelihood of septic arthritis depending on blood markers and clinical features.

Kocher MS, Zurakowski D, Kasser JR. Differentiating between septic arthritis and transient synovitis of the hip in children: an evidence-based clinical prediction algorithm. *J Bone Joint Surg Am* 1999;**81-A**:1662–1670.

Q 2: These are the test results (increased WBC, CRP, ESR, effusion on X-rays and USS). What is the management?
Open washout and drainage.

Some surgeons may argue that you should perform a USS-guided drainage to identify pus or a positive culture but the examiners in this situation want you to describe the approach so will make it a barn door case.

Q 3: Which approach is recommended to perform an open drainage and washout of a child's septic hip and why?
Anterior (Smith Petersen) because the main blood supply to the femoral head is posterior.

You must know this approach for this viva and also the paediatric viva.

Q 4: Describe layers and nerve supply
Supine position
Incision (use part of this) following anterior half of iliac crest to ASIS then curved down vertically 4–5 cm towards the lateral side of the patella.

Externally rotate the leg, identify gap between sartorius (femoral nerve) and tensor fascia lata (superior gluteal nerve) about 5 cm below ASIS, avoid lateral femoral cutaneous nerve which pierces the deep fascia near the interval, incise fascia medial to TFL and retract it downwards and laterally, retract sartorius upward and medially. Ligate the ascending branch of the lateral femoral circumflex artery (crosses gap between sartorius and tensor fascia lata), then develop plane between rectus femoris (femoral nerve) and gluteus medius (superior gluteal nerve). Detach the two origins of rectus femoris (AIIS and superior lip of acetabulum), retract rectus femoris and iliopsoas medially and gluteus medius laterally to expose hip capsule, capsulotomy (longitudinal or T-shaped) and then wash out the hip joint.

This is a pass/fail question and must be known.

Structured oral examination question 3: Henry's/Anterior approach to arm

Q 1: Describe this radiograph. (Figure 13.3.)

It is an X-ray of the right forearm of an adult. There are transverse fractures of the mid shaft of both radius and ulna. They are completely displaced.

You must be able to quickly and concisely describe a fracture as if you were talking to your consultant on the end of a phone and so he can easily imagine the fracture pattern.

Q 2: How would you describe the displacement concisely?

They are off ended.

Q 3: What is the generally accepted surgical treatment for this injury?

Plating of both bones with dynamic compression plates.

Q 4: If you were to approach the fractured radius anteriorly, how would you do it?

Describe Henry's approach, it is acceptable to describe the approach that goes through the bed of flexor carpi radialis (FCR) or a reasonable alternative.

Incise the skin over FCR, aim towards biceps insertion. Develop plane between brachioradialis (radial nerve) and FCR (median nerve) distally and retract FPL. Pronate the arm to expose the insertion of pronator quadratus onto the lateral aspect of

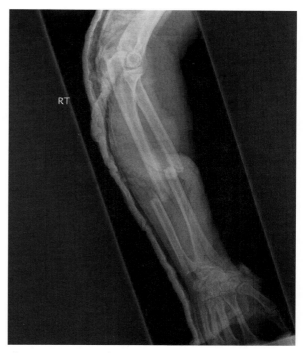

Figure 13.3 Forearm fracture.

radius. Subperiosteally detach pronator quadratus off the radius.

Proximally be aware of recurrent radial artery and fully supinate the arm when releasing supinator muscle to avoid the PIN.

This is a classic approach and (anecdotally) candidates have been failed for not knowing it.

Q 5: How would you extend the exposure proximally?

Proximally the skin incision follows the lateral edge of biceps and then medial edge of deltoid towards coracoid; be aware of the lateral cutaneous nerve of the forearm (branch of the musculocutaneous nerve) interval is between brachioradialis and biceps.

Then the deltopectoral interval.

Q 6: What nerves are at risk during the anterior approach?

Median (distally), posterior interosseous nerve (in proximal forearm), lateral cutaneous nerve of forearm (lateral side of elbow) and radial nerve (upper arm).

Q 7: Where would you apply the plate to the humerus?

There are anterolateral, medial and posterior surfaces of the humerus – a plate is usually applied to the lateral side if performing an anterior approach and the posterior surface if a posterior approach is used. Anterolateral is good from proximal to distal fifth, posterior good for middle and distal fractures. Posteriorly the plate has to slide under the radial nerve.

The AO website has excellent intraoperative drawings and tips on surgical technique.

Q 8: What plate size would you use?

3.5 or 4.5 DCP.

This may lead on to a discussion of what is a plate, what is a screw, what are the features of a screw. You should be able to describe all these pieces of orthopaedic hardware.

Structured oral examination question 4: Posterior approach to the knee

Q 1: A patient is admitted with an injury. Describe your initial steps in management. (Figure 13.4.)
ATLS, neurovascular assessment.

Usually the examiners do not want a great deal of detail about ATLS assessment, they want to get to the orthopaedic details, but be prepared to answer questions on fluid resuscitation in the paediatric patients.

Q 2: The patient has a cold foot, no peripheral pulse and altered sensation. What is the management?

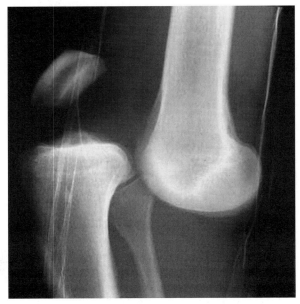

Figure 13.4 Knee dislocation.

Reduce the knee, possibly under sedation.

Q 3: Now what?
Reassess neurovascular status.

Q 4: The patient's foot is still cold with possibly a faint pulse. Any other tests you want to do?
ABPI – need to know what ratio is good/bad (> 0.9 rules out significant arterial injury).
Arteriogram – would you delay surgery if imaging will take 2 hours?

There is some debate about whether all patients should have an arteriogram but there are papers that have demonstrated good outcomes using clinical assessment and selective arteriography.

Try to have evidence to back up your answer, if you can quote a paper such as the one below you will be on your way to a 7.

Stannard JP, Sheils TM, Lopez-Ben RR *et al.* Vascular injuries in knee dislocations: the role of physical examination in determining the need for arteriography. *J Bone Joint Surg Am* 2004;**86-A**:910–915.

Q 5: The vascular surgeon is 1 hour away. He wants you to start the posterior approach to the popliteal fossa.
In reality it would be very rare to have to perform this approach but it is said to be quite commonly asked in the vivas.

Q 6: How do you position the patient?
Prone position.

Q 7: Anything you might do before positioning to make your life easier?
Apply a tourniquet.

Q 8: What landmarks do you use for the skin incision?
The two heads of gastrocnemius muscle from the posterior femoral surface just above the medial and lateral condyles. Semimembranous and semitendinous on the medial border of the popliteal fossa. Curved incision, starting laterally over biceps femoris, obliquely across popliteal fossa, downwards over medial gastrocnemius.

Q 9: What structures are you looking for to guide you in this approach?
Identify the short saphenous vein, on lateral side of the vein is the medial sural cutaneous nerve, trace the nerve to its origin from the tibial nerve in the apex of the popliteal fossa.

At the apex the common peroneal nerve separates from the tibial nerve, identify and protect this. Deep to the tibial nerve are the popliteal artery and vein.

Q 10: Where is the artery in relation to the vein?
The vein lies medial to the artery as it enters the popliteal fossa distally, then it comes to lie posteriorly (superficial) to the artery in the fossa.

Structured oral examination question 5: Posterolateral approach to the ankle

Q 1: Describe this fracture. (Figure 13.5.)
These are AP and lateral views of a right ankle demonstrating a trimalleolar ankle fracture. There is talar shift and significant displacement of the posterior malleolus.

Q 2: What classification systems do you know to describe ankle fractures?
The Weber system.

Q 3: Please expand on this.
The Weber classification describes the fracture in relation to the syndesmosis between the tibia and fibula.

Weber A fractures occur below the syndesmosis.
Weber B fractures occur at the level of the syndesmosis.
Weber C fractures occur above the syndesmosis.

Q 4: Do you know of another classification systems based on mechanism of injury?
That would be the Lauge Hansen system.

Q 5: How would you classify this fracture and what is the sequence of injury to the ankle?
This is a supination external rotation injury.
The first injury is to the anterior tibiofibular ligament, then a fracture of the fibula, followed by rupture of the posterior tibiofibular ligaments and then injury to the medial side, either a fracture of the medial malleolus or rupture of the deltoid ligament.

(b)

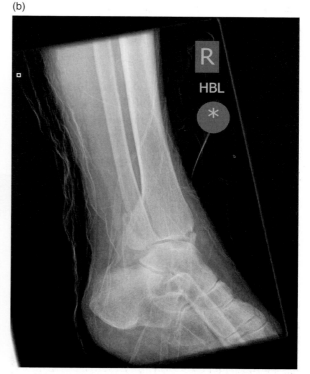

(a)

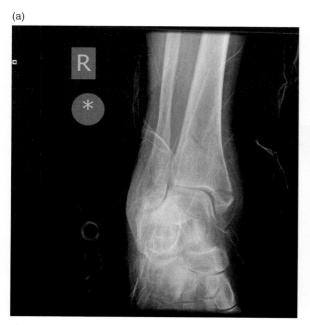

Figures 13.5a and 13.5b Anteroposterior (AP) and lateral radiographs of trimalleolar fractured ankle with a large displaced posterior malleolar fragment.

Q 6: What direction is the fracture of the fibula?
I don't know.

It is important to recognize that the direction of the fibular fracture in an SER injury is distal anterior to proximal posterior. In the pronation external rotation injury the fracture line runs proximal anterior to distal posterior.

Q 7: How would you fix this fracture?
Answer options:

1. Reduce and fix fibula. If post malleolus reduces fix PM with AP screws.
2. Reduce PM through # site. Fix with AP screws.
3. Reduce and fix PM through posterolateral approach.

The posterior malleolus does not reduce when the fibula is reduced therefore you decide to perform a posterolateral approach to the ankle to reduce and fix the fragment under direct vision.

You could say that you are not familiar with this approach and you would prefer to use one of the other approaches above which is acceptable as long as you know it well and how to reduce and fix the fracture using this approach.

Q 8: Describe the steps and NV interval.

Position prone.
Tourniquet.
Skin incision halfway between fibula and Achilles tendon, from tip of fibula to 10 cm proximal.
Preserve the sural nerve and short saphenous veins that run just behind the lateral malleolus.

Incise the deep fascia and identify the peroneal tendons, retract these laterally and anteriorly. Incise the fibres of the flexor hallucis longus over its lateral border and retract it medially, incise the periosteum longitudinally to reach the fracture site.

Q 9: What internervous plane are you utilizing?
Between peroneus brevis (superficial peroneal nerve) and flexor hallucis longus (tibial nerve).

Q 10: Can you extend this approach proximally?
Yes, by extending the skin incision and then developing the interval between the peroneal muscles laterally and the gastrosoleus complex medially.

If you get this far you are getting a good pass.

Structured oral examination question 6: Anterior approach to cervical spine

A patient presents with an 8-week history of severe and worsening pain radiating from his neck down his arm into his hand. He has pins and needles affecting his thumb and index finger.

Q 1: What nerve root is probably affected?
C6.

Q 2: What weakness might you expect to find?
Weakness in wrist extension.

Q 3: Yes, which muscles are weak?
ERCL and ERCB.

Q 4: Where is the most reliable place to test for C6 sensory change?
I'm not sure, on the back of the hand?

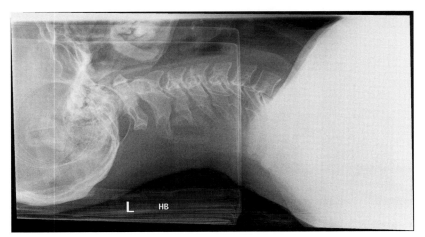

Figure 13.6 Radiograph of a normal cervical spine.

The back of the hand is not precise enough, The American Spinal Injury Association Guidelines and the ATLS guidelines are that the most reliable place is on the volar surface of the proximal phalanx of the thumb.

Q 5:   An MRI scan shows a cervical disc prolapse. What is the standard surgical procedure for treatment of intractable pain resulting from this condition?

Anterior discectomy and fusion.

Q 6:   What is the approach to the anterior cervical spine?

This is another approach that unless you are going to be a spinal surgeon you are unlikely to come across, however it is another classic approach and you should at least know the intervals.

Position – supine with sandbag between shoulder blades, turn head away from incision site, sit the patient by 30°.
Landmarks.
Mandible – C2/3.
Hyoid – C3.
Thyroid cartilage – C4/5.
Cricoid cartilage – C6.
Carotid tubercule – C6.
Skin incision, transverse collar at level of pathology (see levels above) from midline to posterior border of sternocleidomastoid (SCM).
Incise fascia over platysma in line with the skin incision and split the fibres of platysma longitudinally.

Identify the anterior border of SCM and incise fascia immediately anterior to it.
Retract SCM laterally and the strap muscles medially.
    Carotid sheath can now be identified.
Develop a plane between the medial side of the carotid sheath and the midline structures (thyroid, trachea and oesophagus) by cutting the pretracheal fascia on the medial side of the sheath.
Retract the sheath and SCM laterally.
Watch for the superior and inferior thyroid arteries which run transversely and may limit dissection above C3/4.
Develop a plane behind the pretracheal fascia and behind the oesophagus.

Q 7:   What structures are at risk during this approach?

The prevertebral fascia and longus coli muscle should now be seen and after splitting them longitudinally the anterior longitudinal ligament and the cervical vertebra can be identified.
The carotid sheath and its contents.
The vertebral artery.
The recurrent laryngeal nerve and the sympathetic chain.

Q 8:   What is the result of damage to the recurrent laryngeal nerve?

If one side is damaged the patient develops a hoarse voice, if both sides are damaged the patient can be left aphonic and have breathing difficulty.

Pathology

Sunit Patil

Structured oral examination question 1

EXAMINER: A 45-year-old gentleman comes to your clinic with right hip pain. This is the radiograph of his hip. What are your thoughts? (Figure 14.1.)

CANDIDATE: This is an anteroposterior (AP) radiograph of the pelvis with both hips included. There is flattening of the right femoral head with areas of sclerosis and cystic changes in keeping with osteonecrosis. I would like to know the history and clinical findings; in particular, I would want to know if there is a history of alcohol abuse, steroid use, trauma or systemic illness such as sickle cell disease.

EXAMINER: What is the micropathology in osteonecrosis?

CANDIDATE: The micropathology can be divided into three phases:

1. Mechanical phase: This involves intra-osseous occlusion of microvasculature, usually as a result of fat emboli.
2. Chemical phase: These fat emboli are acted upon by lipase resulting in free fatty acid and prostaglandin formation.
3. Thrombotic phase: The prostaglandin formation stimulates focal intravascular coagulation and platelet aggregation.

EXAMINER: How would you manage this patient?

CANDIDATE: The management of this patient would depend on how symptomatic the patient is and the stage of the disease process. In this case subchondral collapse has already occurred with arthritic changes (Ficat stage 4). I would like to get a lateral radiograph as well. My aim of treatment would be to provide a pain-free hip joint. Initial treatment would be in the form of adequate analgesia and use of a walking stick in the opposite hand. If the pain persists and is not controlled with the above measures, I would offer the patient a total hip replacement.

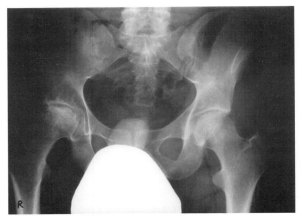

Figure 14.1 Anteroposterior (AP) radiograph pelvis demonstrating AVN right hip.

EXAMINER: Are you aware of any other non-operative treatment in patients with osteonecrosis?

CANDIDATE: Bisphosphonates have been used in patients with osteonecrosis. A paper by Agarwala et al. showed that use of alendronate significantly reduces the progression of osteonecrosis and the need for a hip replacement especially in the pre-collapse phase.[1] In Ficat stage 3 it may delay the need for a hip replacement. However, in this case where arthritis has set in, I do not think bisphosphonates would be of any significant benefit.

EXAMINER: Which hip replacement would you choose in this patient?

CANDIDATE: I would perform a cemented hip replacement: UHMWPE cup with a cemented taper polished stem with a metal-on-polyethylene bearing surface.

EXAMINER: Are you aware of any evidence of results of hip replacement in osteonecrosis?

CANDIDATE: Saito et al. showed that the results of THA in osteonecrosis were much inferior to those in osteoarthritis.[2] However, I am unaware of a good study comparing the two with implants that have a proven good track record. DeKam et al. reported on the use of the Exeter stem in patients under the age of 40 years, many of whom had osteonecrosis, and reported a 100% survival of the stem at a mean 7 years.[3]

Michael Mont has extensively studied AVN. In one paper he reviewed various studies and reported wide differences in failure rates of THA of between 10–50% at 5 years. Furthermore in his systematic review of 27 published series, all except two studies reported a higher rate of failure in patients with AVN than in age matched patients with other disorders.[4]

EXAMINER: Why would you use a cemented cup in a 40-year-old?

CANDIDATE: I am more comfortable using a cemented cup. Moreover, all joint registries, to my knowledge, have shown good results with cemented cups.

EXAMINER: Are you not worried about wear?

CANDIDATE: Yes, wear is a problem. However, results of the low-profile cemented cup show a 15-year survival of 91.7%.[5] The Exeter stem survival has been shown to be excellent, as quoted before.

[DEBRIEF: I thought I did well. The viva started with the basics in osteonecrosis. I tried to bring in the literature I knew, to score points and avoided complicated classifications. I stuck to what I had decided – cemented Exeter THA for almost all cases. You could argue using hybrid or cementless THA.]

1. Agarwala S, Shah S, Joshi VR. The use of alendronate in the treatment of avascular necrosis of the femoral head: follow-up to eight years. J Bone Joint Surg Br 2009; 91–B:1013–1018.

2. Saito S, Saito M, Nishina T et al. Long-term results of total hip arthroplasty for osteonecrosis of the femoral head. A comparison with osteoarthritis. Clin Orthop Relat Res 1989;244:198–207.

3. DeKam DCJ, Klarenbeek RLWA, Gardeniers JWM et al. The medium-term results of the cemented Exeter femoral component in patients under 40 years of age. J Bone Joint Surg Br 2008;90-B:1417–1421.

4. Mont M, Hungerford D. Current concepts review: non-traumatic avascular necrosis of the femoral head. J Bone Joint Surg Am 1995;77-A:459–474.

5. Veitch SW, Whitehouse SL, Howell JR et al. The concentric all-polyethylene Exeter acetabular component in primary total hip replacement. J Bone Joint Surg Br 2010;92-B:1351–1355.

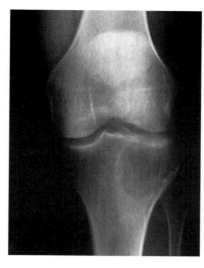

Figure 14.2
Anteroposterior (AP) radiograph knee demon-strating lytic lesion lateral tibial condyle.

Structured oral examination question 2

EXAMINER: Have a look at this radiograph and tell me what you see. (Figure 14.2.)

CANDIDATE: This is an AP radiograph of the knee showing a well-defined eccentric lytic lesion in the metaphysis of the lateral tibial condyle effacing the subchondral bone. This lesion would be classed as IA based on Lodwick's classification as it has a geographic margin with a sclerotic rim (IB is a geographic margin without a sclerotic rim, IC is ill-defined, II is moth-eaten and III is a permeative lesion). There is no obvious matrix I can see within the lesion and no evidence of a periosteal reaction. I would like to see a lateral radiograph and take a full history and examine the patient. (Figure 14.3.)

EXAMINER: The patient has been complaining of a dull ache in the knee for the past 12 months. He was treated with quadriceps-strengthening exercises which did not help. He then underwent an arthroscopy and was told that there was nothing wrong with his knee. On examination he has tenderness over the lateral tibial plateau and a full range of movement. How would you manage him?

CANDIDATE: The aim of treatment here is provide the patient with a painless functional joint. The principles involved here would be firstly to establish the diagnosis and then plan the treatment. I would like to investigate this patient by getting an urgent MRI. I would splint him and keep him non-weightbearing. I would then discuss the images with our local tumour service.

EXAMINER: I do not have the MRI scan here, but it showed that the tumour was contained within the tibia. What is your differential diagnosis?

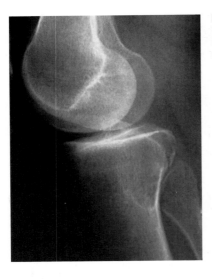

Figure 14.3
Lateral radiograph knee demon-strating lytic lesion.

CANDIDATE: My first differential diagnosis would be a giant cell tumour, followed by aneurysmal bone cyst, chondromyxoid fibroma, non-ossifying fibroma. Other possibilities are fibrous dysplasia, low-grade chondrosarcoma and eosinophilic granuloma, metastatic tumour and Brodie's abscess.

EXAMINER: Do you not think this could be a malignant bone tumour?

CANDIDATE: This is unlikely to be a malignant bone tumour because of a longstanding history, radiological appearances of a well-defined geographic margin with a surrounding rind of sclerosis and no periosteal reaction.

EXAMINER: The local tumour surgeon looks at the scans and tells you that it is a giant cell tumour. What would be your plan of action?

CANDIDATE: The next stage would be to establish tissue diagnosis by means of a needle or open biopsy. This should ideally be performed by the surgeon who is going to carry out the definitive procedure. However the principles are:

Incision should be the shortest possible and longitudinal. It should be sited such that the biopsy site could be excised as a part of the definitive surgical incision.

There should be minimum dissection to avoid contamination of planes.

The biopsy should be performed along the advancing edge of the tumour so that the central area of necrosis is avoided.

Good haemostasis should be achieved. If a drain has to be used, it should be brought out close to the incision and in line with it.

Skin sutures should be placed close to the edges to avoid contamination.

Specimen should be sent for histology as well as culture.

EXAMINER: It is established that this is a GCT. What are the principles of treating it?

CANDIDATE: Surgical treatment consists of curettage and extending the margins with the use of a high-speed burr. Bone graft is then placed in the subchondral region and the cavity is filled with bone cement. This serves two purposes: the heat generated helps in killing the tumour cells and recurrence is easily spotted on radiographs as the cement acts as a contrast.

EXAMINER: What is the risk of recurrence?

CANDIDATE: About 10–15% when margins are extended using a high speed burr (15–55% with simple curettage).[1,2]

EXAMINER: If you do get a recurrence 1 year postoperatively, what would be your plan of action?

CANDIDATE: I would investigate using an MRI scan and assess the status of the joint. If the joint is salvageable, I would repeat the same procedure again. If, however, the joint is not salvageable, then the treatment options are wide excision and knee fusion or tumour knee prosthesis.

[DEBRIEF: This scenario went well. I thought I kept talking for most of the time.]

This is a standard question which should be prepared in great detail by all candidates sitting the FRCS (Tr & Orth).

1. Klenke FM, Wenger DE, Inwards CY, Rose PS, Sim FH. Giant cell tumor of bone: risk factors for recurrence. *Clin Orthop Rel Res* 2011;**469**(2):591–599.

2. Prosser G, Baloch K, Tillman RM, Carter SR, Grimer RJ. Does curettage without adjuvant therapy provide low recurrence rates in giant-cell tumors of bone? *Clin Orthop Rel Res* 2005;**435**:211–218.

Structured oral examination question 3

EXAMINER: You are asked to see a patient in casualty with a 3-year history of backache that has got worse over the past 2 days. The patient has developed increasing right-sided leg pain and urinary incontinence over the past 10 hours. How would you proceed?

CANDIDATE: This patient has got a cauda equina syndrome unless proven otherwise. I would arrange an urgent MRI scan and make plans to take her to theatre as soon as possible.

EXAMINER: Would you not want to examine the patient before getting an MRI?

CANDIDATE: Yes I would. I would examine her spine and carry out a detailed neurological examination including sensory and motor function as well as deep and superficial tendon reflexes.

EXAMINER: Anything you would want to know in the history, particularly in this case?

CANDIDATE: Time since the start of symptoms, previous history of a similar problem, previous back surgery.

EXAMINER: I told you that the patient has developed incontinence over the last 10 hours. What findings would confirm a cauda equina syndrome?

CANDIDATE: Perianal anaesthesia, poor anal tone, weakness in toe and/or ankle dorsiflexors.

EXAMINER: What is cauda equina syndrome and what causes it?

CANDIDATE: Cauda equina syndrome is a condition that results from compression of the nerve roots below the termination of the spinal cord often resulting in bladder dysfunction and loss of perianal sensation. The causes include large disc prolapse, spinal stenosis and fractures to the lumbar spine.

EXAMINER: Any other cause, especially if the patient has a history of cancer?

CANDIDATE: Metastatic lesions.

EXAMINER: This is the MRI scan of the patient. What are your thoughts? (Figure 14.4.)

CANDIDATE: This is a T2-weighted sagittal section of the lumbar spine showing an extruded L5–S1 disc. I would like to see the transverse section.

EXAMINER: Here it is. (Figure 14.5.)

The images show a large extruded L5–S1 disc compressing the cauda equina and the exiting L5 root. This confirms the diagnosis.

EXAMINER: This patient is seen at 22:00 by you at a DGH. What is your management plan?

CANDIDATE: The aim of treatment is to restore normal neurology by relieving the compression caused by the large extruded disc. Ideally this should be performed as soon as possible. I would refer this patient to a spinal surgeon.

EXAMINER: Have you seen this operation?

CANDIDATE: No.

EXAMINER: What are the principles of the operation?

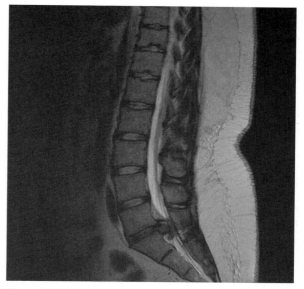

Figure 14.4 T2-weighted MRI sagittal image lumbar spine.

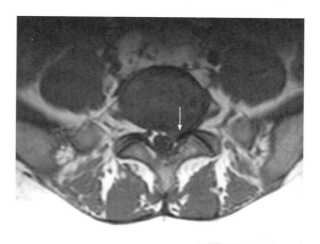

Figure 14.5 T2-weighted transverse MRI image lumbar spine.

CANDIDATE: The principle is to relieve the compression of the cauda.

EXAMINER: How would you position the patient?

CANDIDATE: Prone.

[DEBRIEF: The question did not go well at all.]

If the examiner is doing most of the talking, you are going downhill. If the question is open ended, e.g. 'What do you think ... etc.', seize the opportunity and keep talking in a systematic way. Never jump onto investigations before going through the phrase- 'I would like to take a detailed history and examine the patient.' Here the candidate failed to pick up on the clue of red flag signs in the history. This must be asked in relation to any patient with a spinal problem. In general, examiners do not like the phrase 'I would refer this patient to a subspecialist', except for bone tumours. Have a tactful way of saying it, if you have to, such as: 'I have limited operative experience in this procedure and would like to get help from one of my colleagues who specializes in this procedure. The principles of treatment are: . . .' In this scenario, the ideal answer would have been to start off with taking a good history including red flag signs, clinical examination with special emphasis on perianal sensation and anal tone. This would avoid the regular prompting the examiner had to undertake.

With regards to the operative treatment, if you have not done a spine job, go and see a few discectomies and decompressions. You will be able to describe the procedure much more confidently if you have seen it performed. Current consensus on the timing of surgery is that it should be done as soon as it is safe to do so. Delay beyond 48 hours from onset of symptoms has poor outcome (British Association of Spine Surgeons website).

Structured oral examination question 4

EXAMINER: A 58-year-old lady is brought to A&E with a history of a fall in the bathroom. These are the radiographs obtained in casualty. What are your thoughts? (Figures 14.6, 14.7.)

CANDIDATE: This is an AP and a lateral radiograph of the right hip and proximal femur showing a displaced spiral subtrochanteric fracture. There is a mottled appearance to both the proximal and distal fragments around the fracture indicating that this is most likely a pathological fracture. I would like to take a detailed history and carry out a full clinical examination. In the history I would like to know whether the patient does have a primary malignancy.

EXAMINER: The patient does not have a history of malignancy. She did have some pain in the right hip for the past 4 weeks, but was able to mobilize with the help of a stick. She is otherwise in good health.

CANDIDATE: I would like to know if she noticed any lumps or bumps anywhere in the body, whether she has been losing

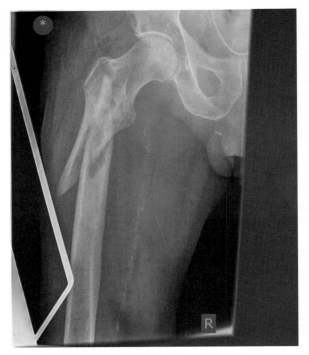

Figure 14.6 Anteroposterior (AP) radiograph right hip demonstrating subtrochanteric fracture femur.

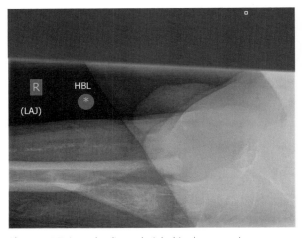

Figure 14.7 Lateral radiograph right hip demonstrating subtrochanteric fracture femur.

weight and whether she has had haematuria, haemoptysis, malena, blood in the stools, altered bowel habits. I would clinically examine her breasts and thyroid, abdomen and chest.

I would provide her with adequate analgesia and apply a Thomas splint. Before moving her to the ward, I would get a full-length view of the femur. I would then admit her and investigate her further in order to establish the cause of her pathological fracture.

The investigations I would request would include:

1. Blood tests: FBC, LFTs, s. Calcium, electrolytes, s. Alkaline phosphatase, electrophoresis for M Band, tumour markers (CA 15–3 for breast Ca, CA125, CEA) only if available.
2. Radiological investigations: CT abdomen and pelvis, CT chest: both to assess the primary and to evaluate metastases if present.
3. Bone scan: This need not be performed if the patient would have to wait for a few days as it usually does not change the management.

EXAMINER: The CT chest and abdomen shows that there is a small cell carcinoma of the lung with metastases to the liver.

CANDIDATE: I would discuss her case in a multidisciplinary team meeting, thereby involving the clinical oncologist, thoracic surgeons and physiotherapists. I would want to know the prognosis of the tumour and whether the primary tumour is operable. Treatment of her femoral shaft fracture would involve maintaining length, alignment and rotation and providing a stable fixation to enable her to mobilize. I would aim to achieve this using a cephalomedullary device.

EXAMINER: Would you consider proximal femoral replacement?

CANDIDATE: Not in this case, as the patient already has systemic metastases. The prognosis from a small cell carcinoma of the lung is usually poor. I would want to get the patient up and about as soon as I can. Femoral fixation is mainly for palliative reasons.

EXAMINER: Are you aware of any evidence comparing proximal femoral replacement/arthroplasty versus fixation of proximal third femoral fractures?

CANDIDATE: Wedin and Bauer noted that endoprosthetic replacement had lower reoperation rate at 2 years than osteosynthesis and therefore should be considered for metastasis from malignancies with a good survival e.g. breast and prostate cancer.[1]

EXAMINER: She was fixed with a Recoin nail with additional circulage fixation around the fracture shaft to aid fracture reduction. These are her II films. (Figure 14.8.)

The examiners are looking for a logical approach. BOA guidelines, though slightly old, are worth mentioning. In an event where despite all investigations no primary is found and there is no evidence of metastasis, MRI +/− biopsy of the lesion is a

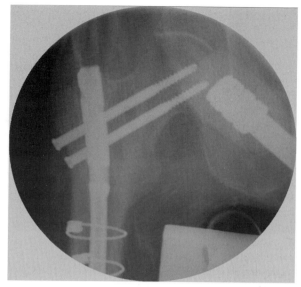

Figure 14.8 II image demonstrating Recoin nail fixation fracture.

reasonable approach after consultation with the tumour service.

1. Wedin R, Bauer HCF. Surgical treatment of skeletal metastatic lesions of the proximal femur: endoprosthesis or reconstruction nail? *J Bone Joint Surg Br* 2005; **87-B**:1653–1657.

Structured oral examination question 5

EXAMINER: This 48-year-old lady came to the clinic with pain in both sides of the groin and a limp. This is her X-ray. (Figure 14.9.)

CANDIDATE: This is an AP radiograph of the pelvis with both hips showing osteoarthritis changes. I would like to see a lateral radiograph and take a detailed history with special emphasis on the severity of pain, night pain, walking distance, need for analgesics and restriction of functional activities. I would examine her hip and assess presence or absence of a fixed flexion deformity, painful hip movements and neurological status.

EXAMINER: Examination confirms painful restricted hip movements. She has normal neurology. She is a very active lady and works as a teacher. The hip pain is restricting her activities significantly and is not controlled with a full dose of codeine and paracetamol. What is your plan of action?

CANDIDATE: I would offer her a total hip replacement on the worse side first. My choice of hip replacement would be a

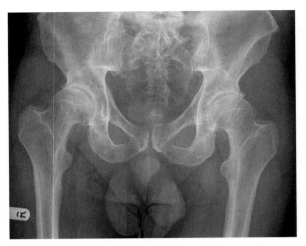

Figure 14.9 Anteroposterior (AP) radiograph demonstrating osteoarthritis.

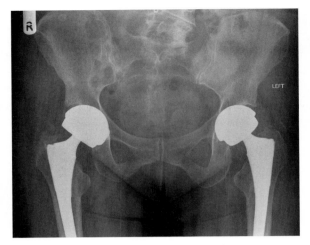

Figure 14.10 Anteroposterior (AP) radiograph demonstrating bilateral THR.

cemented UHMWPE cup and a taper polished collarless cemented stem. The bearing surface would be metal-on-polyethylene.

EXAMINER: The patient wants a long-lasting hip replacement and asks you about the longevity of the hip replacement. What would you tell her about the longevity of your hip replacement?

CANDIDATE: I would explain to her that it is likely that she would need a revision hip arthroplasty at some point in the future. Lewthwaite et al. reviewed 130 Exeter hip replacements in patients younger than 50 years of age.[1] They found that at a mean follow-up of 12.5 years, the stem survival was 100% if aseptic loosening was taken as the end point. Nine cups were revised for aseptic loosening (93.08% survival at a mean 12.5 years). Carrington et al. showed that the survivorship of the universal Exeter stem was 100% at a mean follow-up of 15.7 years.[2] With regards to the cemented polyethylene cup, Veitch et al. showed the survivorship (taking revision for aseptic loosening as the endpoint) at a mean of 15 years was 91.7% with the low/high profile cups.[3] Currently, all joint registries show that the survivorship of the cemented cup is better than that of the uncemented cup. According to the NJR report, the 5-year revision rate after a cemented cup is about 2%.

EXAMINER: Have a look at this radiograph. This lady underwent a bilateral staged total hip replacement. Can you comment on the prostheses used? (Figure 14.10.)

CANDIDATE: This is an AP radiograph of the pelvis with both hips. The patient has undergone a large head metal-on-metal uncemented hip replacement. The cup inclination appears satisfactory on both sides (about 40–45°). There is no lucency around the stem or cup.

EXAMINER: This lady presented to the clinic 3 years following her right THR with a groin swelling and persistent pain in the groin. The radiograph was taken at the time. What are your thoughts?

CANDIDATE: I would be concerned about the possibility of adverse reaction to metal debris (ARMD) as a result of the bearing surface that has been used. The radiograph does not show any osteolysis. I would examine the patient with regards to distal neurovascular status and discuss the case with my radiology colleagues in regard to further imaging.

EXAMINER: There was no neurovascular deficit but her thigh was quite swollen. An ultrasound scan showed that the swelling contained fluid and it arose from the hip replacement. What is your management plan?

CANDIDATE: Firstly, I would like to rule out infection. I would perform a full blood count, CRP, ESR. I would also discuss the scenario with the patient and aspirate her hip in theatre. I would also send her blood for metal ion levels.

EXAMINER: There is no evidence of infection. Blood cobalt and chromium ions are markedly raised.

CANDIDATE: This is a difficult situation. The most likely diagnosis here is ARMD. Given the fact that the patient is symptomatic, I would offer her a revision hip replacement.

EXAMINER: What problems are you likely to encounter?

CANDIDATE: The implants may be well fixed and difficult to explant. There may be large amounts of bone loss on the acetabular side which may necessitate use of bone graft.

EXAMINER: Would you revise both the stem and the cup?

CANDIDATE: If the stem is well fixed, I would not revise it. The aim here is to change the bearing surface. It is thought that the reason for failure of large head metal-on-metal hip replacement is from the wear arising from the trunnion. By replacing the cup and the head, both issues would be addressed.

[DEBRIEF: The viva went well.]

Examiner's thoughts: The candidate had a clear idea of what he would do in a very common day-to-day problem. He straight away volunteered the literature he knew. He was able to talk about ARMD and further management plans.

Each candidate must have a clear management plan for patients with hip OA. You can justify using many prostheses in this situation. It is best to back it up with literature and fight your ground.

1. Lewthwaite SC, Squires B, Gie GA, Timperley AJ, Ling RS. The Exeter Universal hip in patients 50 years or younger at 10-17 years followup. *Clin Orthop Rel Res* 2008;**466**(2):324–331.

2. Carrington N, Sierra R, Gie GA *et al.* The Exeter Universal cemented femoral component at 15 to 17 years: an update on the first 325 hips. *J Bone Joint Surg Br* 2009;**91-B**:730–737.

3. Veitch SW, Whitehouse SL, Howell JR *et al.* The concentric all-polyethylene Exeter acetabular component in primary total hip replacement. *J Bone Joint Surg Br* 2010;**92-B**:1351–1355.

Structured oral examination question 6

EXAMINER: A 62-year-old lady presents to your clinic with a 2-year history of knee pain and deformity. She takes regular paracetamol and codeine but is still woken up every other night with pain. She can walk about 300–400 yards on a bad day and about a mile on a good day after which she has to stop. These are the radiographs of her knee. (Figures 14.11, 14.12.) How would you manage the case?

CANDIDATE: This is an AP and a lateral radiograph of the knee showing arthritic changes predominantly affecting the lateral and patellofemoral compartments. There is a valgus deformity of about 20°. I do not know if these are weightbearing films, but if they are not, I would request them. I would also want to

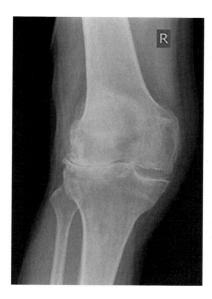

Figure 14.11 Anteroposterior (AP) radiograph demonstrating osteoarthritis right knee.

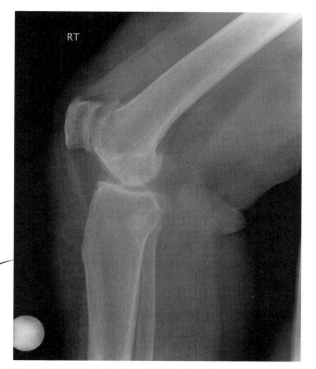

Figure 14.12 Lateral radiograph right knee demonstrating osteoarthritis.

see the skyline view. I would like some more information on the history, particularly with regards to any hip/groin pain, history of rheumatoid arthritis and history of any other medical problems before planning the treatment.

EXAMINER: She is fit and well and has no hip pain.

CANDIDATE: I would like to examine the patient and assess her gait. Presence of a varus thrust would indicate an incompetent medial collateral ligament. I would want to know if there is a fixed flexion deformity in the knee and whether the valgus deformity is correctable. I would assess if the MCL is competent, hip movements are pain free, patellar tracking is normal or not and whether there is any distal neurovascular deficit.

EXAMINER: There is no varus thrust and the MCL is clinically intact. The valgus is partially correctable. Hip movements are normal and there is no distal neurovascular deficit. Patellar tracking is normal. What is your management plan?

CANDIDATE: Given the level of discomfort the patient is in, I would offer her a knee replacement.

EXAMINER: [Interrupts] Describe how you would perform the operation.

CANDIDATE: In an appropriately consented and marked patient, I would perform a team brief explaining to the anaesthetist that the operation would take about 60–90 minutes. I would use a tourniquet and would require prophylactic antibiotics at induction.

EXAMINER: [Interrupts again] What prostheses are you going to use?

CANDIDATE: I would use the AGC knee (Biomet) as I am familiar with it and the literature supports its longevity (97.8% survival at 20 years) and good results.[1] I would have templated the knee to the sizes required. Though I expect to have balanced the knee in this case at the end of the operation, I would ensure that I have the revision system and in the worst-case scenario a rotating hinged knee available.

EXAMINER: Talk me through the steps of the operation.

CANDIDATE: Patient would be supine with a high thigh tourniquet. After the patient is appropriately prepped, I would perform a midline incision over the knee and a lateral parapatellar approach in this case.

EXAMINER: [Interrupts] Why a lateral parapatellar approach?

CANDIDATE: In my experience, I feel that this approach makes balancing a valgus knee much easier as most of the releases are performed as a part of the approach.

I would expose the knee joint and displace the patella medially. I would then use an intramedullary jig to resect the distal femur. Usually, I would use a 5° valgus jig. Once the

distal femur is resected, it is easier to reflect the patella. I normally insert a tibial pin into the tibial tuberosity to avoid avulsion of the patellar tendon. I would then size the femur using posterior referencing, bearing in mind that the lateral femoral condyle would be deficient. I would use the inter-epicondylar axis as well as Whiteside's line to assist me with the rotation.

EXAMINER: What would you do if the femur is between sizes?

CANDIDATE: It depends; if the size is very close to the larger size, I would choose to go with it; if it is too close to the smaller size, I would accept the possibility of a small notch and go with the smaller size. I would however check with the angel's wing before making the cut. If it is truly in between, I would use anterior referencing and downsize the femur. This would avoid notching, but would create a slightly bigger flexion gap. I may be able to counter this by reducing the slope on the tibia.

EXAMINER: Okay, so you have done all your cuts. You now find that the knee is tight laterally (on varus stressing). It is extending completely and is not tight in flexion. What is your next step?

CANDIDATE: As a part of my approach I would have released the iliotibial band and lateral capsule. If these have not been released adequately, I would release them. I would then release the popliteus and the lateral collateral ligament subperiosteally from the lateral femoral condyle. If the knee is not yet balanced, then I would resect the proximal fibula. These steps have been described by Fiddian et al.[2] I have never had to consider the last step.

EXAMINER: You now have noticed that you have been overzealous in your lateral release and the knee is unstable in flexion and extension. You also notice that the MCL is incompetent. What is your next step?

CANDIDATE: In that scenario, I think it may be difficult to balance even with a high tibial post (semi-constrained) knee replacement. I would then decide to go with a constrained rotating hinge knee replacement. The results published by Petrou et al. show a 96.1% survival at 15 years and 91% good-to-excellent results.[3]

[DEBRIEF: The scenario went well, though the examiner kept on interrupting.]

The candidate got out all the information including the literature. This is not an uncommon scenario. You may get asked to describe the steps of a knee replacement, hip replacement, ankle fusion etc. The important thing to remember is to have a sequence and to demonstrate to the examiner that you have done the procedure. So use phrases such as 'I would position the image intensifier in this way, etc.' Lateral parapatellar approach is not used by all. If you are familiar with the medial parapatellar approach, that's fine. Remember, you would be asked finer details about hip and knee replacement.

1. Ritter M. The Anatomical Graduated Component total knee replacement: a long-term evaluation with 20-year survival analysis. *J Bone Joint Surg Br* 2009;**91-B**:745–749.

2. Fiddian N, Blakeway C, Kumar A. Replacement arthroplasty of the valgus knee: a modified lateral capsular approach with repositioning of vastus lateralis. *J Bone Joint Surg Br* 1998;**80-B**:859–861.

3. Petrou G, Petrou H, Tilkeridis C *et al*. Medium-term results with a primary cemented rotating-hinge total knee replacement. *J Bone Joint Surg Br* 2004;**86-B**:813–817.

Structured oral examination question 7

EXAMINER: A 22-year-old basketball player has come to casualty with severe pain in his right shoulder as he reached out to collect the ball. He is unable to move his shoulder. He has had two previous dislocations and feels that this is another one. This is his X-ray. (Figure 14.13.) The A&E SHO is unable to reduce the dislocation and asks you to come over. How are you going to manage this patient?

CANDIDATE: I would firstly make sure that the patient's airway, breathing and circulation are okay. I would ask him whether he has any other injuries.

EXAMINER: This is his only injury.

CANDIDATE: I would examine him for distal neurovascular deficit, particularly looking for sensation in regimental badge area and distal radial pulse.

EXAMINER: Would you expect a brachial plexus injury with this low-velocity injury and in someone who has recurrent dislocations?

CANDIDATE: It would be unusual.

EXAMINER: How would you reduce the dislocation?

CANDIDATE: I have usually tried to reduce these dislocations with the Kocher's manoeuvre. With adequate analgesia, I attempt to externally rotate the adducted arm while keeping the patient engaged in a conversation. I then flex the shoulder in the sagittal plane and then internally rotate the shoulder.

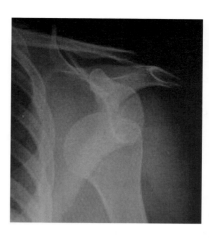

Figure 14.13 Anteroposterior (AP) radiograph dislocated right shoulder.

This usually works well in recurrent dislocations and when the patient is relatively relaxed.

EXAMINER: You still cannot reduce the dislocation. The patient has just had a sandwich as he was waiting in the A&E reception. What would you do next?

CANDIDATE: I would ensure that the patient has adequate analgesia on board. I would be tempted to use intra-articular lidocaine to provide adequate analgesia if it was not already given. An RCT by Miller *et al.* showed that this is a safe and effective method.[1] A systematic review concluded that this should be the first method to be used.[2]

I would then use the traction–countertraction method described by Matsen. I would apply traction in abduction as my colleague uses a sheet around the chest wall and axilla as countertraction. Gentle internal rotation would aid reduction.

EXAMINER: Despite this you cannot reduce the joint.

CANDIDATE: My last option before taking the patient who is not nil by mouth to theatre would be to consider the Stimson technique. I would lay the patient prone and attach a weight of about 10 pounds to his wrist. Over a period of 5–10 minutes the joint often relocates.

EXAMINER: The shoulder does eventually relocate. This is the check X-ray done when you see him in your clinic in a week's time. Describe the X-ray. (Figure 14.14.)

CANDIDATE: This is an AP radiograph of the glenohumeral joint. It does show that the joint is well reduced. There appears to be a Hill–Sach's lesion.

EXAMINER: What is your management plan?

CANDIDATE: I would examine the patient again with special emphasis on axillary nerve and rotator cuff function. I would

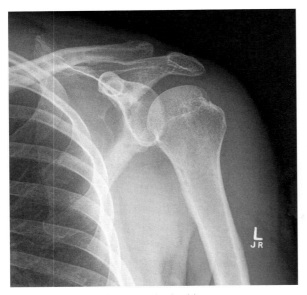

Figure 14.14 Post-relocation right shoulder.

initially refer the patient to our physiotherapist for establishing the full range of motion. I would then examine the patient about 2–3 weeks following the dislocation for anterior instability. I would perform a Beighton's score to make sure that the patient does not have hyperlaxity. I would explain to the patient that there are two options: non-operative and operative. With the non-operative option there is a high chance of his shoulder dislocating repeatedly in the future. Decision on what operative treatment to perform would depend on whether his Hill–Sach's lesion is engaging or not.

EXAMINER: So what is your next step?

CANDIDATE: I would prefer to perform an examination under anaesthesia (EUA), arthroscopy of the shoulder and if the Hill–Sach's lesion is non-engaging, perform an arthroscopic Bankart repair for anterior instability. If however, the Hill–Sach's lesion is engaging, I would not perform any operative procedure at that time but discuss various options with him at a later date in the clinic. In this situation my preferred surgical option would be the Bristow–Latarjet procedure.

This is a classic scenario. It starts off with a simple question, which you would be expected to answer. Remember, the initial setting question is aimed at mark 6. If you falter, you would be given easier questions, but then you go down to mark 5, which is a fail. The questions normally get more difficult and are aimed to assess whether you have a clear thought process ('higher order thinking').

1. Miller SL, Cleeman E, Auerbach J, Flatow EL. Comparison of intra-articular lidocaine and intravenous sedation for reduction of shoulder dislocations: a randomized, prospective study. *J Bone Joint Surg Am* 2002;**84-A**:2135–2139.
2. Fitch RW, Kuhn JE. Intraarticular lidocaine versus intravenous procedural sedation with narcotics and benzodiazepines for reduction of the dislocated shoulder: a systematic review. *Acad Emerg Med* 2008; **15**(8):703–708.

Structured oral examination question 8

EXAMINER: A 12-year-old girl presents to your clinic with an 8-week history of pain and swelling over her right ankle. The pain is worse in the evening. She is finding it difficult to walk for more than 300–400 yards without pain. This is her X-ray. What are your thoughts? (Figure 14.15.)

CANDIDATE: This is an AP radiograph of the distal tibia and fibula. The growth plates are still open. There is a periosteal reaction over the distal tibia with some lytic lesions in the distal tibial metaphysis. There are some areas of sclerosis in the metaphysis. The epiphysis does not show any obvious changes. Ankle joint appears normal. I would like to see the lateral X-ray and get a detailed history and examine the patient.

EXAMINER: I do not have the lateral X-ray with me. It did not show any breach of the cortex. What else do you want to know in the history?

CANDIDATE: History of night pain, previous infection/ osteomyelitis, history of weight loss/systemic illness.

EXAMINER: She has woken up at night on a couple of occasions. There is no history of a diagnosed infection, but the mother recalls that about 2 years ago she developed some redness in the area, which did settle with antibiotics. There is no history of weight loss, but the girl feels generally unwell.

Given these facts, what is your differential diagnosis?

CANDIDATE: My differential diagnosis would be: osteomyelitis, Ewing's sarcoma, osteosarcoma, lymphoma, leukaemia/other haematological malignancy.

I would like to investigate further in order to establish the diagnosis and plan further management. Firstly, I would request a FBC, U&E, LFTs, s. Ca, ESR and CRP. I would also request an urgent MRI with contrast.

The MRI would give us an idea of whether it is an infection or a tumour. However, at times it may be very difficult to establish the diagnosis. In that situation I would discuss the case with my oncology colleagues.

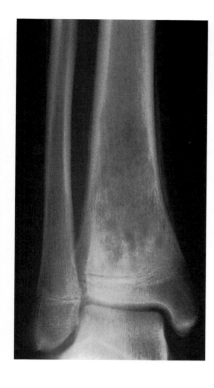

Figure 14.15
Anteroposterior
(AP) radiograph
distal right tibia and
fibula.

EXAMINER: The oncology colleagues think it is an infection and ask you to perform a biopsy.

CANDIDATE: I would perform a needle biopsy under image intensifier control in the operating theatre. I would take all precautions as I would do for a tumour biopsy [see the section on giant cell tumours].

EXAMINER: Where and how would you send the biopsy?

CANDIDATE: I would send off the biopsy in a formalin container for histological examination as well as in a dry container for culture and sensitivity.

EXAMINER: The culture results are back showing a growth of *Staphylococcus aureus* sensitive to flucloxacillin. The biopsy does not show any evidence of malignancy.

CANDIDATE: The MRI scan would give an idea of whether there is a sequestrum and/or a soft tissue abscess. The aim of the treatment would be to eradicate the infection. This would involve excision of the dead bone and soft tissue along with administration of local and systemic antibiotics.

EXAMINER: If there was a sequestrum apparent on the MRI, what would you do?

CANDIDATE: It would not be possible to eradicate the infection without excising the dead bone fragments. I would make a

window in the cortex and excise the dead bone. If necessary, I would use a spanning external fixator to stabilize the bone.

Always have an open mind. Biopsy whatever you culture and culture whatever you biopsy. Infection is an important differential diagnosis of Ewing's sarcoma.

Structured oral examination question 9

EXAMINER: A 35-year-old lady presents to your clinic with a 10-week history of a pain behind the knee. She was referred for quadriceps-strengthening exercises, which did not relieve the pain. On examination, she has a bony lump palpable just proximal to the popliteal fossa. She has no ligamentous instability and a full range of movement of the knee. This is the lateral radiograph of her knee. Describe the radiograph. (Figure 14.16.)

CANDIDATE: The lateral radiograph shows evidence of well-defined new bone formation on the posterior aspect of the distal femur. The proximal extent appears to be about 10 cm proximal to the knee joint line. The medullary canal appears to be unaffected and the knee joint is normal. I would like to take a detailed history and thoroughly examine the patient. Looking at the radiographs and the brief history my differential diagnosis would be: parosteal osteosarcoma or heterotopic ossification.

EXAMINER: Does this lesion look malignant to you?

CANDIDATE: The appearances are in keeping with a slow-growing tumour which could be a low-grade malignancy or a benign lesion.

EXAMINER: How would you manage this case?

CANDIDATE: Firstly, I would investigate the patient. This would include blood tests including FBC, U&Es, LFTs, ESR and CRP. I would organize a MRI and CT scan to assess the extent of the tumour and to confirm that it is a surface lesion. (Figure 14.17.) I would also get a CT of the chest and abdomen. I know that it is uncommon for parosteal osteosarcomas to metastasize, but I would still like to be sure.

I would then discuss the case with my oncology colleagues and further management would be based on a multidisciplinary team discussion. This should include the orthopaedic oncologist, clinical oncologist, pathologist and physiotherapist.

The aim of the treatment is to obtain a permanent cure from the osteosarcoma with minimal loss of function. Prior to

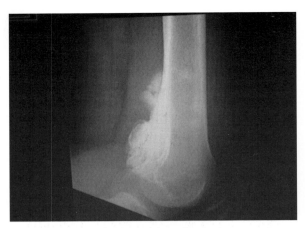

Figure 14.16 Lateral radiograph knee demonstrating new bone formation distal femur posteriorly.

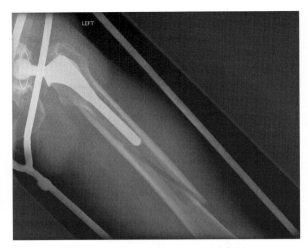

Figure 14.18 Anteroposterior (AP) radiograph left hip demonstrating periprosthetic fracture.

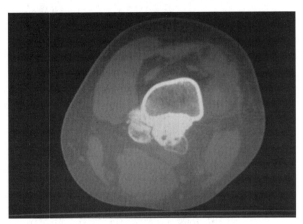

Figure 14.17 CT scan axial image distal femur.

consideration of any treatment a tissue diagnosis is essential. This should ideally be carried out by the surgeon who would be carrying out the definitive treatment [further details have been mentioned in structured oral question 2]. If the diagnosis of parosteal osteosarcoma is confirmed, the treatment is wide surgical excision. Chemotherapy is generally not of much use.

This was a short scenario to assess whether the candidate is aware of the diagnosis of parosteal osteosarcoma and that its treatment is different from that of the conventional osteosarcoma.

Structured oral examination question 10

EXAMINER: A 70-year-old man underwent a total hip replacement for a fractured neck of femur 10 years ago. He was

doing well until he sustained a fall at an underground station and sustained a femoral fracture. This is his X-ray. Please comment on it. (Figure 14.18.)

CANDIDATE: This is an AP and a lateral radiograph of the hip and femur showing a Vancouver type B peri-prosthetic fracture that extends from around the tip of the prosthesis distally. The hip replacement is of a reverse hybrid type with a cemented cup and an uncemented stem. It is difficult to say whether the stem is loose or not. However, given the fact that the patient was asymptomatic, and that there is no lysis on the radiograph, I think that the stem is well fixed. I would like to see a lateral as well as a full-length view of the femur to assess the status of the cortices and the canal distally. I would also like to take a full history particularly with regards to wound healing and/or infection at the time of the hip replacement and general health and function of the patient. I would examine the patient and assess the distal neurovascular status and the condition of the skin.

EXAMINER: The patient suffers from rheumatoid arthritis, but is otherwise well. I don't have an X-ray of the distal femur, but the fracture ends about 15 cm above the knee joint. What is your management plan?

CANDIDATE: I think this is a Vancouver B1 fracture and hence my plan A would be to perform an open reduction and internal fixation of the fracture. I would aim to provide absolute stability by using inter-fragmentary screws. I would use a pre-contoured distal femoral plate extending proximally. I would use 3–4 cables proximally and also unicortical locking screws proximally. Distally I would use a combination of locking and non-locking screws. Intraoperatively, I would be able to see the stem through the fracture site. I would assess whether it is loose. If it is loose, my plan B would be to perform a revision THR with a distal fix long stem. The stem I am familiar with is the Echelon stem. This would be a much bigger operation. Hence, prior to proceeding to theatre, I would discuss the case with one of my revision arthroplasty colleagues and seek his or her help.

EXAMINER: This is what was done. What are your thoughts? (Figures 14.19, 14.20.)

CANDIDATE: The AP radiograph of the femur and the hip shows that the fracture was fixed using a broad DCP with multiple cables and interfragmentary screw fixation. The fracture appears to have united on this view.

EXAMINER: Yes, the patient was doing well, until about 10 months down the line, he developed redness and swelling around the distal part of the wound. This burst open and he developed a sinus discharging pus. He was systemically well. What would you do now?

CANDIDATE: I take a detailed history and assess if he had wound problems in the postoperative period or whether he had an infection elsewhere in the recent past. I would examine the patient and assess if there was an abscess. I would request a FBC, CRP, ESR, U&E. I would get a new radiograph and an ultrasound if there was a collection. My aim would be to be aggressive and try to eradicate the infection. I would aim to debride the wound and obtain deep tissue samples for culture and sensitivity. At the time of debridement, I may consider inserting gentamicin beads.

EXAMINER: Would you take out the plate?

CANDIDATE: I would be very reluctant to take the plate out within a year of the fracture being fixed. This is a difficult situation. It is possible that the patient developed a postoperative infection, which may have been suppressed by the drugs taken for rheumatoid arthritis. It may be that he has developed a haematogenous spread of the infection. In either case, I would wait for a year before taking the plate out.

EXAMINER: The plate was taken out at about 16 months post-fixation. The fracture had healed. But now he has grown *Staphylococcus aureus* from his hip and the wound, and the wound is still discharging. This is his current X-ray. What is your plan now? (Figure 14.21.)

CANDIDATE: This is a very difficult situation now. The radiograph shows that the fracture has healed. There are areas of sclerosis

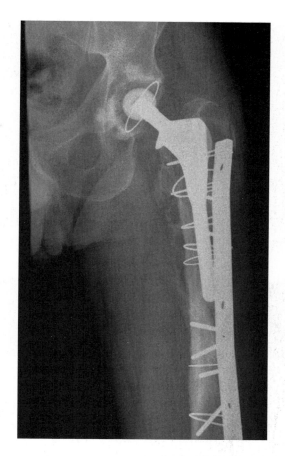

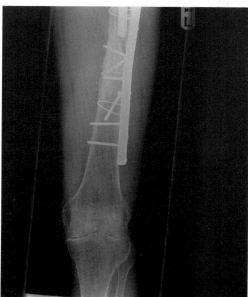

Figures 14.19 and 14.20 Anteroposterior (AP) radiographs demonstrating plate fixation periprosthetic fracture left femur.

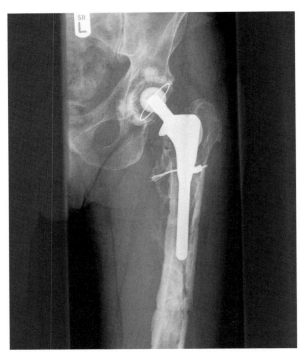

Figure 14.21 Anteroposterior (AP) radiograph left femur following plate removal.

around the fracture. I would like to obtain a view of the full femur. Also, I would like to know if the patient is systemically well and would want to know his inflammatory markers. An MRI scan of the femur would help assess the extent of the osteomyelitis. I would discuss two options with the patient. One is to use suppressive antibiotic therapy to control the infection, accepting the fact that we would never be able to eradicate the infection. The other is to consider major one- or two-stage revision to a possible total femur replacement.

EXAMINER: Would you consider a one-stage or a two-stage revision in this scenario?

CANDIDATE: Though I would be more comfortable with a two-stage revision, in this particular scenario, I would consider a

single-stage revision to a total femoral replacement. This is because it would be difficult to create a spacer after the first stage and the causative organism is known.

EXAMINER: Do you know of any evidence of single-stage versus two-stage revision for infected hip replacement?

CANDIDATE: The failure rate of a two-stage revision with an antibiotic cement spacer after the first stage has been reported to be 11% by Biring *et al.*[1] The reported failure rate of single-stage revision using antibiotics in the allograft has been reported at 8.1% by Winkler *et al.*[2] However other studies have shown a higher failure rate with single-stage revision (12.4%) as compared with two-stage revision (3.5%).[3]

The scenario went well. It started with a common scenario of a periprosthetic fracture and ended up with a difficult situation that may need a total femoral replacement. The other paper that could be quoted is Stockley *et al.* where he used a two-stage revision without parenteral antibiotics and was successful in eradicating infection in 87.7% of the cases.[4]

1. Biring G, Kostamo T, Garbuz DS, Masri BA, Duncan CP. Two-stage revision arthroplasty of the hip for infection using an interim articulated Prostalac hip spacer: a 10- to 15-year follow-up study. *J Bone Joint Surg Br* 2009;**91-B**:1431–1437.

2. Winkler H, Stoiber A, Kaudela K, Winter F, Menschik F. One stage uncemented revision of infected total hip replacement using cancellous allograft bone impregnated with antibiotics. *J Bone Joint Surg Br* 2008; **90-B**:1580–1584.

3. Elson R. Exchange arthroplasty for infection. Perspectives from the United Kingdom. *Orthop Clin North Am* 1993;**24**(4):761–767.

4. Stockley I, Mockford B, Hoad-Reddick A, Norman P. The use of two-stage exchange arthroplasty with depot antibiotics in the absence of long-term antibiotic therapy in infected total hip replacement. *J Bone Joint Surg Br* 2008;**90-B**:145–148.

Chapter

Biomaterials and biomechanics

Iain McNamara and Andrew P. Sprowson

Structured oral examination question 1

EXAMINER: This is a plain radiograph of a total knee replacement of a patient that presented in pain to my clinic.

What do you think of the radiograph? (Figure 15.1.)

CANDIDATE: [This was the first viva – I took a deep breath and described the radiograph.]

This is a plain AP radiograph of a total knee replacement. The obvious features are likely mal-positioning of the tibial component with a large zone of osteolysis underneath the base plate. The base plate has subsided and there is a possible fracture through the lateral cortex of the tibia. The femoral component appears to be of an appropriate size but might have some early osteolysis as well.

EXAMINER: Fine. What are the potential causes for this picture?

CANDIDATE: The main areas that I would be concerned about are osteolysis secondary to polyethylene debris or infection. Other causes would be . . .

EXAMINER: [interrupts] What would make you think clinically that this might be osteolysis?

CANDIDATE: I would want to know how long the joint replacement had been in situ, whether the patient had any predisposing factors for infection, such as diabetes; the medications that the patient was on, e.g. steroids or immunosuppressants; whether the postoperative course had been complicated with wound problems such as leakage or dehiscence; whether the patient had had

(a)

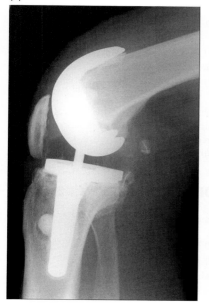

(b)

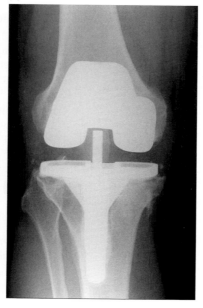

Figure 15.1 AP and lateral radiographs of total knee replacement (TKR).

any intercurrent illness, such as a UTI or tooth abscess prior to presentation ... [at this point I was interrupted again].

EXAMINER: I can tell you that the diagnosis is osteolysis secondary to polyethylene debris. Why does this happen?

CANDIDATE: Essentially the polyethylene base plate is subject to wear ... [the examiner jumped in]

EXAMINER: What modes of wear do you know?

CANDIDATE: There are four modes of wear: (1) the generation of debris from two articulating surfaces that are intended to rub together; (2) the wear between an articulating surface and a non-articulating surface; (3) third-body wear; and (4) the wear between two non-articulating surfaces, such as backside wear [trying to lead the examiner].

EXAMINER: Which is this type?

CANDIDATE: There is probably a combination of type 1 and type 4 wear.

EXAMINER: Fine. What are the predisposing factors for wear in this case?

CANDIDATE: Firstly I can see a large amount of soft tissue shadowing, so I can propose that the patient is overweight. Patients with a BMI greater than 40 kg/m^2 have demonstrated increased wear compared to patients with lower BMIs.[1]

Secondly, the tibial tray appears to be in varus, this leads to overload of the medial compartment and predisposes to failure.[2]

EXAMINER: Okay, I think that is all we can deduce from the radiograph. Here are the retrieved components, what more can you tell me?

CANDIDATE: The polyethylene has fractured and the femoral component has been articulating on the tibial base plate. The polyethylene component itself is a mobile bearing ...

EXAMINER: Good, a mobile bearing. What does this mean?

CANDIDATE: In essence, rather than the poly being either moulded or fixed into the tibial tray it rotates around a central post that theoretically allows greater conformity during movement which has theoretical advantages in reducing contact stresses and wear. However, there are disadvantages that there is a second surface that articulates and produces wear particles – i.e. backside wear. Retrieval studies have demonstrated that in a comparison of fixed to mobile bearings, the fixed bearing had greater high-grade wear on the articulating surface and minimal on the backside of the

components, whereas the mobile bearing had less high-grade wear on the articulating surface but an increased low-grade wear on the backside.[3] Clinically there has never been any difference proven.[4]

EXAMINER: You referred to the patient's size earlier, what difficulties might you encounter during revision surgery?

CANDIDATE: The exposure might be difficult, with great difficulty everting the patella ...

EXAMINER: Yes, and what would you do about that?

CANDIDATE: I would elongate the incision, if that didn't work then I would create a pocket for the patella to sit in to allow eversion, I might consider a lateral release or possibly a rectus snip or quads turn down.

EXAMINER: Which way do you cut for a rectus snip?

CANDIDATE: Erm, into the rectus ... laterally from the medial parapatella incision.

[I think that we were both running out of material!]

EXAMINER: Fine, let's move on.

1. Amin AK, Clayton RA, Patton JT *et al*. Total knee replacement in morbidly obese patients. Results of a prospective, matched study. *J Bone Joint Surg Br* 2006;**88-B**:1321–1326.

2. Wong J, Steklov N, Patil S *et al*. Predicting the effect of tray malalignment on risk for bone damage and implant subsidence after total knee arthroplasty. *J Orthop Res* 2011;**29**(3):347–353.

3. Lu YC, Huang CH, Chang TK *et al*. Wear-pattern analysis in retrieved tibial inserts of mobile-bearing and fixed-bearing total knee prostheses. *J Bone Joint Surg Br* 2010;**92-B**:500–507.

4. Smith TO, Ejtehadi F, Nichols R *et al*. Clinical and radiological outcomes of fixed-versus mobile-bearing total knee replacement: a meta-analysis. *Knee Surg Sports Traumatol Arthrosc* 2010;**18**(3):325–340.

Structured oral examination question 2

EXAMINER: Tell me about synovial fluid.

CANDIDATE: Synovial fluid is a dialysate of blood plasma, without clotting factors or erythrocytes. It contains hyaluronate and plasma proteins. The main function of synovial fluid is to facilitate low-friction joint lubrication.

EXAMINER: Tell me about joint lubrication.

CANDIDATE: There are two main hypotheses surrounding joint lubrication in synovial joints.

The first is fluid-film lubrication, in this hypothesis the joint surfaces are separated by a fluid film which fully supports the applied load, preventing contact between the surfaces. The minimum thickness of the fluid film must exceed the surface roughness of the bearing surfaces by a factor of three.

The second is boundary lubrication. In this situation the bearing surfaces are in contact but separated by a very thin layer of fluid that decreases the friction of the surfaces.

It is thought that fluid-film lubrication dominates in synovial joints. However, realistically, both fluid-film and boundary lubrication occur in synovial joints, depending on the joint in question and the type of loading applied.

EXAMINER: Can you tell me about the different types of fluid-film lubrication?

CANDIDATE: There are a number of different types of fluid-film lubrication.

The first is hydrodynamic (HD) lubrication. In hydrodynamic lubrication there is no contact between the joint surfaces. The surfaces are separated by a thin fluid film which supports the load. In simple terms, the movement of the joint surfaces creates a thin wedge-shaped fluid film between the surfaces to prevent them from contacting one another.

A model that is more likely in synovial joints is elastohydrodynamic (EHD) lubrication. In this model the cartilage is not considered to be rigid, as it is in the previous model, rather it is elastic and can deform. In elastohydrodynamic lubrication, elastic deformation of the bearing surface enlarges the surface area and traps the fluid. This in turn increases the ability of the fluid-film to carry load and decreases stress within the cartilage.

A modification of the elastohydrodynamic model of lubrication is micro-elastohydrodynamic lubrication (MEHD). The micro-elastohydrodynamic lubrication model assumes that the asperities of articular cartilage are deformed under high loads. This smoothes out the bearing surface, . . .

. . .[The examiner was bored, which was a shame because I knew quite a lot about this!]

EXAMINER: You mentioned the load across joints, can you tell me what the difference is between the anatomical and the mechanical axis of the knee joint?

CANDIDATE: The anatomical axis passes down the shaft of the femur into centre of the knee joint and then down the axis of the tibia into the centre of the ankle joint. By contrast the mechanical axis passes from the centre of the femoral head, through the centre of the knee joint and then down the long axis of the tibia into the centre of the ankle joint. The anatomical axis is usually between 5° and 7° of valgus compared with the mechanical axis in the femur. In the tibia the mechanical and anatomical axes are identical.

EXAMINER: Do you know how these terms are important in total knee replacement?

CANDIDATE: The weightbearing surfaces of the total knee replacement (TKR) are parallel to one another and orthogonal to the mechanical axis. The cuts for the femoral component of the TKR are determined by the native anatomical axis, an intramedullary rod is passed up the femur and the distal femoral resection is usually made between 5° and 7° of valgus to recreate the anatomical axis. The tibial resection is made perpendicular to both the anatomical and mechanical axis. The femoral cut is usually made in 3° of external rotation (or the femoral component has 3° of ER built in, like the Genesis 2). This is necessary as the tibia has a 3° varus slope, if all of the cuts were made with the same rotation then the extension and flexion gaps would not be equal, rather the extension gap would be a rectangle and the flexion gap would be a rhomboid. The 3° of ER matches both flexion and extension gaps as rectangles.

EXAMINER: What do you know about bone graft?

CANDIDATE: Bone graft can be defined by its source or type. The main sources are allograft and autograft, the main types are cancellous, corticocancellous and cortical.

EXAMINER: What do you mean by these terms that you have just used?

CANDIDATE: Autograft is a graft from the same individual, allograft is from a different individual of the same species.

EXAMINER: In terms of biomechanical properties, is there a difference between cancellous and cortical bone?

CANDIDATE: Cortical bone is much stiffer with a Young's modulus of 20 GPa, whereas cancellous bone has a Young's modulus of 1 GPa.

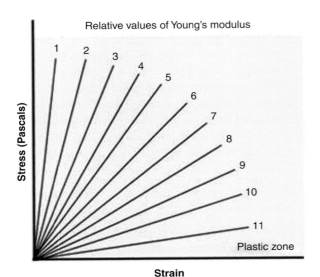

Relative values of Young's modulus

Figure 15.2 Diagram stress–strain curve and Young's modulus.

EXAMINER: Good, can you draw the relative moduli on a graph and compare them with materials for joint reconstruction?

[I was drawing and talking – the examiner kept on asking me the approximate values for the different materials.]

1. Ceramic (Al_2O_3).
2. Alloy (Co-Cr-Mo).
3. Stainless steel.
4. Titanium.
5. Cortical bone.
6. Cancellous bone.
7. PMMA.
8. Polyethylene.
9. Matrix polymers.
10. Tendon/ligament.
11. Cartilage.

EXAMINER: How would you define bone graft on a biomechanical basis?

[I took this to be the same question as talking about the mechanical properties of bone – just a different spin.]

CANDIDATE: Bone graft exhibits elastic, plastic and viscous behaviour depending upon the applied stress.

EXAMINER: What do you mean by these terms that you have just used?

CANDIDATE: Elastic means that there is no permanent deformation of the bone with the application of a stress.

Plastic means that there is a permanent deformation of the bone with the application of stress, which remains once the stress is removed.

Viscous means that the response to an applied stress is dependent upon the amount of stress applied, the rate of strain application and the bone exhibits hysteresis.

EXAMINER: What do you mean by stress and strain?

CANDIDATE: Stress is force applied per unit area, strain is change in length divided by original length.

EXAMINER: Do you know any other materials that can be used to fill bone defects in elective or trauma surgery?

CANDIDATE: Synthetic bone graft substitutes can be used for both purposes.

EXAMINER: Do you know any examples?

CANDIDATE: The commonest materials are hydroxyapatite or beta tricalcium phosphate.

EXAMINER: Fine, what can you tell me about them and how do they differ from autograft?

CANDIDATE: Autograft is still considered the gold standard as it is osteoconductive, osteoinductive and osteogeneic. Despite excellent clinical results there are problems associated with its use, such as donor site morbidity and limits to the supply. Both hydroxyapatite and beta tricalcium phosphate are synthetically produced. They have chemical similarities to the mineral in bone. They are osteoconductive but not osteoinductive or osteogenic.

EXAMINER: Do you know how osteoinductive behaviour is determined? [A stinker of a question!]

CANDIDATE: I think that it is determined by its ability to form bone in a muscle pouch in an animal. [I had read it somewhere and took a punt.]

EXAMINER: So, going back to what we were talking about, what would the stress–strain curve for hydroxyapatite look like?

CANDIDATE: Well [deep breath] it is stiffer than bone, more brittle . . .

EXAMINER: Draw it, draw it . . .

[The drawing began.] (Figure 15.3.)

CANDIDATE: So it will be stiffer and hence it has a steeper line than the bone. It is more likely to fracture rather than undergo plastic deformation.

EXAMINER: What does that make it . . . ?

CANDIDATE: More brittle.

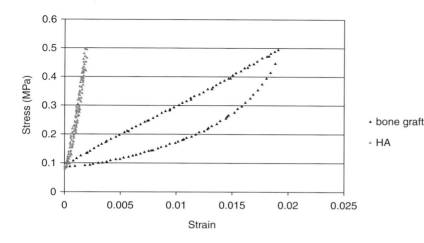

Figure 15.3 Stress–strain curve for hydroxyapatite (HA) and bone graft.

EXAMINER: Other than the type of material, what changes are there that affect the rate of bone formation in bone graft substitutes?

CANDIDATE: The materials differ in their porosity; it is thought that an increase in both the macro- and microporosity affects the rate of bone formation.

EXAMINER: Do you know of any figures of porosity that are important?

CANDIDATE: A macroporosity of 60% affects the rate of ingrowth.

A viva that seemed quite testing but actually just asked very basic principles that are in most basic science textbooks – it was just a slightly abstract way of testing simple concepts.

Structured oral examination question 3

EXAMINER: Tell me about your approach to the fixation of this fracture. (Figure 15.4.)

CANDIDATE: Firstly I would assess the patient, the soft tissue and then consider the fracture. I would start with ATLS ...

EXAMINER: Yes, yes, there are no tricks in this question, everything is fine with the patient, this is a question about the biomechanics of fracture fixation.

CANDIDATE: Right, okay, this is a plain radiograph of a comminuted displaced, intra-articular fracture of the tibial plateau. The principles regarding the fixation of this fracture are anatomical reduction and absolute stability of the articular block and then the restoration of length, axis and rotation of the lower limb by attaching the articular block onto the shaft of the tibia by utilizing a bridging plate and relative stability.

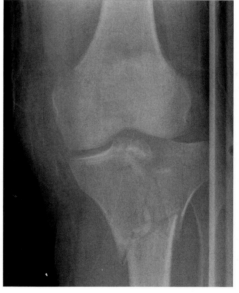

Figure 15.4 Anteroposterior (AP) radiograph of left knee demonstrating tibial plateau fracture.

EXAMINER: Tell me about how you would achieve a stable fixation of the articular surface.

CANDIDATE: I would open the joint and reduce the articular fragments under direct vision. I would apply a peri-articular clamp to hold the fragments reduced and to compress the fragments. If necessary I would use K-wires as a temporary fixation device. I would then use 6.5 mm partially threaded cancellous screws to act as both a subchondral raft and also to compress the fracture fragments.

EXAMINER: Okay, I think that you misunderstand the AO principles of compression of a fracture. In this case we are not

Not

using the screws as a compression device but applying them so that after removal of the peri-articular clamp the implant ends up in tension.

[I am still not sure that there is much difference in this, except in terms of semantics.] However, why do you want to achieve absolute stability?

CANDIDATE: As it is an intra-articular fracture, the healing of the bone should be by primary bone healing without the formation of callus. In order for this to happen there has to be no movement at the fracture site. The lack of movement means that the osteoclasts involved in the remodelling of bone will essentially ignore the fracture site and proceed directly across the fracture site using cutting cones, therefore healing by primary bone healing without the formation of callus.

EXAMINER: How does a screw work?

CANDIDATE: A screw converts rotational movement into longitudinal advancement. With a lag screw, the screw is partially threaded therefore as the distal threads bite in the fracture fragment, the proximal smooth barrel can slide over the proximal fragment and so as it is tightened the distal fragment is pulled towards the proximal and compression of the distal piece against the proximal cortex occurs.

EXAMINER: What do you, as the surgeon, have to be particularly careful of when using lag screws in this fracture?

CANDIDATE: Getting a good reduction?

EXAMINER: Yes, but in multifragmentary fractures of both the medial and lateral tibial plateaus, one must be careful in using lag screws so as not to narrow the proximal tibia by overtightening.

EXAMINER: You mentioned restoration of length, axis and rotation. How do you do that?

CANDIDATE: I would establish the mechanical axis of the limb by holding a diathermy lead from the centre of the femoral head and stretching it taut onto the centre of the ankle. The line of the diathermy cable should pass through the centre of the knee, thus checking the axis. Rotation can be checked by looking at the symmetry with the other leg and also using the thickness of the cortex on the II to check the rotation.

EXAMINER: It's not easy, is it? And you also mentioned that you would aim to use your plate in a bridging mode – what do you mean by that?

CANDIDATE: There are a number of modes by which a plate can be used . . .

EXAMINER: Can you name them?

CANDIDATE: Buttress, bridging, compression, tension band, protection.

EXAMINER: So why would you use this one in bridging mode?

CANDIDATE: There is a large amount of comminution in the metaphysis therefore it is impossible to compress the fracture fragments. If the other features of length, axis and rotation are correct then the fracture would be expected to heal by secondary bone healing with callus formation.

EXAMINER: Fine, if this was a simple fracture then how would you use the plate?

CANDIDATE: I would probably use the plate as a protection plate. In such an instance I would try to achieve interfragmentary compression by using a lag screw and then apply the plate to neutralize the forces acting on the screw, thus protecting while the bone healed.

EXAMINER: So why apply different biomechanical principles to the two fracture configurations?

CANDIDATE: Sorry, how do you mean?

EXAMINER: Well, why not use the plate in bridging mode for a simple fracture?

CANDIDATE: Oh right, sorry. For bones to heal there should be the correct strain environment. As bones heal there is a reduction in the strain that can be tolerated across a fracture. In a simple fracture the movement of the two fracture ends is across a very small gap, however, if the bone ends are not compressed then the strain across this gap is very large. A large strain can either delay or prevent bone healing. This in turn can lead to delayed or non-union. By contrast, if there is a large segment of comminuted bone then the same movement across the fracture is distributed over a much larger segment. This means that the strain across the fracture site is much lower and therefore the bone can heal by secondary bone healing and callus formation.

EXAMINER: Fine, so how does an unlocked tibial nail compare with a bridging plate in its mode of action?

CANDIDATE: A bridging plate acts as a load-bearing device and the nail in this situation acts as load-sharing device.

EXAMINER: So, how does one alter the design of a nail to alter its biomechanical properties?

CANDIDATE: The stiffness of a nail depends upon its working length, the diameter of the nail, the material from which the nail is constructed.

EXAMINER: Do you know how the stiffness of the nail is related to its length and diameter?

CANDIDATE: The rigidity of an IM nail under torsion varies with the fourth power of radius. The stiffness of a nail in bending is also proportional to the fourth power of the radius.

EXAMINER: And finally, with regard to external fixators, what factors affect the stiffness of a construct using an external fixator?

CANDIDATE: The important factors are: diameter of the pins, diameters of the bars, number of bars, working length, proximity of the bars to the base of the pins, angle of the pins, material from which the external fixators is constructed.

EXAMINER: And ...

CANDIDATE: Erm ...

EXAMINER: The most important – the quality of the reduction with the bone ends in apposition.

CANDIDATE: Of course.

[Nothing too taxing – all had been covered on the AO advances course and in a basic sciences book. I quite enjoyed it.]

Ruedi TP, Buckley R, Moran CG. *AO Principles of Fracture Management.* New York: Thieme Medical Publishers, 2007.

Ruedi TP, Buckley R, Moran CG, Perren SM. Evolution of the internal fixation of long bone fractures. The scientific basis of biological internal fixation: choosing a new balance between stability and biology. *J Bone Joint Surg Br* 2002;**84-B**:1093–1110.

Structured oral examination question 4

EXAMINER: What are these? (Figure 15.5.)

CANDIDATE: The hip replacement on the left is an Exeter hip replacement and the one on the right looks like a Charnley hip replacement.

EXAMINER: Good, what are the differences between the two?

CANDIDATE: The Exeter hip replacement is a collarless, polished double taper cemented hip replacement. By contrast the Charnley has a collar to prevent subsidence and is not as smooth.

EXAMINER: By what biomechanical principles are they supposed to work?

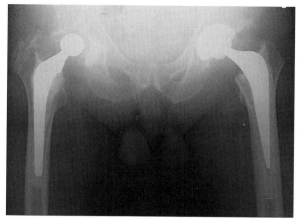

Figure 15.5 Anteroposterior (AP) pelvis demonstrating bilateral THR: an Exeter hip replacement and a Charnley hip replacement.

CANDIDATE: The Exeter works by utilizing a taper slip design and controlled subsidence. It is implanted within a cement mantel and the highly polished nature and the taper allows controlled subsidence of the stem within the cement mantel. This taper means that the hoop stresses which are perpendicular to the long axis of the implant remain applied to the bone as the hip subsides.

By contrast the Charnley works in a composite beam manner with the loading passing though the collar and onto the proximal femur in that manner. It is not designed to subside.

EXAMINER: What is cement?

CANDIDATE: Cement in a hip replacement acts as a grout. It functions to fill the defect in between the stem and the bone, act for load transfer, allows modulus matching between implant and bone and in the case of the taper slip stems, allows controlled subsidence of the stem.

EXAMINER: What are the design principles behind the use of uncemented joint replacements?

CANDIDATE: The uncemented joint replacement can be put in in two ways. The first is a press-fit design, the second is a line-to-line fixation. In the press fit, the femoral canal is prepared to match the orientation of the eventual stem but the broach is slightly smaller than the stem. When the stem is inserted it is therefore a tight fit. As it is inserted, the viscoelasticity of the bone allows the slightly larger stem to be inserted and then the stem is gripped by the bone. Theoretically, no additional fixation is required. In line-to-line fixation, the bone is prepared to be the same size as the eventual implant, e.g. an uncemented cup. A cup the same size as the prepared acetabulum is inserted but in this case additional fixation, such as screws, is frequently required.

EXAMINER: What can you tell me about the surface finish of the implant?

CANDIDATE: The surface finish is usually roughened to encourage bone ingrowth. There are two main ways of doing this: the first is by grit blasting, the other is by introducing porosity into the surface of the stem.

In grit blasting, the stem is roughened to allow bone on growth onto the surface. By contrast the porous surface allows bone ingrowth into the pores on the surface.

EXAMINER: Do you know anything about the design of the pores?

CANDIDATE: The porosity of the stem should not be greater than 50% otherwise there is the possibility of the pores shearing off.

EXAMINER: Okay.

EXAMINER: What is shown in this photograph?

CANDIDATE: This is an ASR hip replacement which has been explanted.

EXAMINER: How does this differ from the other two hip replacements?

CANDIDATE: This is a resurfacing hip replacement whereas the others are total hip replacements. In addition this is a metal-on-metal hip replacement and utilizes a large head.

EXAMINER: What are thought to be the advantages of a metal-on-metal hip replacement?

CANDIDATE: Metal-on-metal was thought to have a number of advantages. The large head meant that there was a large effective radius which generates high angular velocity, also the metal can be polished very smooth and therefore the radial clearance is very small. The favourable wear characteristics of the metal mean that it is much more likely that fluid–film lubrication can be achieved and there is exceptionally low wear.

EXAMINER: So what are the problems with it?

CANDIDATE: Well, there is a run-in period which generates large numbers of metal ions, these are potentially carcinogenic and their effect upon a developing fetus is unknown. In addition, some people are developing a reaction, thought to be secondary to metal debris that affects the soft tissue around the hip.

EXAMINER: What is the name of that reaction?

CANDIDATE: ALVAL – aseptic lymphocytic vasculitis associated lesion.

EXAMINER: Nearly, I think that you mean aseptic lymphocyte-dominated vasculitis-associated lesion.

Who is meant to be predominantly affected?

CANDIDATE: Overweight women with small bones.

EXAMINER: Well sort of, it is amazing how they always come in saying that they are large boned ... I always hate to disappoint them! Anyway ... how do these patients present?

CANDIDATE: Normally with groin or knee pain or deteriorating gait.

EXAMINER: Okay. Do you know of any tests that might be able to diagnose ALVAL?

CANDIDATE: It is possible to measure serum ion levels ...

EXAMINER: Which ones?

CANDIDATE: Erm ...

EXAMINER: Cobalt and chromium, and do you know of any levels that might be considered significant?

CANDIDATE: Sorry, no.

EXAMINER: It is not known exactly but recent guidelines dictate that significant values are thought to be levels of chromium or cobalt more than 7 parts per billion, although we do not fully know the significance of the levels.

Can we image the hips?

CANDIDATE: Erm ... MRI [a guess].

EXAMINER: Correct – one scan is a MARS (metal artifact reduction sequence) which can show the characteristic fluid collections and soft tissue damage associated with these reactions.

I think that you would benefit from reading the latest Medical Device Alert report. I think that this is something that you need to have at your fingertips if you are going to be a lower limb surgeon. [A reasonable viva. All fairly obvious and topical stuff, there had been a decent review article in the *Journal of Bone and Joint Surgery* which I had read a week or so before which was fairly useful.]

Breusch SJ, Malchau H. *The Well-cemented Total Hip Arthroplasty: Theory and Practice.* Berlin: Springer.

Chapter

16

Tissues of the musculoskeletal system

Andrew P. Sprowson and Iain McNamara

Introduction

Knowledge of tissues of the musculoskeletal system is a difficult topic to grasp on face value, as it appears removed from the average orthopaedic surgeon's practice, but it pervades many aspects of clinical practice and therefore must be understood. Well, at least until you pass FRCS (Tr & Orth) viva!

You may be asked questions in a general manner or in more detail; you need to cover both bases. This chapter will provide examples of longer structured oral sections along with common topics and examples. In certain sections we have also given a rough marking scheme, so you can gauge your level.

Recommended books – This one, and a good basic science book. That's it.

Structured oral examination question 1

EXAMINER: This is a coronal MRI through the thigh. Can you tell me what has happened? (Figure 16.1.)

CANDIDATE: [I was not sure exactly sure what I was looking at initially!] There appears to be a tendon pulled off the bone, along with an associated haematoma.

[This is just using your basic understanding of MRI.]

EXAMINER: Appears to be, or actually is?

CANDIDATE: There is a definite avulsion of tendon from the bone.

[Be confident.]

EXAMINER: What's the function of the bone attachment?

CANDIDATE: [I really didn't know where to go, so I gave a very basic answer!] It represents an interface between bone and tendon.

EXAMINER: But what is the function?

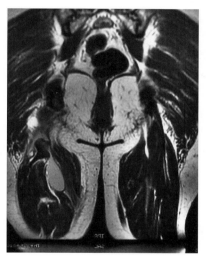

Figure 16.1
Coronal T1 MRI image of thigh.

CANDIDATE: It allows a load to be transferred from muscle to bone and stores energy.

[As you can see I've not read much on this and gave short answers so I didn't get into trouble.]

EXAMINER: What type of load?

CANDIDATE: Tensile?

EXAMINER: What is the difference in general terms between ligaments and tendons?

CANDIDATE: [I started to talk about ligaments attaching bone to bone!]

Mark 4

EXAMINER: No, I mean structurally!

CANDIDATE: [Finally I can get going now.] Collagen content is higher in tendons and can be up to 80–90% in extremity tendons.

Postgraduate Orthopaedics: Viva Guide for the FRCS (Tr & Orth) Examination, ed. Paul A. Banaszkiewicz and Deiary F. Kader. Published by Cambridge University Press. © Cambridge University Press 2012.

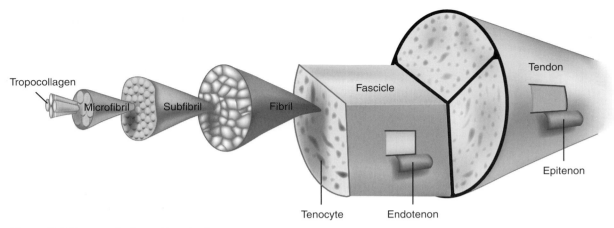

Figure 16.2 Diagram of collagen hierarchical structure.

[BEST ANSWER: up to 99% of dry weight. Remember that tendons and ligaments are made up from 80% ECM and 20% cells.]

EXAMINER: What are the cells found in tendons and ligaments?

CANDIDATE: Fibroblast represents the vast proportion of cells, at about 20% of total mass.

EXAMINER: You mentioned collagen, which is the common type?

CANDIDATE: Type I represents the most common type.

Mark 5

EXAMINER: That was a little guarded, give me a figure.

CANDIDATE: 90%.

EXAMINER: Tell me about Type I collagen.

CANDIDATE: Type I collagen consists of three polypeptide chains, two alpha and one beta. [This was wrong: it's two (alpha 1) and one (alpha 2).] They combine to form a triple helix, which provides the tensile strength.

Mark 6 – Pass

If you can't talk at this stage you will fail this section, you must have a broad knowledge base.

EXAMINER: How does this structure retain its stability?

CANDIDATE: There is cross linking which is allowed to occur due to hydrogen bonds.

EXAMINER: Can you draw a picture of collagen in a ligament and tendon and explain how they differ?

CANDIDATE: [I drew a longitudinal section basically with a well aligned pattern for a tendon and more haphazard for a ligament. I explained that the less parallel structure in a ligament means it takes tension in one direction, but can also take stresses in other directions. In each layer they are parallel, but in subsequent layers the collagen is at a slightly different angle.]

EXAMINER: Can you draw a schematic of this hierarchical structure? (Figure 16.2.)

CANDIDATE: [I talked about the layers as I drew, only got to the fibril and he was bored!]

Remember that there are lots of different ways to draw this diagram, just use one and learn how to draw it and talk. It is the principles, not the details, which are important!

EXAMINER: So, what makes up the extracellular matrix?

CANDIDATE: This essentially is a proteoglycans matrix, with plasma proteins and glycoprotein. These proteoglycans bind water and provide a gel-type matrix. The proteoglycans are glycosaminoglycans which bind to a protein core, linked to a hyaluronic acid chain which proves a very high molecular weight.

Mark 7 – Good pass

EXAMINER: Can you draw the stress–strain curve for tendons and ligament and talk through it? (Figure 16.3.)

You can get this from any of the basic science books, just learn it!

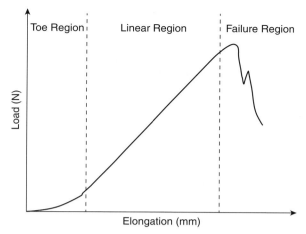

Figure 16.3 Stress–strain curve for tendon and ligament.

CANDIDATE: There are three major regions of the stress–strain curve: (1) the toe or toe-in region, (2) the linear region and (3) the yield and failure region. In physiological activity, most ligaments and tendons exist in the toe and somewhat in the linear region. These constitute a non-linear stress–strain curve, since the slope of the toe-in region is different from that of the linear region.

In terms of structure–function relationships, the toe-in region represents 'un-crimping' of the crimp in the collagen fibrils. Since it is easier to stretch out the crimp of the collagen fibrils, this part of the stress–strain curve shows a relatively low stiffness. As the collagen fibrils become uncrimped, then we see that the collagen fibril backbone itself is being stretched, which gives rise to a stiffer material. As individual fibrils within the ligament or tendon begin to fail damage accumulates, stiffness is reduced and the ligament/tendons begin to fail. Thus a key concept is that the overall behaviour of ligaments and tendons depends on the individual crimp structure and failure of the collagen fibrils.

Mark 8 – Excellent pass

This is an example of a question which is based on one specific topic, which is great if you know it well, but very bad if you don't. This emphasizes the fact you must be able to talk to a basic level on all topics, or you may flounder very early on in the question. This question will be in your basic science viva and last 5 minutes.

Structured oral examination question 2

EXAMINER: Which cells reside in bone?

CANDIDATE: Osteoblasts, osteoclasts, osteocytes and undifferentiated mesenchymal stem cells.
[Don't forget the mesenchymal stem cells.]

EXAMINER: What do they all do?

CANDIDATE: Osteoblasts are large cells responsible for the synthesis and mineralization of bone during both initial bone formation and later bone remodelling. Osteoblasts form a closely packed sheet on the surface of the bone, from which cellular processes extend through the developing bone. An osteocyte lies within the matrix bone. It occupies a lacuna, which is contained in the calcified matrix of bone. Osteocytes are derived from osteoblasts, or bone-forming cells, and are essentially osteoblasts surrounded by the products they secreted. Cytoplasmic processes of the osteocyte extend away from the cell toward other osteocytes in canaliculi. These canaliculi allow nutrients and waste products to be exchanged to maintain the viability of the osteocyte.
[Examiner cut me off, as he realized I would sit and regurgitate up the whole book!]

EXAMINER: Where are osteoclasts derived from?

CANDIDATE: Osteoclast precursor is a member of the monocyte/macrophage family, and, although the resorptive cell can be generated from mononuclear phagocytes of various tissue sources, the principal precursor resides in the marrow.
[A lot of candidates get confused in this section.]

EXAMINER: Tell me about mesenchymal stem cells.

CANDIDATE: Mesenchymal stem cells are multipotent stem cells that can differentiate into a variety of cell types. Cell types that MSCs have been shown to differentiate in vitro or in vivo include osteoblasts, chondrocytes, myocytes and adipocytes.
[And, as described lately, beta-pancreatic islets cells.]

EXAMINER: What types of cartilage do you know about?

CANDIDATE: There are three types of cartilage: hyaline cartilage, fibrocartilage and elastic cartilage.
[Elastic cartilage exists in the epiglottis and the Eustachian tube.]

EXAMINER: Draw a cross-section of cartilage. (Figure 16.4.)

This is one of the commonest questions to get asked in the basic science viva, know it well. Fail to be able to draw this diagram at your peril! Practise the drawing and discussion of it at least 10 times.

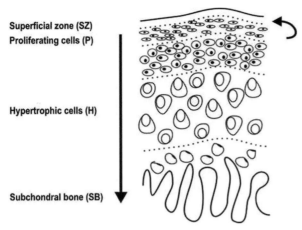

Superficial zone (SZ)
Proliferating cells (P)

Hypertrophic cells (H)

Subchondral bone (SB)

Figure 16.4 Diagram cross-section of cartilage.

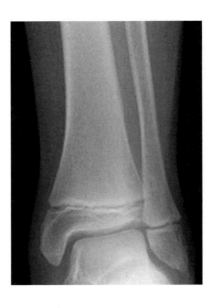

Figure 16.5
Anteroposterior
(AP) radiograph
ankle.

EXAMINER: What are the differences between articular cartilage and meniscus?

CANDIDATE: Articular cartilage is 68–85% water, 10–20% (Type I) collagen and 5–10% proteoglycans. Meniscus is 60–70% water, 15–25% (Type II) collagen and 1–2% proteoglycans.

EXAMINER: Can you draw a picture of collagen and proteoglycans?
[Draw the standard picture seen in many textbooks.]

EXAMINER: What's the importance of water?

CANDIDATE: 30% of the total water exists between the collagen fibres and this is determined by the negative charge of the proteogylcans which lie within the collagen matrix. Because the proteogylcans are bound closely, the closeness of the negative charges creates a repulsion force that must be neutralized by positive ions in the surrounding fluid. The amount of water present in cartilage depends on the concentration of proteoglycans and the stiffness and strength of the collagen network. The proteoglycan aggregates are basically responsible for the turgid nature of the cartilage and in articular cartilage they provide the osmotic properties needed to resist compressive loads. If the collagen network is degraded, as in the case of OA, the amount of water in the cartilage increases, because more negative ions are exposed to draw in fluid. The increase in fluid can significantly alter the mechanical behaviour of the cartilage.

That is a very specific question, but common theme.

EXAMINER: Bearing in mind what we have discussed, what do you want to talk about next?

CANDIDATE: Growth plates.

EXAMINER: Correct answer! Tell me about any classifications you know of specific to the growth plate?

CANDIDATE: Salter–Harris fractures are classified from Types I through V in the order of prognosis, with Salter–Harris Type V having the poorest prognosis and the greatest impact on potential deformity. Type I is a slipped growth plate, II the fracture lies metaphyseal, III is epiphyseal, IV both metaphyseal and epiphyseal and in V the physis suffers a compression injury. Salter–Harris Type II fractures are the most common. When all types of Salter–Harris fractures are considered, the rate of growth disturbance is approximately 30%. However, only 2% of Salter–Harris fractures result in a significant functional disturbance.

The fracture types described later, also less common, include Type VI (injury to the perichondral structures – rare), Type VII (isolated injury to the epiphysis only), Type VIII (isolated injury to the metaphysis) and Type IX (an injury to the periosteum which could interfere with membranous growth). I would not mention any of this unless asked. You may end up speaking to an orthopaedic paediatric professor!

EXAMINER: Draw me a growth plate. (Figure 16.6.)

CANDIDATE: [I drew a simple schematic like this one.] Zone I is the reserve or resting zone with low rates of proliferation, proteoglycan synthesis and Type IIB collagen. These cells have a high lipid body and vacuole content which is involved with

ZONE

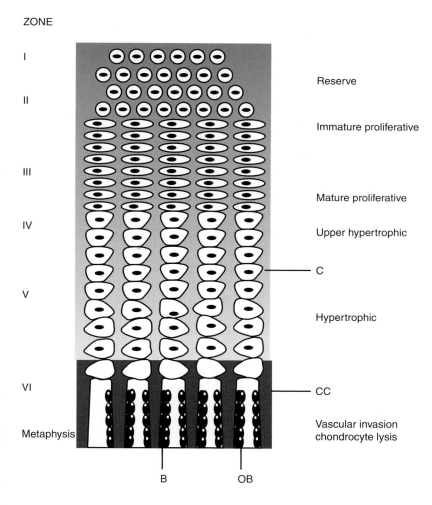

I

II

III

IV

V

VI

Metaphysis

B   OB

Figure 16.6 Diagram of a growth plate. B = bone, OB = osteoblast, CC = calcified cartilage, C = cartilage matrix.

Reserve

Immature proliferative

Mature proliferative

Upper hypertrophic

C

Hypertrophic

CC

Vascular invasion chondrocyte lysis

storage for later nutritional requirements. This is not a germinal layer of 'mother cartilage cells'.

Zone II is the upper proliferative or columnar region. The function of the proliferative zones is matrix production and cell division that result in longitudinal growth. Chondrocytes are flat and are arranged longitudinally. The zone is the true germinal layer of the growth plate and Type II collagen synthesis is increased.

Zone III is the mature proliferating zone, morphologically similar to zone II, but with less DNA synthesis.

Zone IV is the hypertrophic zone, where cell size increases and the columnar arrangement is less regular. Metabolic activity is high, with matrix synthesis approximately threefold compared with the proliferative zone. The main matrix components synthesized are types II and X collagen and aggrecan.

[I got stopped at this point, but will continue for completeness.] Zone V is the zone of the matrix calcification as this calcified matrix becomes the scaffolding for bone deposition in the metaphysis. High levels of alkaline phosphatase synthesis of type X and type II collagen cell death by hypoxia.

Zone VI is the junction of the growth plate with the metaphysis, the region where the transition from cartilage to bone occurs. Type I collagen, a marker of the osteoblast phenotype, is immunolocalized to this area.

There are a lot more facts in many textbooks, but if you know roughly about each zone that will be fine for a pass, more detailed knowledge will equal a good pass.

EXAMINER: How is the growth plate regulated?

CANDIDATE: Insulin-like growth factor (IGF) is one of the most potent growth factors for skeletal tissue previously known as somatomedins. They have significant effects on the growth plate chondrocytes, and IGFs retained in bone matrix are important in the regulation of bone remodelling. IGFs stimulate osteoblast and chondrocyte proliferation, induce differentiation in osteoblasts and maintain the chondrocyte phenotype.

Transforming growth factors (TGFs) have an important role in skeletal tissue, particularly certain members of the TGF-b gene family which includes the bone morphogenetic proteins involved in morphogenesis and regulation of endochondral ossification and in bone remodelling. BMPs are the only molecules so far discovered capable of independently inducing endochondral ossification in vivo.

Urist, 1965 is the paper to quote.[1] Be able to mention something about BMP2 and 7.

Fibroblast growth factor stimulates proliferation of mesenchymal cells in the developing limb that leads to limb outgrowth; this group are also involved in later stages of bone growth.

Platelet-derived growth factor plays a role in bone development and growth, being important in the regulation of bone and cartilage cells, although little is currently known of their role in normal endochondral ossification.

Tumour necrosis factors stimulate bone and cartilage resorption, division and reversibly inhibit ectopic bone formation in animal models.

If you get to this stage it's a good pass. Other growth factors to think about are: interleukin 1, 6, 8, interferons, colony-stimulating factors, parathyroid hormone-related peptide and calcitonin gene-related peptide.

1. Urist MR. Bone: formation by autoinduction. *Science* 1965;**150**(3698):893.

Structured oral examination question 3

EXAMINER: What can you see in this X-ray? (Figure 16.7.)

CANDIDATE: The anteroposterior (AP) pelvis radiograph demonstrates a right intracapsular fractured neck of femur.
[I was desperately looking for something else, but it was that simple.]

EXAMINER: What is a common reason for a fracture?

CANDIDATE: Mechanical fall, confusion, seasonal conditions . . .

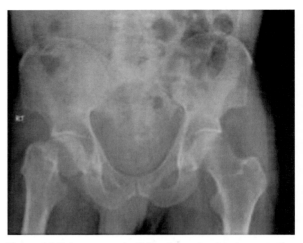

Figure 16.7 Anteroposterior (AP) radiograph pelvis demonstrating intracapsular fractured neck of femur.

EXAMINER: No, I mean with the bone?

CANDIDATE: Osteoporosis is a common cause.

EXAMINER: Define osteoporosis.

CANDIDATE: The World Health Organization (WHO) has established criteria for making the diagnosis of osteoporosis, as well as determining levels that predict higher chances of fractures. These criteria are based on comparing the BMD of the patient with that of a typical healthy, young female.

BMD values that fall well below the average for the healthy, young females (stated statistically as 2.5 standard deviations below the average) are diagnosed as osteoporotic. If a patient has a BMD value less than the healthy, young female, but not 2.5 standard deviations below the average, the bone is osteopenic. Osteopenic means decreased bone mineral density, but it's not as severe as osteoporosis.

This is the WHO definition and it's wrong in a lot of books.

EXAMINER: Any issue with this system?
[I was not sure if he was getting at DEXA or my answer, so I thought I could give the easy answer first and then move onto DEXA, if needed.]

CANDIDATE: Yes, they were based on a Caucasian female, so there will be differences when these levels are applied to non-Caucasian females, children or to males in general. Despite this flaw, BMD measurement is still a common method.

EXAMINER: How is this improved?

CANDIDATE: By using T- and Z-scores. The T-score compares your bone density with the optimal peak bone density for your gender. It is reported as number of standard deviations below the average. A Z-score is used to compare your results with others of your same age, weight, ethnicity and gender. This is useful to determine if there is something unusual contributing to your bone loss. Factors include thyroid abnormalities, malnutrition, medication interactions and tobacco use. [I could not remember any more.]

Pass

This comes up constantly, so know it well, as it's easy to get muddled up with all the scores.

Structured oral examination question 4

EXAMINER: Draw a cross-section of a nerve and nerve fibre. (Figure 16.8.)

CANDIDATE: [I talked about the three layers and the only four components of a nerve fibre I knew.]

EXAMINER: How are these classified?

All you need to know is Seddon[1] and Sunderland.[2]

CANDIDATE: Seddon classified the injury originally into three types and Sunderland defined these into six. Seddon defined neuropraxia as ionic block with possible segmental demyelinization (Sunderland 1), axonotmesis with axon severed but endoneurial tube intact (Sunderland 2), endoneurial tube torn (Sunderland 3) or only epineurium intact (Sunderland 4). Finally, neurotmesis with loss of continuity (Sunderland 5) or a combination of above (Sunderland 6).

[At this point I could not remember exactly what the implications of all the Sunderland classifications were, so I did not offer them.]

Basically, Sunderland 1 and 2 are full recovery, 3 are incomplete, 4 is neuroma, 5 are none and 6 is unpredictable. The easiest way to get this down is to draw a box diagram and get used to filling it in.

EXAMINER: If you cut the median nerve during surgery, what factors affect long-term results?

CANDIDATE: The age of the patient is the single most critical factor in sensory recovery after nerve repair and a good result is adversely affected by associated injuries to muscle, arteries, tendons, and bone. In children I believe you get good results in 50% and 40% in adults.

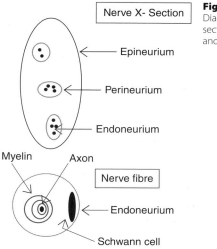

Figure 16.8
Diagram of cross-section of a nerve and nerve fibre.

The good results in children are actually 75% and 50% in adults, although this drops on a yearly basis year on year. The examiner either didn't know or decided to leave this point. Just be a bit careful of using percentages, as they may ask where this information originates, which you may well not know.

EXAMINER: What will you do if there is a 2 cm gap?

CANDIDATE: If there is going to be tension on the graft, I would either use a nerve graft or a conduit.

[I don't offer any further information at this point as my knowledge is limited! Unfortunately this strategy does not work very well.]

EXAMINER: What nerve grafts are available for use?

CANDIDATE: Sural nerve, which has up to 20 cm, medial or lateral antebrachial cutaneous nerve.

EXAMINER: What about nerve conduits?

CANDIDATE: I have never seen a nerve conduit, but they may allow up to 2 cm of nerve growth.

[I had never seen a conduit graft, and knew virtually nothing about them, so I justified my answer. The examiner was happy with this and admitted it would be unfair to ask anything further since I had not seen the procedure. Lucky escape.]

1. Seddon HJ. Three types of nerve injury. *Brain* 1943;**66**(4):238–288.
2. Sunderland S. Advances in diagnosis and treatment of root and peripheral nerve injury. *Adv Neurol* 1979;**22**:271–305.

Structured oral examination question 5

EXAMINER: What is the purpose of the spine?

CANDIDATE: The primary purpose of the spine is to provide protection for the spinal cord and an axial support system to allow locomotion and function of limbs. It has three natural curves which provide an s-shape.

[I genuinely didn't know what to say at this stage, which can be seen by the rather pathetic statement above.]

EXAMINER: Okay, what is the primary site of movement in the spine?

[The penny drops!]

CANDIDATE: Much of the ability to rotate and move within the spinal column is possible due to the intervertebral discs.

EXAMINER: Tell me about the anatomy of the intervertebral disc.

CANDIDATE: Essentially the disc is made up as two parts, the outer annulus fibrosus and the nucleus pulposus. In the C and L spine the discs are thicker anteriorly and in the T spine the disc is equal. The largest disc is at the level of L5/S1.

[Largest disc is actually L4/5, but the examiner either didn't know this or didn't want to push me at this stage.]

Classic paper to quote and read is Coventry *et al.* There are three parts to this.

EXAMINER: Okay, can you tell me about the structure in more detail?

CANDIDATE: The annulus fibrosus makes up the peripheral portion of disc structure and is predominantly made up from fibrocartilage and Type I collagen. The fibres run obliquely and are arranged primarily in concentric layers. The orientation of the fibres varies in successive layers and alternates at about 45°. The nucleus pulposus is predominantly Type II collagen and has a high water content which enables it resist compressive loads. With age the water content declines which reduces its resilience.

EXAMINER: What is the nerve supply?

CANDIDATE: The majority of the nerve supply lies in the outer rings of annulus fibrosus, with supply from the sympathetic chain interiorly.

EXAMINER: And posterior?

CANDIDATE: I can't recall!

[Sinus vertebral nerve dorsally.]

EXAMINER: Why is discitis common in children then?

CANDIDATE: Blood vessels occur in the annulus up to late teens, and into the cartilage endplates until 8 years, which is why discitis occurs in this specific paediatric group.

Coventry MB, Ghormley RK, Kernohan JW. The intervertebral disc: its microscopic anatomy and pathology. Part 1. Anatomy, development and physiology. *J Bone Joint Surg* 1945;**27**:105–12.

Rudert M, Tillmann B. Lymph and blood supply of the human intervertebral disc. Cadaver study of correlations to discitis. *Acta Orthop Scand* 1993;**64**(1):37–40.

Buzz topics which commonly arise in the VIVA

These are the rest of the topics you need to know well to pass. All these topics are covered in various FRCS review and revision books – this just gives you a list of areas to prioritize.

Blood supply to bone

You need to be able to explain the three separate blood supplies that occur in bone. Remember that the skeletal system actually receives 10% of the cardiac output in an adult. In brief the three systems are:

- High-pressure system which is the nutrient artery entering the nutrient foramen with ascending and descending branches. Remember that the end arterioles run on the Volkmann canals which drain into the Haversian system and finally drain back into the central venous sinus and out via the nutrient vein.

- The low-pressure system supplies the outer third of the bone cortex. The normal direction is centrifugal, however following endosteal damage this system is reversed to centripetal. This is the dominant system in children which allows their circumferential growth.

- Peri-articular vascular system which is the series of anastomoses with the medullary system.

Fracture healing

Primary and secondary bone healing comes up repeatedly and you need to be very clear about the distinction between primary and secondary healing and need to understand the relevance to clinical practice. Key points of what you need to know are as follows:

Primary bone healing

- Requires anatomical reduction and interfragmentary compression.
- Absolute stability.
- This system will not tolerate strain.
- Gap healing.
- Briefly describe cutting cones.

Secondary bone healing

- Relative stability, this system *does* requires strain
- Periosteal bone callus – bone formation with *no cartilage*.
- Fibrocartilaginous: fibrocartilage develops at the bone ends and this is subsequently calcified and replaced by woven bone or osteoid.
- All stages of callus formation, hematoma and inflammation, soft callus, hard callus and finally remodelling.

This topic is frequently introduced by the examiners as a clinical question, and you can quickly lead them into this bone biology section by mentioning bone stability. This is guaranteed easy points if you can talk about it for 5 minutes.

Bone grafts

Three levels of bone grafts, which have varying ability to support bone growth and differentiation.

- Osteogenesis (autograft): contains all the living cells and some of the growth factors to allow differentiation into bone.
- Osteoinduction (fresh frozen allograft): contains many of the growth factors that allow activation of osteoprogenitor cells, which can differentiate to cartilage and bone.
- Osteoconduction (various 3D scaffolds): provide structural support and allow both growth factors and mesenchymal stem cells to infiltrate and differentiate into bone and cartilage.

You need to have an understanding of differences between different types of graft which include allograft, autograft and vascularized grafts.

Tendon/ligament insertion to bone

The gradual change in tissue composition from tendon/ligament to bone is to aid in the efficient transfer of load between the two materials. Four zones to know:

- The **first zone** consists of normal tendon, and has properties similar to those found at the tendon mid-substance. This zone consists of well-aligned Type I collagen fibres with small amounts of proteoglycan.
- The **second zone** consists of fibrocartilage and represents the beginning of the transition from tendinous material to bony material. This zone is predominantly composed of Types II and III collagen, and small amounts of the proteoglycan aggrecan.
- The **third zone** contains mineralized fibrocartilage, indicating a transition towards bony tissue. The predominant collagen is Type II, and there are significant amounts of type X collagen.
- **Zone four** consists of bone, which is made up predominantly of Type I collagen with a relatively high mineral content.

Types of muscle contraction

- **Concentric contractions**: Muscle shortens during contraction. When a muscle is activated and lifts a load which is less than the maximum tetanic tension it can generate, the muscle begins to shorten. This is known as concentric contractions. An example is bicep curl.
- **Eccentric contraction**: Muscle actively lengthening as it contracts. As the load on the muscle increases, it finally reaches a point where the external force on the muscle is greater than the force that the muscle can generate. Therefore the muscle is forced to lengthen due to the high external load.
- **Isometric contraction**: Muscle held at a fixed length. The muscle contraction is activated, but instead of being allowed to lengthen or shorten, it is held at a constant length. Example, carrying an object in front of you.
- **Passive stretch**: Muscle passively lengthening. The muscle is lengthened while in a passive state (i.e. not contracting). Example is the pull felt in hamstrings while touching your toes.

This is not an exhaustive list, but will provide you with a taster of the standard and the format the viva will take for basic science.

Other things to know about

- Perren's strain theory.
- Problems with bone graft.
- Graft substitute (you need to know at least three).
- Bone banking.
- Understand donor consent, screening and processing.
- Calcium metabolism.
- Phosphate metabolism.
- Vitamin D.
- Parathyroid hormone.
- Calcitonin.

Chapter

17

Evidence-based practice

Sattar Alshryda and James Mason

Introduction

Evidence-based practice has become an integral part of routine trauma and orthopaedic practice. You apply evidence of many kinds in your daily practice and this has been reflected in the FRCS (Tr & Orth) exam. In the MCQ part, candidates are given a paper to appraise and answer related questions. Although evidence-based practice may be applied in each exam station, you may be specifically asked about different points of evidence-based practice and be probed to assess the depth of your understanding of these aspects, their strengths or limitations. In the structured oral exam, quoting evidence to support your views is perceived highly and can raise your performance and pass grade. This chapter will cover, in a series of questions, the common scenarios you may face. It has been based on real exam questions that have appeared in the FRCS (Tr & Orth), the EBOT and SICOT exams. The answers are deliberately expanded for comprehension and to help address potential follow-up questions.

Station 1: Level of evidence and grades of recommendations

Q 1:   Look at Table 17.1 and fill in the blanks.

1. Systematic review (SR) of randomized controlled trials (RCT) with homogeneous findings.
2. Individual RCT with narrow confidence interval (CI).
3. All-or-none studies.
4. Absolute SpPins and SnNouts.
5. Expert opinion.
6. Analysis based on clinically sensible costs of alternatives; systematic review(s) of the evidence; and including multi-way sensitivity analyses.

Q 2:   What is a systematic review and meta-analysis? What is meant by homogeneity or heterogeneity?

For many surgical procedures, there have been a number of clinical studies and it would seem natural to want to combine them to get the most comprehensive overview of the effect of treatment. A review locates and summarizes the findings of studies. A systematic review is a rigorous and pre-structured approach to conducting a review. The researchers decide beforehand on their inclusion and exclusion criteria, how they will search the literature, extract data, synthesize and analyse them. The meta-analysis attempts to combine data from different studies statistically with a view to get a combined and more precise estimate of the intervention effectiveness. This is not always possible due to data limitations.

When comparing study findings, these are expected to vary naturally due to the play of chance (i.e. within the bounds of sampling error). However, findings may also vary due to different methodologies (randomized or not, how allocation is concealed, blinding etc.); patients (inclusion and exclusion criteria); interventions (type, dose, duration etc.); outcomes (type, scale, duration of follow-up and usage). Such variations can introduce heterogeneity into study findings (variation greater than that expected by chance). Heterogeneity is formally tested using the chi-squared heterogeneity test (or Q statistic). A statistically significant Q test suggests heterogeneity, and that the overall finding is unreliable because findings are inconsistent with a single underlying treatment effect. Homogeneity conversely means that the results of each individual trial are compatible with a single underlying treatment effect.

Cochrane software (RevMan) produces I^2 which is the proportion of variation that is due to heterogeneity rather than chance. Roughly, I^2 values of $< 50\%$

Postgraduate Orthopaedics: Viva Guide for the FRCS (Tr & Orth) Examination, ed. Paul A. Banaszkiewicz and Deiary F. Kader. Published by Cambridge University Press. © Cambridge University Press 2012.

Table 17.1 Levels of evidence.

Level		Intervention	Prognosis	Diagnosis	Economic and decision analyses
1	a	1-	SR (with homogeneity) of inception cohort studies	SR (with homogeneity) of Level 1 diagnostic studies	SR (with homogeneity) of Level 1 economic studies
	b	2-	Individual inception cohort study with ≥ 80% follow-up	Validating cohort study with good reference standards	6-
	c	3-	All or none case-series	4-	Absolute better-value or worse-value analyses
2	a	SR (with homogeneity) of cohort studies	SR (with homogeneity) of either retrospective cohort studies or untreated control groups in RCTs	SR (with homogeneity) of Level >2 diagnostic studies	SR (with homogeneity) of Level >2 economic studies
	b	Individual cohort study (including low quality RCT; e.g. < 80% follow-up)	Retrospective cohort study or follow-up of untreated control patients in an RCT	Exploratory cohort study with good reference standards	Analysis based on clinically sensible costs or alternatives; limited review(s) of the evidence, or single studies; and including multi-way sensitivity analyses
	c	'Outcomes' research; ecological studies	Outcomes research		Audit or outcomes research
3	a	SR (with homogeneity) of case–control studies		SR (with homogeneity) of 3b and better studies	SR (with homogeneity) of 3b and better studies
	b	Individual case–control study		Non-consecutive study; or without consistently applied reference standards	Analysis based on limited alternatives or costs, poor-quality estimates of data, but including sensitivity analyses incorporating clinically sensible variations
4		Case-series	Case-series	Case–control study, poor or non-independent reference standard	Analysis with no sensitivity analysis
5		Expert opinion	Expert opinion	5-	Expert opinion

indicate low, 50–75% indicate moderate, > 75% indicate high heterogeneity.

Q 3: What are the important design aspects to be considered when designing a clinical trial?

A clinical trial is an experiment in humans where subjects are allocated to one of two (or more) treatment groups. The trial is conducted to an ethically approved protocol that prospectively sets out its rationale, conduct and plan of analysis. Important design considerations include:

1. A literature search to establish current knowledge, thus refining the research question and trial methods to take knowledge forward and avoid unnecessary research. Trials are often very expensive and sometimes adequate answers can be found either from the literature or alternative study designs.

2. Sample selection and generalizability: It is vital that participants are representative of the population of interest. Thus inclusion and exclusion criteria are important trial design

features. Thought is needed about non-participation (will patients take part, will only certain patients take part?) and loss to follow-up (how will the analysis cope if many patients fail to provide outcome data at the end of the study?). Adequate patient involvement at the design stage, piloting and use of appropriate incentives are some of the design solutions.

3. Sample size (power). Study power refers to the ability of a trial to find a clinical difference with statistical significance if it truly exists. For example if treatment A truly is better than B, a study with 90% power will get the correct result nine times out of ten. A sample size is calculated to provide an adequate chance of finding a clinically worthwhile difference between treatments, where over-recruitment is undesirable as being uneconomic and unethical (exposing more patients to an 'unnecessary' experiment when the answer has been established within reasonable bounds). Sample size is usually calculated for the primary outcome and has four design elements:

   - Chosen significance level (usually 5%).
   - Study power (typically 80% or 90%).
   - Chosen clinically important difference in the primary outcome.
   - The variability in response (standard deviation in the primary outcome).

4. Bias refers to systematic error in trial design, conduct, analysis or reporting. The true effect of the treatment under investigation is systematically under- or overestimated. For example:

   - Question bias: e.g. comparing a new treatment with the most poorly performing alternative will inflate the apparent benefit of the new treatment.
   - Sampling bias: patients with significant comorbidity are excluded from a trial or decline to participate, limiting the generalizability of findings.
   - Selection bias: patients with underlying prognosis are systematically assigned in larger numbers to one treatment than another.
   - Information bias: including any of a range of factors that distort the recording of data e.g. measurement error, recall bias, work-up bias, interviewer bias, misconduct.

   - Windowing: where the investigators' prejudices influence the selection and presentation of findings.
   - Publication bias: Studies with negative or no difference are less likely to be submitted, published, quoted or even read.

5. Randomisation: if adequately conducted, randomization reduces the chance of selection bias since unknown and unknown prognostic influences are distributed by chance among the different treatment groups.

6. Blinding (masking): If researchers or patients have a preference for a particular treatment, this can introduce bias. Blinding is an important design feature to manage both explicit and implicit prejudice although it is not always possible.

7. Outcome measures: A trial will normally have a primary outcome (around which the trial is designed) and a number of secondary (or supportive) outcomes. They should be clinically relevant, valid, reproducible and sensitive to detect changes.

8. Analysis: This is conducted according to a protocol agreed prospectively before any analysis has begun. Analysis is by intention-to-treat meaning that participants are analysed according to the group allocated regardless of whether they continued with that treatment. These two steps are essential for valid statistical inference – changing the primary analysis after seeing the results or non-intention to treat analyses give invalid conclusions. Practically, there often emerge problems to do with inclusion criteria, trial procedures and loss to follow-up: the findings need to be interpreted in the light of these limitations.

9. Logistics (ethics approval, local approval, building and training a research team).

Q 4: Why is a narrow confidence interval important in level Ib?

A confidence interval (CI) shows the range within which the true treatment effect is likely to lie while a p value is calculated to assess whether treatment effect is likely to have occurred simply through chance. CIs are preferable to p values, as they tell us the range of possible effect sizes. Confidence intervals aid inter-pretation of clinical trial data by putting upper and lower bounds on the likely size of any true effect. A CI that includes no difference between treatments indi-cates that the treatment under investigation is not significantly different from the control. If the confidence interval is narrow, capturing only a small range of effect sizes, we can be quite confident that any effects far from this range have been ruled out by the study. This situation usually arises when the size of the study is large and, hence, the estimate of the true effect is quite precise.

Q 5: What is the difference between a pragmatic and an explanatory trial?

Explanatory trials generally measure efficacy – the outcomes of treatments under ideal conditions, often using carefully defined subjects. Pragmatic trials measure effectiveness – the benefit the treatment produces in routine practice: more relevant to clinicians.[1]

Q6: What is meant by equivalence trials?

Normally we conduct superiority trials, i.e. we are trying to demonstrate the additional value of one treatment over another. Sometimes, however, we may want to demonstrate that two treatments are similarly effective (within certain limits) for which we would use an equivalence design. Alternatively we might want to show that a new treatment is no worse than an existing treatment, for which we could use a non-inferiority design. There are increasing numbers of new and effective treatments for many diseases making placebo comparisons unethical when there is already an established treatment. Thus these study designs always involve comparison against an alternative active therapy; hence they are sometimes called active control equivalence or non-inferiority studies (ACES, ACNS).

Q 7: What do you understand by all-or-none studies?

In an all-or-none study, the treatment causes a dramatic change in outcomes (for example, all patients died when they did not receive the treatment). Such a finding would preclude further study in a controlled trial. Antibiotics for meningitis, surgical intervention for leaking aneurysm and chest decompression for tension pneumothorax are examples.

Q 8: What do you understand by the term sampling error?

In research we explore research questions by sampling, as it is not usually possible to study a whole population. Suppose a random sample of patients with hypertension is sampled from the population of all patients with hypertension. The mean blood pressure in the sample will not exactly match the population because they have been drawn at random from the population. Each random sample will be slightly different, but the answers will cluster round the true population value. This variation is called sampling error. The size of sample error is controlled by the sample size. As sample size increases so the effect of sampling error is reduced and we get more precise estimates. A statistic expressing the size of sampling error is called the standard error (SE), estimated as the standard deviation (SD) of the characteristic (e.g. blood pressure) divided by the square root of the sample size (N) i.e. $SE = SD/(\sqrt{N})$.

Q 9: What do you understand by the null hypothesis?

Within research we formulate and test hypotheses: we make an assertion and see if the observed data support or falsify our assertion. The null hypothesis is normally the default position, it is easier to prove a statement false than true. For example, if you want to prove that 'all hands have five fingers', and you show 1000 hands with five fingers, there is still doubt that a a hand somewhere has 4 fingers. But once you show me one hand only with 4 fingers, the hypothesis of 'all hands have five fingers' is rejected.

The null hypothesis is paired with a second alternative hypothesis, e.g. there is a difference between treatments.

To test our hypotheses, we apply an appropriate statistical test to our observations (which depends on the type of data). The null states that any pattern in our data occurs purely by chance. Conventionally we say the test is statistically significant when the test probability is less than 5% and we reject the null hypothesis in favour of the alternative – the pattern in the data is unlikely to be a chance occurrence.

Formally, the null hypothesis cannot be proven: the observed data either reject the null hypothesis or fail to reject it. Failure to find a statistically significant difference between treatments does not prove they are the same, just that your data do not support rejecting the null hypothesis.

Q 10: Could you possibly reject the null hypothesis when you should not?

Yes, this is possible. Suppose that there really is no difference between two treatments. Setting the significance level at 5%, we accept that if we could repeat a study many times we would reject the null hypothesis incorrectly in 5% of studies. This error rate is called Type I error (or α) and can be reduced by requiring a tougher test of significance (e.g. $p < 1\%$). A Type I error can occur because of sampling error (you simply got an unusual sample by chance) or because of bias (subjects were selected in a non-random manner).

Q 11: What is meant by study power, and why does it matter?

There is a converse risk of accepting the null hypothesis when there is a true difference between the treatment groups, called Type II error (or β). The statistical power in a study is defined as $1-\beta$, i.e. the ability of a study to find a true difference between treatments.

Ensuring a study is adequately powered means that the study sample size is large enough, given the kinds of outcomes that are being measured, to be unlikely to miss a real difference between treatments. Ultimately if we make every study infinitely large we will get precise answers to every question but this would be uneconomic and unethical (since patients would continue to be researched long after an adequate answer was known). Thus study power is an ethical issue: adequate numbers are included so that a robust answer is obtained to inform future care while not exposing additional patients unnecessarily to research. Most researchers accept 80% and above power for their tests as a standard for adequacy.[2]

Q 12: What is meant by the phrase 'absolute SpPins and SnNouts'?

An absolute **SpPin** is a diagnostic finding whose **S**pecificity is so high that a **P**ositive result rules-**IN** a particular diagnosis. An absolute **SnNout** is a diagnostic finding whose **S**ensitivity is so high that a **N**egative result rules-**OUT** the diagnosis.

Q 13: What is a cohort study and how does it defer from a case–control study?

A cohort study is an observational design where patients are selected on the basis of an exposure variable. This is in contrast with a case–control design where patients are selected on the basis of an outcome. Here is an example:

Cohort study: An orthopaedic surgeon recruited 3000 women who were using bisphosphonate and a similar number of women who were not using bisphosphonate. The researcher followed both groups for 10 years and recorded numbers of fragility fractures in each group.

Case–control study: One hundred and fifty patients with Dupuytren's disease were obtained from the James Cook University Hospital waiting list. Controls were obtained from elective hand clinic. The researcher examined the relationship between smoking and development of Dupuytren's disease in the two groups.

Q 14: The following was copied from a paper on treating slipped upper femoral epiphysis. Can you tell me what is meant by the grades (B, C and D)? (Figure 17.1.)

These refer to the grades of recommendation, based on levels of evidence. Several schemes have been published. I follow the one recommended by the Oxford Centre for Evidence-Based Medicine in which grade A is used for good evidence, grade B for fair evidence, grade C for poor evidence and grade D for insufficient or conflicting evidence.[3] (Table 17.2.)

1. Roland M, Torgerson DJ. What are pragmatic trials? *Br Med J* 1998;**316**(7127):285.

2. Ramachandran M. *Basic Orthopaedic Sciences. The Stanmore Guide*. London: Hodder Arnold, 2007.

3. Grades of Recommendation. *Oxford Centre for Evidence-based Medicine*, 2009. Available from: http://www.cebm.net/?o=1025.

Recommendation for Treating Slipped Capital Upper Femoral Epiphysis

Although a rare condition, slipped upper femoral epiphysis or slipped capital upper femoral epiphysis (SCUFE) is one of the most common types of paediatric and adolescent hip disorder. SCUFE involves instability of the growth plate at the junction between the head and neck of the thigh bone (femur) resulting in the head of the femur slipping backwards and downwards from the femoral neck. About 30% of patients subsequently developed bilateral SCUFE with the other hip slipping as well [1–3]. With increasing severity, SUFE is associated with increasing pain and disability. Stable SUFE is best treated with single central screw fixation (grade B, C) [4–8]. If a realignment osteotomy is selected for secondary reorientation of a SUFE, the flexion type rather than the Southwick type should be used (grade C) [9–12]. Unstable SUFE treatment is very controversial and our recommendation is urgent gentle repositioning, 1–2 cannulated screw fixation, joint decompression, and protected weightbearing (grades D, C) [13–16].

Figure 17.1 Recommendation for treating slipper upper femoral epiphysis.

Table 17.2 Grades of recommendation.

Grades	Strength	Descriptions
A	Good	Consistent level I studies for or against recommending intervention
B	Fair	Consistent level II or III studies or extrapolations from level I studies
C	Poor	Level IV studies or extrapolations from level II or III studies not allowing a recommendation for or against intervention
D	Insufficient	Level V evidence or troublingly inconsistent or inconclusive studies of any level

Station 2: Statistics and data interpretation

Q 1: This table is from a systematic review and meta-analysis of the effect of tranexamic acid on blood transfusion rate in total knee replacement. Can you comment on the findings?

This is a forest plot of 14 studies comparing tranexamic acid (TXA) with control. The forest plot consists of several columns:

1. The first column lists the names of the studies and the date of publication. These can be ordered alphabetically (as in this example) or the year of publication, the weight of the studies or the treatment effects.
2. The fourth column represents the events in the TXA group. In the plot, it is the number of patients who received a blood transfusion.
3. The fifth column represents the number of participants in the TXA group.

Table 17.3 The effect of tranexamic acid on blood transfusion rate in total knee replacement.

Study or subgroup	Control Events	Total	Tranexamic acid Events	Total	Weight	Risk ratio M-H, Fixed, 95% CI	Risk ratio M-H, Fixed, 95% CI
Alvarez 2008	6	49	1	46	1.3%	5.63 [0.70, 45.01]	
Benoni 1996	24	43	8	43	10.3%	3.00 [1.52, 5.92]	
Camarasa 2006	23	68	1	35	1.7%	11.84 [1.67, 84.06]	
Ellis 2001	7	10	1	10	1.3%	7.00 [1.04, 46.95]	
Engel 2001	3	12	0	12	0.6%	7.00 [0.40, 122.44]	
Good 2003	14	24	3	27	3.6%	5.25 [1.71, 16.08]	
Hiippala 1995	12	13	10	15	12.0%	1.38 [0.94, 2.05]	
Hiippala 1997	34	38	17	39	21.6%	2.05 [1.41, 2.98]	
Jansen 1999	13	21	2	21	2.6%	6.50 [1.67, 25.33]	
Molloy 2007	11	50	5	50	6.4%	2.20 [0.82, 5.87]	
Orpen 2006	3	14	1	15	1.2%	3.21 [0.38, 27.40]	
Tanaka 2001	26	26	47	73	32.7%	1.53 [1.28, 1.83]	
Veien 2002	2	15	0	15	0.6%	5.00 [0.26, 96.13]	
Zohar 2004	12	20	3	20	3.9%	4.00 [1.33, 12.05]	
Total (95% CI)		**403**		**421**	**100.0%**	**2.56 [2.10, 3.11]**	
Total events	190		99				

Favours control   Favours Tranexamic acid

Heterogeneity: Chi-square = 51.97, df = 13 (p <0.00001); I^2 = 75%.
Test for overall effects Z = 9.44 (p <0.00001).

4. The second column represents the events in the control group.

5. The third column represents the number of participants in the control group.

6. The sixth column is the weight that is given to each study. The weight reflects the importance of the study in terms of its number of patients and events and thus influence in the meta-analysis (combined result). Thus Tanaka 2001 is the most influential study

7. The seventh column represents the treatment effect estimate. In this example it is the risk ratio which is equal to (events/total of the control) divided by (events/total in the TXA group). The risk ratio is one of several ways of analysing proportions: others are odds ratios and risk differences. Continuous outcomes such as height, weight, blood loss are analysed in meta-analysis using either a mean difference or a standardized mean difference. Meta-analysis can be conducted using a number of software packages, including Review Manager (RevMan 5) as used by Cochrane library. The Mantel–Haenszel (M–H) method is used to combine studies using a fixed-effects model – i.e. assuming there is a true underlying answer which each study estimates.

8. The last column provides a plot of the measure of effect for each study. Each study is represented by a square which is proportional in area to the study's weight in the meta-analysis. On each side of the square there is a horizontal line representing the confidence interval. The study findings are distributed and referenced against a vertical line representing the no-effect line. Depending on the outcome of each study, it can be on either the left or right side of the no-effect line. The further away from the line, the more profound is the effect. If a study confidence interval crosses the no-effect line, then it indicates that the treatment effect is not statistically significant. More influential studies give more precise results, having tighter confidence intervals and thus are given greater weight in the combined result. The combined estimate from the weighted study findings is represented by a diamond. Similarly, if the diamond overlaps the line of no effect, then it indicates that the combined estimate of treatment effect is not statistically significant.

TXA has reduced the risk of transfusion by 2.56 times with 95% CI (2.10 to 3.11) and p-value 0.00001. However there is significant heterogeneity as evident by a high I^2 value of 75%.

Q 2: How does this heterogeneity affect your interpretation of the findings?

My interpretation for the above finding is that there is evidence that TXA does reduce the risk of blood transfusion (a statistically significant finding), but the range of trial findings is too great to explain by chance alone and other factors are varying between trials (so the RR of 2.56 can't be applied simply to an 'average' patient). I expect the authors to explore this heterogeneity further. There are several options:

1. Report the forest plot without the combined estimate, and report that heterogeneity limits the interpretation of a simple meta-analytic approach. A report of the range of study findings may still be informative.

2. Separate trials into subgroups by defined characteristics, e.g. trials using low- and high-dose TXA. Limitations are that only characteristics that have been consistently reported can be explored, and that each smaller group provides a less precise answer because it has smaller patient numbers and events contributing. However this approach may reduce heterogeneity by comparing groups that are more similar.

3. Change the statistical assumptions. In this example, the authors used the fixed effect model for combining studies. Using the random effects model allows for heterogeneity by assuming a distributed rather than single answer but it doesn't explain the cause of heterogeneity.

4. Investigate causes of heterogeneity using meta-regression. Meta-regression is potentially an improvement upon subgroup analyses in that it allows the effects of multiple factors to be investigated simultaneously on all the trials (rather than a subset). It is similar in concept to other regressions, in which an outcome variable is predicted according to the values of one or more independent variables. In the above example, the outcome variable is the effect estimate (RR). The independent variables are characteristics of studies that might influence the RR such as dose, timing of administration, the use of heparin, the use of transfusion protocol etc.

5. Patient-level analysis. This commonly involves the original trial investigators agreeing to share patient-level data to permit more refined statistical analysis.

Q 3: Can you elaborate more on fixed- and random-effects models?

Fixed-effects models are based on the assumption that every study measure the same single (fixed) treatment effect. In other words, if we were doing a meta-analysis of risk difference, we would assume that every study is estimating the same risk difference; and this might not be true.

A random-effects model makes the assumption that individual studies are estimating different treatment effects. These treatment effects have a distribution with some central value (such as mean, median) and some degree of variability (range). The random effects model deals with the central value of the distribution of effects. There is a debate among researchers about whether it is better to use a fixed- or random-effect meta-analysis.

Q 4: What is meant by the term categorical data?

Data in general are divided into various types. These can be summarized as:

1. Categorical data: The objects being studied are grouped into categories based on some qualitative trait (hence, sometimes called qualitative data). This is furthered classified into:

   a. Nominal: categories without order e.g. gender, smoking status, marital status etc.

   b. Ordinal: categories with order e.g. social status, Ficat grading and pain score (mild, moderate, severe) etc.

Categorical variables with just two categories are called binary variables.

2. Measurement (numerical) data: The objects being studied are measured based on some quantitative trait. Hence, sometimes are called quantitative data. These are further classified into:

   a. Discrete: Only certain values are possible (there are gaps between the possible values) e.g. number of admissions to orthopaedic ward, number of spinal metastases, number of patients transfused.

   b. Continuous: Theoretically, any value within an interval is possible with a fine enough measuring device e.g. age, height, weight, blood loss.

Q 5: Why is it important to distinguish between different types of data?

The type(s) of data collected in a study determine the type of presentation and statistical analysis used. Categorical data are commonly summarized using percentages or proportions and tested using non-parametric tests whereas measurement data are summarized using means, range, standard deviation etc. and may be tested by parametric tests if parametric assumptions are met.

Q 6: What is the difference between parametric and non-parametric tests?

How we test for statistical significance depends upon the assumptions we make about how our test variable is distributed in the population, for example whether the distribution of patient BMI is normally distributed (or bell-shaped). In statistical analysis, parametric significance tests are only valid if such assumptions are met. To compare the BMI of two groups of patients on different weight-loss programmes we can use a t-test if the distribution of BMI values in each group is approximately normal. If they are not, a non-parametric test can be used, which makes no distributional assumptions (e.g. for the BMI data the Mann–Whitney U test). It is desirable to use a parametric test when possible since they are more powerful. Table 17.4 summarizes statistical testing in different situations.

Q 7: How can you tell that the data are normally distributed?

There are several ways to check data for normality. Plotting normally distributed data using a histogram produces a symmetrical bell-shaped curve. Real-world data (being a sample from a bigger population) are never perfectly bell-shaped. There are two quantities that can be calculated from the data to assess normality: skewness and kurtosis (Figure 17.2).

Skewness examines the horizontal distortion (left or right) from a normal curve, kurtosis examines the vertical distortion (pointed, squashed). Data that are positively skewed have more values greater than the mean. Graphically, the curve has a tail pointing to the right. A negatively skewed distribution has a tail pointing to the left. Positive kurtosis indicates a peaked curve (leptokurtosis) while negative kurtosis indicates a flat curve (platykurtosis).

Table 17.4 Levels of evidence.

Testing	Normal distribution	Non-normal distribution	
		Ordinal, measurement data	Nominal data
Data description – central tendency (spread)	Mean (SD)	Median (Range)	Proportion
Comparison of two different treatment groups (such as placebo vs. treatment)	Unpaired t-test	Mann–Whitney U test	Chi-square (Fisher's test for sample samples of < 5)
Comparison within one group or between matched groups (e.g. Oxford hip or knee scores before and after joint replacement)	Paired t-test	Wilcoxon signed rank test	McNemar's test
Comparison of two or more groups	ANOVA	Kruskal–Wallis test	Chi-square test
Repeated comparison over time of two or more groups e.g. pain measured at 3, 6 and 12 months	Repeated measures ANOVA	Friedman test	Cochran's Q test
Association between two variables (e.g. recurrent falls and number of fractures)	Pearson correlation	Spearman correlation	Contingency coefficients
Simple regression (one independent variable, one dependent variable)	Simple linear or non-linear regression	Non-parametric regression	Simple logistic regression
Multiple regression analysis (multiple independent variables, one dependent variable)	Multiple linear or non-linear regression		Multiple logistic regression

A perfectly normal distribution will have a skewness and kurtosis statistic of zero. This can be formally tested using the Kolmogorov–Smirnov test or Shapiro–Wilk's test for normality.

Q 8: What to do if data are not normal?

A violation of normality does not preclude running parametric tests. However, when violation occurs in conjunction with violations of equality of variance, the use of non-parametric statistical alternatives or transformation of the data (to make it normal) may be useful.

A new technique which is getting more popular is the bootstrapping technique which involves random sampling of data with replacement to build a large number of data for parametric testing.

Q 9: You mentioned earlier odds ratio, risk ratio and risk difference. What are they and why choose one over the other?

These are common measures of the size of an effect. They are used in case–control studies, cohort studies, clinical trials and increasingly in systematic reviews and meta-analyses. Risks and odds are just ways of expressing chance in numbers. For example: Group A includes 24 trained skiers who ski a course during which six fall down:

(Quick revision: $25/100 = 25\% = 0.25$ = one quarter, these four are all identical.)

The risk = number with an event (fall)/total number of subjects = $6/24 = 0.25$.

The odds = number with an event (fall)/ number without an event (no fall) = $6/18 = 0.33$.

A second group of 24 untrained skiers complete the course and 12 fall down:

The risk = falls/subjects = $12/24 = 0.5$.

The odds = falls/no falls = $12/12 = 1$.

- Relative risk or risk ratio (they mean the same thing and are both abbreviated as RR) is simply the risk of the event in one group divided by the risk of the event in the other group. RR value of 1 means no difference between the two groups. The

(a)

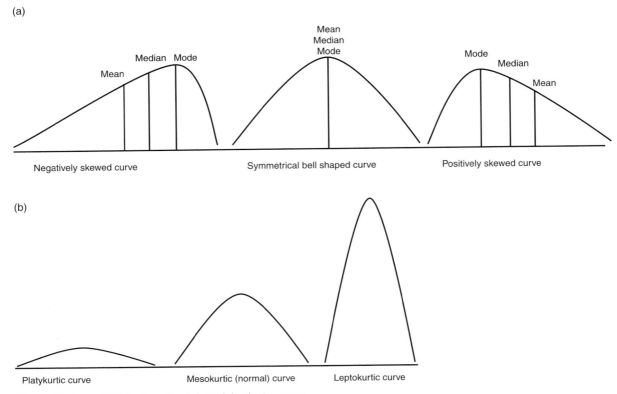

Figures 17.2a and 17.2b Normal and skewed distribution curves.

RR of a fall with training is 0.25/0.5 = 0.5, a halving of the risk of falling.

- The risk difference (RD) is (as the name suggests) the difference between two groups in the risk of falling. The RD is 0.25–0.5 = −0.25 i.e. a 25% *reduction* in the risk of falling. An RD value of 0 means no difference between the two groups. Sometimes we report the absolute risk reduction (ARR) by removing the minus sign. The ARR = 0.25.
- The number needed to treat (NNT) is how many people would need to be trained to prevent one fall: the inverse of RD. Here it is 1/0.25 or four people.
- The odds ratio (OR) is the odds of the event occurring in one group divided by the odds of the event occurring in the other group. OR value of 1 means no difference between the two groups. In our example OR = 0.33/1 = 0.33.

Odds ratios are hard to understand, and are often misinterpreted. Risk differences (and derivatives like NNT) are more clinically useful than relative risks and odds ratios. However relative measures tend to

be more useful in meta-analysis because of their statistical properties. Risk differences tend to vary with duration of follow-up (benefits grow over time for chronic disease and treatment) and with underlying prognosis (more severely ill patients may show greater benefit). Relative measures may be less sensitive to time or severity.

Q 10: **The following plot is from the same above systematic review and meta-analysis of the effect of tranexamic acid on blood transfusion rate in total knee replacement. Can you comment on the findings? (Figure 17.3.)**

This is called a funnel plot which is a simple scatterplot of the treatment effects (RR) estimated from individual studies (horizontal axis) against the precision of the studies represented by standard error (SE). The vertical dotted line shows the estimated combined RR from the meta-analysis. The diagonal dotted lines show the range in which studies might be distributed by chance given the size (and thus precision) of each study.

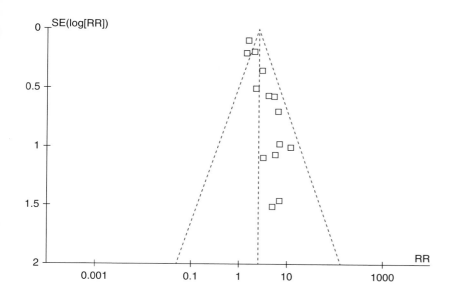

Figure 17.3 The effect of tranexamic acid on blood transfusion rate in total knee replacement.

Thus larger (big sample size), more precise (smaller standard error) studies should be closely distributed either side of the pooled effect and smaller studies should be distributed more widely giving the classic inverted symmetrical funnel. If the studies are not distributed randomly (due to sampling error) around the combined RR estimate then some other influence is suggested.

The funnel plot shows trials scattered asymmetrically around the pooled RR with smaller trials reporting a greater effect than larger ones. Two possible explanations are: smaller trials of lower methodological quality tend to overestimate true effect; publication bias has led to the smaller negative trials remaining unpublished.

Q 11:   The following plot is from the Norwegian joint registry about the effect of cement type on Charnley stem revision. Can you describe the findings? (Figure 17.4.)

This is a survival analysis of Charnley femoral prostheses using different types of cements (high viscosity, low viscosity and Boneloc). There is a statistically significant difference between the three groups (no overlaps in the confidence interval and p value < 0.0001). The high viscosity cement seems to provide a higher survival rate where about 97.5% survived to 6 years.

Q 12:   Can you tell me more about survival analysis? What do these bizarre lines represent?

Survival analysis is a special kind of analysis of time-to-event data, which includes *censoring*. For example,

we are interested in how many years a prosthesis will function for before it fails. However, to wait for complete follow-up of every patient until they die would involve waiting many years for the answer. Instead we follow patients for a limited (and often varying) period of time: either the prosthesis fails at a certain time during this period or the patient is *censored* at the end of the period (because we don't know what may happen afterwards). In a survival analysis each hip either has a fail date or a censor date. The survival curves (called Kaplan–Meier curves) show the progress of failing hips. If the analysis is conducted at one point in time on patients receiving surgery over a number of years, then it will include progressively fewer patients with longer periods of observation. Many patients provide 1 year of follow-up but far fewer provide 6 years in the example. Due to censoring or events the number of patients contributing diminishes with time, thus the confidence intervals become wider and wider.

Station 3: Epidemiology and screening

Q 1:   What is the difference between incidence and prevalence?

Incidence refers to the frequency of development of a new disease in a population at risk in a certain period of time (usually 1 year). Prevalence is the actual number of cases alive with the disease, either during a period of time (period prevalence) or at a particular point in time

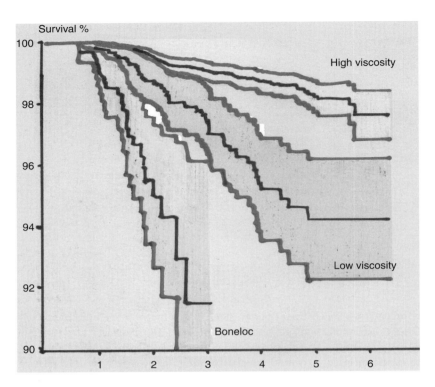

Figure 17.4 Survival curves of Charnley femoral prosthesis with high viscosity, low viscosity and Boneloc cement.

(point prevalence). Incidence is important for understanding and managing trends while period prevalence informs about the disease burden in a population.

Q 2: **Name one disease in orthopaedics which is suitable for screening. What are the characteristics of a good screening test?**

There are a few conditions in orthopaedics suitable for successful screening such as developmental dysplasia of the hip, osteoporosis and scoliosis. There are certain features for a successful screening programme. These features can be roughly divided into:

1. Disease features:
   i. Disease with significant impact on community.
   ii. Natural history of the disease is known.
   iii. Detection occurs before a critical point (before it is too late).

2. Screening test features:
   i. Accepted and tolerated by patients.
   ii. High sensitivity is essential to rule out effectively those testing negative.
   iii. High specificity is also desirable to reduce false unnecessary positive result.
   iv. Cost-effective.

3. Screened population features:
   i. Disease has high enough prevalence to allow screening.
   ii. Patients willing to undergo further evaluation and treatment.
   iii. Accepted and effective treatment is available.

Q 3: **So do you think developmental dysplasia of the hip is a suitable disease for screening?**

Yes. It has most of the criteria for suitability for screening test. It has a well-known natural history; there is a very sensitive and relatively specific test for it (ultrasound) and if it is detected early, there is an effective, cheap treatment. If not treated early, it may lead to long-term disability. However, cost-effectiveness is the issue. To train sonographers, provide the equipment for universal screening and education is costly. One solution to increase the cost-effectiveness of the DDH screening programme is to screen an at-risk population only such as newborns with family history, breech presentation, postural foot/neck deformity or oligohydramnios. The limitation is that only one-third of cases of dislocated hip have these risk factors.[1] Similar points can be made about screening for osteoporosis.

Table 17.5 Contingency table of test outcomes.

	Disease positive	Disease negative
Test positive	True positive (TP)	False positive (FP)
Test negative	False negative (FN)	True negative (TN)

Q 4: You mentioned sensitivity and specificity of screening tests, can you elaborate more on these and other features of screening tests?

Test properties for a simple screening test or confirmatory test can be tabulated (Table 17.5).

There is one pre-test feature:

Prevalence: the probability of having disease before testing.

Prevalence = disease positive/(disease positive + disease negative).

There are six features of this test:

1. Sensitivity (Sn): the probability of correctly identifying all cases of disease.
   Sn = true positive/(true positive + false negative).
2. Specificity (Sp): the probability of correctly excluding all cases without disease.
   SP = true negative/(true negatives + false positives).
3. Accuracy (A): the probability of correct identification of a disease.
   A = (true positive + true negative)/total number.
4. Positive predictive value (PPV): the probability of disease when testing positive.
   PPV = true positives/(true positives + false positives).
5. Negative predictive value (NPV): the probability of no disease when testing negative.
   NPV = true negatives/(true negatives + false negatives).
   Predictive values interact (change) with the prevalence of disease in the population. Clearly the higher the prevalence (pre-test probability of disease), the higher the PPV (post-test probability of disease) regardless of the value of the test. Screening tends to involve high-sensitivity, low-prevalence contexts which provide good rule-out tests when they exclude the large majority of those being screened. Patients testing positive are then a relatively small group at higher risk and go forward for more definitive (and possibly invasive) testing.

6. Likelihood ratio (LR): the ratio of the chances of truly having a disease to not having it, given that a positive test result was obtained. Clearly, the larger the value of LR, the better the test.
   LR = Sn/(1−Sp).

To decide when a test is positive requires determining a cut-off or threshold value in the test measure. Tests are seldom perfect so the test values of diseased and undiseased patients overlap. Suppose the probability of disease increases with test score. We can increase specificity (make negative results more accurate by increasing the threshold value – we mislabel fewer undiseased people) but then we reduce sensitivity by missing more true cases of disease. A receiver operating characteristic (ROC) curve is used to explore the trade off between sensitivity and specificity as the test threshold value increases. If there is no overlap between the test results of diseased populations then any test value in-between would be a perfect test: 100% sensitive and 100% specific. If the two distributions of test results lie exactly on top of one another the test is useless (a straight diagonal line). In practice tests are not perfect or useless. A ROC curve rising quickly to the upper left corner of the graph and then flattening suggests a very good test and a ROC curve not very different from a straight diagonal is a poor test (Figure 17.5). The surgeon or experimenter decides how to use the test by choosing a cut-off value. Different cut-off values result in a balanced test, or a test that is optimized for use in screening or confirmation (Figure 17.6). Note once more, high-sensitivity, negative test rules out (SnNout) is desired for screening.

1. Paton RW. Screening for hip abnormality in the neonate. *Early Hum Dev* 2005;**81**(10):803–806.

Station 4: Outcome measures

Q 1: What do you understand by PROMs?

PROMs stands for patient reported outcome measures. They are short, self-completed questionnaires, which measure the patients' symptoms, functional ability and health-related quality of life from the patient perspective rather than the clinician perspective.

In the past, clinician-based outcome measures (CBOMs) were considered objective when the clinician was assessing patient progress using 'hard signs'

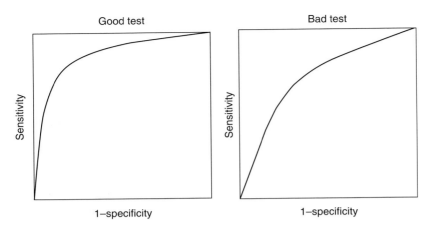

Figure 17.5 Receiver operating characteristic (ROC) curves of two different tests.

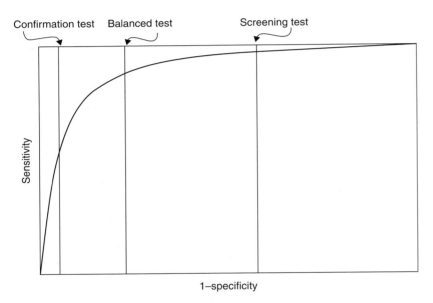

Figure 17.6 A receiver operating characteristic (ROC) curve; different cut-off values for different uses.

such as range of motion, strength, swelling etc. Objectivity was dependent on the reliability or reproducibility of the clinicians' assessments. In contrast, PROMs were considered as subjective and soft and there was reluctance to use them. Now, it is generally agreed that the health-status information collected from patients using PROM questionnaires before and after an intervention provides a valuable indication of outcomes or quality of care delivered to patients.

PROMs are further classified into generic and disease-specific measures. The generic measures are designed to give a general overview of health-related quality of life. The European Quality of life measure (EuroQol), Short Form (SF) 36, SF 12 and Nottingham Health Profile (NHP) are examples of generic outcome measures. Disease-specific measures, on the other hand, focus on aspects of health that are specific to that particular disease, for example: the Oxford Hip Score (OHS) for hip arthritis, The Oxford Knee Score (OKS) for knee arthritis, Disability of the Arm and Shoulder and Hand (DASH) for upper limb.

From 1 April 2009, all NHS hospitals have been required to collect PROMs for four clinical areas: hip replacements, knee replacements, hernia and varicose veins. The OHS and the EuroQol are used for hip replacement. The OKS and EuroQol are used for knee replacement.

Q 2: Why do you think these scores or outcome measures are chosen?

There are several reasons why one might prefer one outcome measure instead of others. One obvious consideration is that the measure is being used for its designed purpose and patient group. More detailed considerations are how carefully the measure was designed, developed and validated. This can be summarized as follows:[1]

1. **Content (are the contents of the measure relevant to your population?).**
    A. Type:
        i. Clinician-based outcome measure (CBOM).
        ii. Patient-based outcome measure (PROM).
    B. Scale: What questions make up the outcome? How are they are scored?
    C. Interpretation: Do higher scores indicate a better outcome?

2. **Methodology.**
    A. Validity: Does it measure what it is supposed to measure?
        i. Construct validity: quantitative assessment of validity.
            1. Divergent: Two measures do not correlate highly if they measure different things.
            2. Convergent: Two measures have a high correlation with each other when measuring the same thing.
            3. An outcome measure must show both convergent and divergent validity as evidence of construct validity: neither alone is sufficient.
        ii. Content validity (face validity) – Are the contents comprehensive and relevant? This is established by content experts: clinicians in the case of CBOMs and patients or both in the case of PROM.
        iii. Criterion validity: correlation with the golden standard.
            1. Predictive validity: ability to predict the future state of health e.g. patients with low score will do badly.

2. Concurrent validity: accurately predict current state of health when compared with other measures.
    B. Reliability: consistent measurement of a condition.
        i. Internal consistency: How consistent are the questions in measuring the same outcome; that is why there are several questions to measure a single dimension.
        ii. Reproducibility: produce the same results when there are no changes.
            1. Intra-observer (test–retest): consistency when used on the same patient on two different occasions (with no change in patient condition).
            2. Inter-observer: agreement between two or more observers using the same measure on the same patient at the same time.
    C. Responsiveness: ability of the measure to change when the status of the patient changes.

3. **Clinical utility.**
    A. Patient friendliness (acceptability): easy to complete by patients, clear questions, easy to understand, does not take too long to complete etc.
    B. Clinician friendliness (feasibility): easy to use and administer, issues include need for licensing or special software, cost, time etc.

Q 3: How should you measure inter-observer agreement in outcome measures?

A simple way is for two or more observers to complete a questionnaire, test or measure then compare findings. There will be some level of agreement by chance even if the observers were just guessing. Thus it is conventional for statistical tests to measure the level of agreement over and above that expected by chance.

The Kappa (K) statistic is used to measure inter-observer agreement between two observers for categorical outcomes (mainly nominal data) and a value of 1 reflects a perfect agreement, a value of 0 means no better than chance and a negative value is disagreement. For more than two observers, Fleiss' K is used.

The intra-class correlation coefficient (ICC) is used to measure inter-observer agreement for continuous data. The range of the ICC may be between 0 and 1 with 1 reflecting perfect agreement.

Cronbach's alpha is a coefficient of reliability which is usually used to measure internal consistency. Its range is 0–1 and it generally increases as the correlations among test items increase. Most health professionals require a reliability of 0.70 or higher before they will use an outcome measure.

1. Suk M, Hanson BP, Norvell DC, Helfet DL. *AO Handbook. Musculoskeletal Outcome Measures and Instruments*. Basel: Thieme, 2004.

Chapter

18

Imaging and investigative techniques

Rajesh Kakwani and Mike Newby

General radiology viva advice

In the FRCS (Tr & Orth) structured oral exam it is probably unlikely that you will be asked a full-blown 5-minute radiology question. It is possibly too much detailed knowledge for the average candidate (and examiner) to stretch out for a 5-minute discussion. That said, sometimes dangerous assumptions can be made and we know candidates who have had very detailed questioning on the radiological/imaging principles, and it is advisable to be well enough prepared to answer questions which may relate to physics, image acquisition or interpretation of all mainstream radiological modalities.

The other aspect of radiology, which is extremely important and can certainly set you apart from the average candidate, is image interpretation. This needs to be accurate, relevant and succinct, with a recommendation for further imaging if felt necessary. To approach such questions well, the candidate must fully appreciate the potential benefits and limitations which relate to any particular imaging technique. This is not always an easy skill to acquire so our suggestion would be to arrange one or two tutorials from a local friendly radiologist who will be able to put you on the spot in describing various scans and radiographs. Going on a viva course, closely observing and making mental notes of how other candidates describe various radiographs is another way in which you can refine this technique. If all else fails then practise out loud describing radiographs and scans from a book.

Structured oral examination question 1: Radiographs

EXAMINER: What are X-rays? (Figure 18.1.)

CANDIDATE: X-rays are electromagnetic radiations of wavelength: 10–0.01 nm.

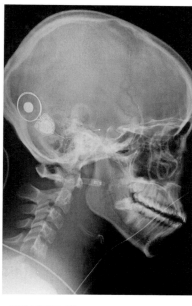

Figure 18.1 X-ray – cervical spine lateral (C5–6 dislocation).

EXAMINER: How are X-rays generated?

CANDIDATE: X-rays are released on heating a fine tungsten filament to around 2200 °C in a vacuum.

EXAMINER: How does digital radiography work?

CANDIDATE: Digital radiography uses a phosphor compound detector plate instead of the conventional photographic emulsion film. The detector generates a digital image that can either be printed or sent to a PACS (picture archiving and communication system).

EXAMINER: What measures will you take to minimize radiation exposure to staff whilst using an image intensifier?

CANDIDATE: The main source of radiation for the surgeon and the team is the scattered radiation from the patient. Measures to minimize the radiation exposure to staff are summarized as TDS (Time/Distance/Shielding):

Postgraduate Orthopaedics: Viva Guide for the FRCS (Tr & Orth) Examination, ed. Paul A. Banaszkiewicz and Deiary F. Kader. Published by Cambridge University Press. © Cambridge University Press 2012.

1. Time: keep the radiation time exposure As Low As Reasonably Achievable (ALARA principle).
2. Distance: The inverse square law. The amount of scatter radiation is inversely proportional to the square of the distance from the X-ray source. The distance between the X-ray source and the patient should be maximized i.e. keep the image-intensifier as close to the patient as possible. (Staff to stay 1 metre away from the X-ray source.)
3. Shielding: Lead aprons (0.25 mm thick), thyroid shields and protective goggles.

EXAMINER: What is collimation?

CANDIDATE: Reduction in the size of the window through which the X-rays are emitted leads to sharper radiographs as well as reduction in radiation dose.

EXAMINER: What is the maximum safe dose of occupation-related radiation exposure?

CANDIDATE: A whole-body exposure of 20 mSv over a year is the maximum acceptable radiation dose (averaged over 5 years).

Additional notes

1. Natural background radiation: 0.01 mSv/day (UK – 2.2 mSv/year).
2. Cosmic radiation during high-altitude flights: 0.001–0.01 mSv/hour.
3. X-ray chest: 0.1 mSv.
4. CT head: 1.5 mSv.
5. CT abdomen: 9.9 mSv equivalent to 500 chest X-rays.

Ramachandran M. *Basic Orthopedic Sciences*. London: Hodder Arnold, 2007.

Structured oral examination question 2: Ultrasound

EXAMINER: What is the physics behind ultrasound imaging?

CANDIDATE: The passage of electric current through a piezoelectric crystal causes deformation of the crystal surface, in turn producing sound waves. When the transducer is then applied to the patient's skin using a lubricating jelly, these waves are then transmitted into the patient's body. The reflected waves when received back by the transducer cause distortion of the crystal surface, producing a voltage, which is then converted to an image. The duration between the sound wave emission and detection reflects the depth of the tissue being studied.

EXAMINER: Tell me a few of the practical applications of ultrasound in orthopaedics.

CANDIDATE: A few uses of ultrasound in orthopaedics include:

1. Hip:
   a. Diagnosis and treatment monitoring in developmental dysplasia of the hip. (The viva can drift to Graf's classification of DDH from here.)
   b. Detection and guided aspiration of hip effusion (especially in children).
2. Shoulder: To diagnose impingement and rotator cuff tears.
3. Tendons: To detect tendon ruptures, swelling/edema (Achilles/tibialis posterior).
4. Soft tissue swelling – size, extent, solid or cystic +/− guided biopsy.

Ramachandran M. *Basic Orthopedic Sciences*. London: Hodder Arnold, 2007.

Structured oral examination question 3: CT scanners

EXAMINER: How does a CT scanner work? What are the principles of a CT scanner?

CANDIDATE: The X-rays are liberated from the axially rotating X-ray tube. After passing through the patient, they are received by a circle of stationary detectors. The data collected are processed by the computer and digital images are reconstructed. The scanning gantry rotates helically around the patient allowing continuous acquisition of data. With modern multi-detector CT transverse (or axial) anatomical sections can be produced with high resolution, and reformatted to create reconstructions in any plane.

General information

1. CT was discovered by Sir Godfrey Hounsfield (Hayes, UK) and the first patient brain scan was done in 1971. Sir Hounsfield was awarded the Joint Nobel Prize (with Allan McLeod Cormack of Massachusetts) in 1979.
2. Hounsfield units are a measure of the attenuation coefficient of the tissue being scanned. (Bone = 1000 HU.) Bone windows are usually centred on 300 HU with a width of 1200.

3. Limitations:
   a. Radiation dose.
   b. Artifact from orthopaedic metalware reduces image quality.
   c. Soft tissue detail is limited.

EXAMINER: Give some orthopaedic indications for CT scan.

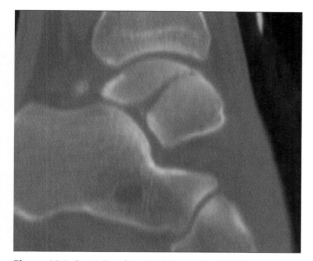

Figure 18.2 Sagittally reformatted image of ankle CT demonstrating talar body fracture.

CANDIDATE:

1. Complex peri-articular fractures – for example, fractures of the acetabulum, tibial plafond, tibial plateau, proximal humerus, talus, calcaneum and vertebrae. (Figure 18.2.)
2. Polytrauma patients – head, chest and abdominal scanning.
3. CT arthrography/myelography (if MRI contraindicated).
4. Assessment of union: scaphoid.
5. Drilling/ablation of osteoid osteoma.

Structured oral examination question 4: MRI scanners

EXAMINER: Please describe the findings (Fig. 18.3).

CANDIDATE: This is an MRI scan of the lumbo-sacral spine of ... Dated ... Age ...

EXAMINER: Is it a T1-weighted image or T2?

CANDIDATE: The image to the right is a T1 image as it has a TR (time to repetition) value of < 1000 ms, whereas the image on the left is a T2 image (TR > 1000 ms).[1]

[Don't rely on fluid/fat signals for judging the type, as they can be confusing in STIR or fat-suppressed images.]

Most imaging protocols will use a combination of different sequences to optimally evaluate the structures and pathologies in question by providing both anatomical and pathological information.

(a)

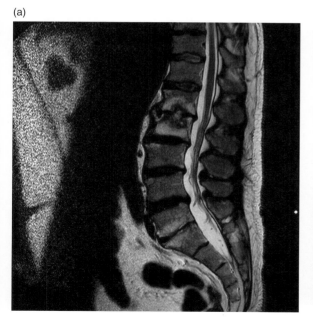

(b)

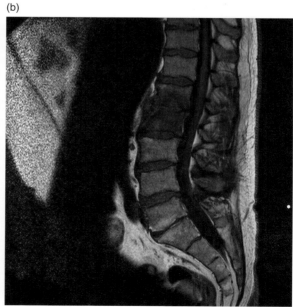

Figure 18.3 Sagittal T2 (a) and sagittal T1 (b) images of the lumbar spine. This demonstrates L1/2 disc space abnormality with adjacent endplate oedema. It could represent either disc space infection or acute inflammatory discovertebral lesion as might be seen in spondylitis.

MRI can be utilized in any plane, and this is sometimes crucial in providing additional information.

EXAMINER: What are the differences between T1- and T2-weighted images?

CANDIDATE:

	T1 weighted	T2 weighted
TR	< 1000	> 1000
TE	Short (< 80)	Long (> 80)
Definition	Time constant of exponential growth of magnetism	Time constant of exponential decay of signal following the excitation impulse
	Fat is bright	Water is bright/Fat is bright too
	Anatomy	Pathology

EXAMINER: What contrast is generally used with MRI?

CANDIDATE: Chelated gadolinium. It enhances the oedematous tissues on T1 images.

An important but rare complication of gadolinium is nephrogenic systemic fibrosis (a fibrosing dermopathy), which has been reported to occur rarely in patients with Stage 4 renal failure.

Current guidance is that if the eGFR < 30, gadolinium should not be administered.

EXAMINER: What are the contraindications for MRI scan?

CANDIDATE:
(1) Implanted pacemaker and defibrillators.
(2) Internal hearing aids/cochlear implants.
(3) Implanted nerve stimulators.
(4) Metal objects in orbit of the eye.
(5) Intra-cranial metal clips.
(6) Aortic stent graft.
(7) Mechanical heart valve.

Most coronary stents and many other vascular stents are not contraindications for MRI, but will require a pre-MRI check regarding their compatibility. MRI is usually used with extreme caution within the first 6 weeks postoperatively when any metallic clip (including skin clips) or implant has been utilized.

EXAMINER: What are the indications for MR arthrograms?

CANDIDATE:
1. Shoulder: Suspected capsular/labral tears.
2. Hip: Labral tears/impingement.
3. Knee: Post-meniscectomy for recurrent tear.
4. Wrist: Scapholunate dissociation, TFCC tear.

EXAMINER: What is the basic principle of an MRI scanner?

CANDIDATE: The MRI scan involves exploiting the magnetic moment/nuclear spin property of the hydrogen nucleus (in the tissues) when placed in a strong magnetic field. Radio waves (64 MHz) are then applied using the transmitter coil. Following the cessation of the radio waves, the individual magnetic moments then precess and the response is recorded in the receiver coil.

EXAMINER: What do the terms PD, STIR and FAT SAT sequences mean?

CANDIDATE:
PD is a proton density weighted image. It is commonly used in knee protocols to image the menisci.

FAT SAT and STIR are both sequences used to improve tissue contrast by suppressing the response from fat in tissues.

FAT SAT is an abbreviation for fat saturation (spectral fat saturation). It can be applied to T1/T2/PD sequences. T1 fat-saturated sequences are commonly used in MR arthrography and after the administration of contrast, and both PD and T2 fat-saturated sequences are commonly utilized to identify pathology.

STIR stands for short tau inversion recovery. This is a very robust, commonly used sequence, which is very sensitive to abnormal fluid or oedema and so ordinarily demonstrates pathological processes well.

EXAMINER: What is TE?

CANDIDATE: Time to echo. When a second radiofrequency pulse is applied after the first one is turned off, the time duration between the first wave and the echo formation is termed TE. TE is a controllable factor as timing of application of the second radiofrequency pulse is at the discretion of the user.

EXAMINER: What is extremity MRI?

CANDIDATE: Extremity MRI involves placement of only the involved extremity in the magnetic bore of a very compact MRI scanner, whilst the rest of the body remains outside.[2]

ADVANTAGES ARE:
1. Reduced cost.
2. Improved patient comfort and reduced claustrophobia.
3. Facilitated sitting.
4. Reduced patient risk.

DISADVANTAGE: Only the distal two-thirds of the extremity can be scanned.

EXAMINER: What is your option if the patient is claustrophobic in an MRI scanner?

CANDIDATE: Open MRI scanner, or consider alternative imaging modalities.

1. Miller MD. *Review of Orthopaedics*. 5th Edition. Philadephia, PA: Saunders Elsevier, 2008.
2. Einhorn TA, O'Keefe RJ, Buckwalter JA (Eds). *Orthopaedic Basic Science: Foundations of Clinical Practice*. 3rd Edition. Rosemont, IL: American Academy of Orthopaedic Surgeons, 2007.

Structured oral examination question 5: Bone densitometry

EXAMINER: What is bone densitometry?

CANDIDATE: Bone densitometry includes all techniques used to quantify the amount of bone in the skeleton.

The WHO guidelines for interpretation of bone densitometry results (T-score):

Normal	Score not more than one standard deviation below the average value of young adult
Osteopaenia	Score more than 1 standard deviation below the young adult average, but not more than 2.5 standard deviations below
Osteoporosis	More than 2.5 standard deviations below the average value for young adult
Severe osteoporosis	Osteoporosis + Fragility fracture/s

EXAMINER: What are its uses?

CANDIDATE: The clinical applications of bone densitometry include:
1. Assessment of bone status in primary and secondary osteoporosis.
2. Assessment of the effect of treatment for osteoporosis.
3. Fracture risk assessment (What is FRAX score?).
4. Evaluation of preventive measure for bone loss associated with ageing/metabolic disorders.
5. Measure periprosthetic bone loss (particularly cementless hip arthroplasty).

EXAMINER: Name some techniques used to measure bone density in the axial skeleton.
[The same question can be asked regarding appendicular skeleton.]

CANDIDATE: Techniques that can be used to measure bone density in the axial skeleton are:
1. DEXA: Dual energy X-ray absorptiometry.
2. Quantitative CT (rarely used).
3. Quantitative MRI (rarely used).

EXAMINER: Does DEXA measure true bone density or apparent?
[A rather pointed question.]

CANDIDATE: DEXA measures apparent density (obviously) as it is a two-dimensional measurement quantified in g/cm^2. Quantitative CT gives a volumetric (three-dimensional) true representation of bone density in g/cm^3. Even quantitative CT can give false low readings as it also measures intravertebral fat.

EXAMINER: Which of the bone density measurement techniques can differentiate between cortical and trabecular bone?

CANDIDATE: Quantitative CT and quantitative MRI.

EXAMINER: What is a FRAX score?

CANDIDATE: FRAX (Fracture Risk Assessment Tool) is the tool used to assess 10-year probability of hip/major osteoporotic fracture of patients. It integrates clinical risk factors with bone mineral densitometry for femoral neck. Treatment for osteoporosis is recommended if the FRAX score for hip fracture is more than 3% or that for major osteoporosis-related fracture is more than 20% (National Osteoporosis Foundation 2008).[1]

EXAMINER: What is the Singh and Maini index for osteoporosis?[2] (Figure 18.4.)

CANDIDATE:

Grade 6 (Normal)	All the normal trabecular groups are visible and the upper end of the femur seems to be completely occupied by cancellous bone
Grade 5	The structure of principal tensile and principal compressive trabeculae is accentuated. Ward's triangle appears prominent
Grade 4	Principal tensile trabeculae are markedly reduced in number but can still be traced from the lateral cortex to the upper part of the femoral neck

Grade 3	There is a break in continuity of the principal tensile trabeculae opposite the greater trochanter. This grade indicates definite osteoporosis
Grade 2	Only the principal compressive trabeculae stand out prominently, the others have been resorbed more or less completely
Grade 1	Even the principal compressive trabeculae are markedly reduced in number and are no longer prominent

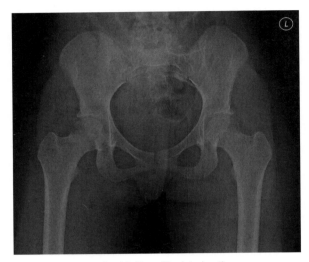

Figure 18.4 Normal pelvis X-ray (Singh Index 6).

The candidate should be able to mark on a radiograph all the trabeculae: primary compressive, primary tensile, secondary compressive, secondary tensile, greater trochanteric trabeculae and Ward's triangle.

1. Kanis JA. Diagnosis of osteoporosis and assessment of fracture risk. *Lancet* 2002;**359**:1929–1936.
2. Singh M, Nagrath AR, Maini PS. Changes in trabecular pattern of the upper end of the femur as an index of osteoporosis. *J Bone Joint Surg Am* 1970;**52-A**:457–467.

Structured oral examination question 6: Bone scanning

EXAMINER: What are the principles of bone scanning? How does a bone scan work?

CANDIDATE: A bone scan involves the intravenous injection of ^{99m}T-MDP (technetium methylene diphosphonate compound). The technetium gets adsorbed onto the hydroxyapatite crystals in bone and emits gamma rays, which are then received using a scintillation gamma camera. The gamma camera contains sodium iodide crystals, which absorb ^{99m}T gamma rays. The received signal is amplified using photomultiplier tubes and processed using a computer to produce an image. It reflects blood flow and osteoblastic activity.

Some features of ^{99m}T-MDP that could be asked by the examiners:

1. Half-life: 6 hours.
2. Excretion: Urine – 70% of the administered dose is excreted within 24 hours.
3. Dose: 500–600 MBq.
4. Emits only gamma rays (not alpha or beta).

EXAMINER: What is a SPECT scan and give any particular uses?

CANDIDATE: Single photon emission tomography involves obtaining tomographic images on a bone scan. The scans are obtained with an arc of 360° around the patient. The images can then be reconstructed in axial, coronal and sagittal planes. The SPECT scan is especially useful to study the posterior spinal elements and to look for areas of decreased uptake in osteonecrosis.

EXAMINER: What is a PET scan and what is it used for?

CANDIDATE: Positron emission tomography is mainly used for tumour diagnosis. It involves injection of ^{18}F-fluorodeoxyglucose (FDG), which is a glucose analogue. FDG is transported into cells by a method similar to that of glucose but is not metabolized. Hence it accumulates in areas of high metabolic activity. Successful chemotherapy can cause a decrease in uptake compared with scans before starting chemotherapy.

EXAMINER: What is the duration for which a bone scan can be positive following a fracture?

CANDIDATE: The bone scan usually becomes positive within 24 hours to 3 days following a fracture. The dynamic flow component can remain positive for as long as 2–3 weeks following the fracture before returning to normal. The blood pool scan remains positive for approximately 8 weeks. The delayed static scan is usually positive for 6 months to 2 years due to continuing bone healing and remodelling. In cases of malunion, it can remain positive indefinitely due to continued bone remodelling.

EXAMINER: What are the phases of a bone scan?

CANDIDATE:

Name	Timing following injection	Significance	Use
Dynamic/ blood flow	1–2 minutes	Perfusion	-
Blood pool	3–5 minutes	Extent of bone/soft tissue hyperaemia	Inflammatory lesions: cellulitis and osteomyelitis Vascular soft-tissue abnormalities such as tumours Dating of traumatic lesions such as fractures or myositis ossificans
Static bone phase	4 hours	Displays sites at which tracer accumulates in skeletal structures when urinary excretion has decreased the amount of the radionuclide in soft tissues	Occult bone or joint pain Metastatic disease Infection: Cellulitis, osteomyelitis, multifocal osteomyelitis Trauma: Occult, stress fractures Tumour: Osteoid osteoma and osteoblastoma, especially spine Primary malignant bone tumours, benign bone tumours Painful joint arthroplasty Avascular necrosis Paget's disease
Delayed	24 hours	-	-

EXAMINER: What is a 'Flare phenomenon' in a bone scan?

CANDIDATE: The paradoxical increase in uptake and size on a bone scan following chemotherapy for metastatic lesions, despite clinical improvement. This can last for up to 6 months following commencement of chemotherapy. This occurs as a result of bone repair following successful chemotherapy.

EXAMINER: Why is a bone scan not the best investigation to study the extent of a bone tumour?

CANDIDATE: The malignant neoplastic lesions may show increased update beyond the actual extent of the tumour due to the presence of hyperaemia and bone oedema occurring beyond the actual extent of the tumour.

[NB: Bone scan can be false negative in up to 50% of cases of multiple myeloma.]

EXAMINER: How does ^{67}Gallium localize in sites of infection?

CANDIDATE: No clue.

Answer: Gallium localizes in sites of infection due to the following factors:
1. Gallium is taken up by neutrophils as well as bacteria.
2. Binding to lactoferrin/plasma transferrin.
3. Increased vascularity.
4. Increased capillary permeability.

EXAMINER: What advice will you give the patient after a bone scan?

CANDIDATE:
1. Drink plenty of fluids for the rest of the day and go to the toilet often. Flush the toilet twice.
2. Avoid contact with pregnant women.
3. If travelling abroad in the 7 days following the scan, to take a doctor's note along as ports and airports have very sensitive radiation detectors which may pick up tiny amounts of radioactivity remaining after the scan.

EXAMINER: Describe the role of bone scan in the investigations for a painful arthroplasty.

CANDIDATE: In cases of cemented hip replacements and total knee replacements, the bone scan can remain positive for up to 1 year following the operation. In a case of uncemented THR there can be increased uptake around the distal tip of the femoral stem for many years postoperatively.

Painful arthroplasty, more than 1-year postoperative:
In case of suspected periprosthetic infection with radiographs showing no evidence of loosening, bone scan generally shows an increased uptake in the

delayed static phase as well as hypervascularity in the blood-flow and blood-pool phases.

Mechanical loosening: Bone scan shows increased uptake in the region of loosening in the delayed bone phase due to the increased bone turnover. Blood-flow and blood-pool phases are normal.

Although technetium bone scan is sensitive for diagnosing infection, it is not specific. Gallium and indium-labelled white blood cell scans are more specific for infection.

Structured oral examination question 7: Nerve conduction studies

EXAMINER: Tell me some of the uses of nerve conduction studies. What are the indications for nerve conduction studies?

CANDIDATE:
1. To determine the presence and severity of any (large myelinated) peripheral nerve dysfunction.
2. Its localization.
3. Distribution.
4. Pathophysiology.

EXAMINER: What is latency, amplitude and conduction velocity?

CANDIDATE:
Latency is the time between the application of stimulus and the onset of response in milliseconds.

Amplitude is the size of response (millivolts) (baseline to negative peak). Conduction velocity (m/s) = distance (mm) between proximal and distal stimulating sites/proximal latency (ms) – distal latency (ms).

EXAMINER: What is the normal conduction velocity?

CANDIDATE: Normal conduction velocity for the upper limb is 50–70 m/s and that for the lower limb is 40–50 m/s. At birth, the values are about 50% of the adult values, increasing to about 75% by 12 months and 100% by 4–5 years. Hypothermia reduces conduction velocity.

EXAMINER: What is supramaximal stimulation?

CANDIDATE: The standard stimulus is a 0.1–0.2 ms square wave pulse, slowly repeated at a rate of 1–2 per second. The intensity is gradually increased to get the maximal response and then increased by 20–30%. This is referred to as supramaximal stimulation and is used to ensure activation of all the nerve fibres.[1]

EXAMINER: What are orthodromic and antidromic potentials?

CANDIDATE: Orthodromic potentials are ones that follow the physiological route i.e. sensory potentials towards the spinal cord and motor potentials away from the spinal cord.

Orthodromic potentials are generally triphasic with an initial downward (positive) deflection. Antidromic potentials are generally biphasic with an initial upward (negative) deflection.

EXAMINER: What are F waves?

CANDIDATE: Supramaximal stimulation of a peripheral nerve causes an antidromic passage of impulse to the spinal cord and then in turn an orthodromic impulse down the spinal cord to the muscle via the α motor neurone. This long latency motor response is termed the F wave.

Significance:
1. Evaluation of proximal (nerve root/plexus/proximal segment) lesions of peripheral nerves.
2. Evaluation of patients with demyelinating polyradiculoneuropathy (Guillain–Barré syndrome).

EXAMINER: What is the 'H' reflex?

CANDIDATE: A submaximal stimulation of the 1a afferent fibres (from muscle spindle) of a mixed nerve leads to a monosynaptic spinal cord reflex contraction of the corresponding muscle. This is termed the 'H' reflex.

The clinical application of H reflex:
1. In cases of unilateral sciatica, it helps to differentiate S1 (unilateral abnormality of soleus H reflex) from a L5 radiculopathy.
2. In evaluation of demyelinating neuropathies.
3. In the absence of bilateral S1 radiculopathy, it is a very sensitive indicator of peripheral polyneuropathy (bilateral abnormality H reflex present).

EXAMINER: How does the H reflex differ from the M wave?[1]

CANDIDATE:
1. The threshold of stimulus required to elicit an H reflex is much lower than that needed for an M wave.
2. Its amplitude is often higher than the M wave for low intensity stimuli.
3. The latency and wave form of an H reflex tends to remain constant at a fixed stimulus intensity.

4. After the age of 1 year, the H reflex tends to persist only in the calf muscle and FCR (flexor carpi radialis).

1. Einhorn TA, O'Keefe RJ, Buckwalter JA (Eds). *Orthopaedic Basic Science: Foundations of Clinical Practice*. 3rd Edition. Rosemont, IL: American Academy of Orthopaedic Surgeons, 2007.

Structured oral examination question 8: Electromyography (EMG)

EXAMINER: Describe 'endplate activity' on EMG.

CANDIDATE: In healthy muscle at rest, the only activity measured on EMG is at the endplate region. The 'endplate activity' is of two types:

1. Endplate noise: The random release of transmitter from the motor nerve terminal causes a non-propagated endplate depolarization. It is an irregular hissing sound. Monophasic (negative).

2. Endplate spike: Non-propagated single muscle fibre discharges caused by excitation of intramuscular nerves. Irregular. Crackling sound. Biphasic (initial negative).

EXAMINER: What is 'insertional' activity on EMG?

CANDIDATE: The single burst of activity recorded on insertion of the needle into the muscle that generally lasts for 300–500 ms is called 'insertional' activity.

Increase: polymyositis, myotonic disorders and some myopathies.

Decrease: prolonged denervation.

EXAMINER: What types of 'spontaneous' activity are there in a relaxed muscle?

CANDIDATE: Any abnormal activity in a relaxed muscle that is not from the endplate and continues after the insertional activity has ceased is called 'spontaneous' activity.

Types of spontaneous activity:

1. Fibrillations:
   a. Action potentials that arise spontaneously from single muscle fibres.
   b. Rhythmic.
   c. Biphasic or triphasic (initial positive spike).
   d. High-pitched clicks.
   e. Possibly caused by oscillations of the resting membrane potential in denervated fibres.

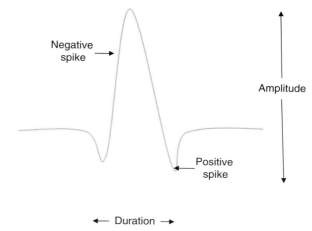

Figure 18.5 Motor unit action potential.

2. Positive sharp waves:
   a. Found in association with fibrillations.
   b. Precede fibrillations in appearance following a nerve lesion.
   c. Arise from single fibres.
   d. Biphasic or triphasic.
   e. Initial positive phase followed by a slow prolonged phase. Much lower in amplitude.
   f. Dull popping sound.

3. Fasciculation potentials:
   a. Spontaneous discharges of a group of muscle fibres representing part/whole muscle unit.
   b. Visible twitching of muscle.
   c. Occurs in diseases of anterior horn cell.

4. Myokimic discharges:
   a. Group fasciculation potentials resulting from discharge of multiple units.
   b. Found in amyotrophic lateral sclerosis, progressive spinal muscular atrophy, poliomyelitis and demyelinating motor nerve fibres.

5. Complex repetitive discharges.

EXAMINER: Draw and describe a motor unit action potential. (Figure 18.5.)

CANDIDATE: A MUAP is the summated electrical activity of the muscle fibres innervated by a single motor neurone. It is generally biphasic or triphasic. It makes a sharp and crisp sound.

Additional note: EMG findings in the following conditions:

1. Upper motor neurone lesion: Lower firing frequency during maximal contraction.
2. Myopathy: The motor units are smaller in myopathy, hence a greater number of units are recruited to produce a given submaximal force. In advanced myogenic disorders, recruitment patterns are similar to those in neurogenic disorders due to loss of entire motor units.

Chapter

19

Diagrams for the FRCS (Tr & Orth)

Asir Aster and Muthu Jeyam

There are three components to drawing out diagrams for the FRCS (Tr & Orth) exam. These are:

- To be able to quickly draw the diagram out to a reasonable artistic standard.
- To explain what you are drawing out while you are doing so.
- To be able to answer questions thrown at you by the examiners while you are drawing the diagram.

In some instances instead of drawing a diagram you may be handed a laminated photograph of it instead (e.g. growth plate). You would need to identify areas/parts of the diagram and probably answer questions from the examiners in a slightly more detailed fashion.

So the advice would be to draw, draw and then draw again until you are comfortable drawing out the diagram subconsciously. After this you should practise out loud describing what you are drawing when drawing and think about possible questions the examiners may ask you.

You need to fully understand the concept of the diagram and you should try to summarize the picture into a few short paragraphs.

Questions

1. Nerve

What is 1? How would you perform a repair of a peripheral nerve? What is the most important factor affecting the growth of a repaired nerve? What is the average growth of a repaired nerve in an adult?

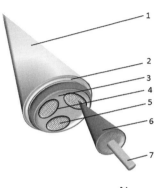

Nerve

2. Nerve cell

Describe this structure. What are the different types of nerve injury? What is 6? What is the function of this structure? How long do the motor end plates of a denervated muscle stay intact?

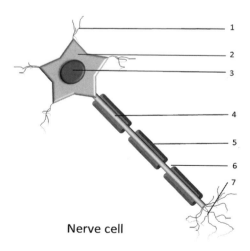

Nerve cell

Postgraduate Orthopaedics: Viva Guide for the FRCS (Tr & Orth) Examination, ed. Paul A. Banaszkiewicz and Deiary F. Kader. Published by Cambridge University Press. © Cambridge University Press 2012.

267

3. Bone architecture

See colour plate section.

What is 6? What is 4 and what are its functions? Which type of collagen is in the bone? What happens to the collagen fibres in osteogenesis imperfecta?

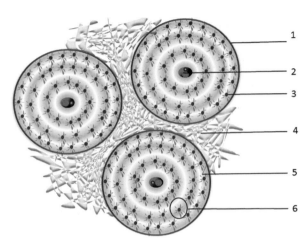

Bone architecture

4. Proteoglycan

See colour plate section.

Describe the structure of proteoglycan.

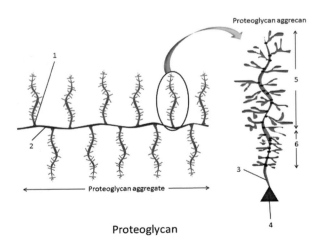

Proteoglycan

5. Skeletal muscle

See colour plate section.

What is 4? What happens at 10 during exercise?

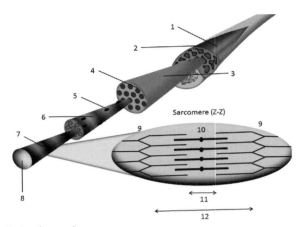

Skeletal muscle

6. Tendon vasculature

See colour plate section.

How would you classify the tendons by their vascular supply? How does the difference in vascular supply affect the tendon healing?

Tendon vasculature

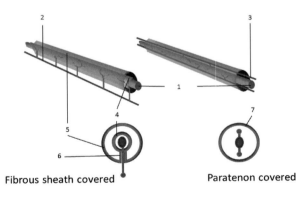

Fibrous sheath covered   Paratenon covered

7. Immunoglobulin

See colour plate section.

What would be the clinical manifestation of each of these pathologies? How would you treat them?

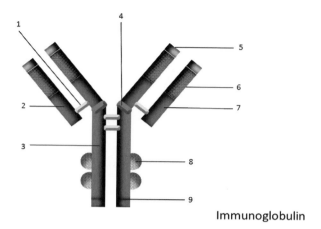

Immunoglobulin

8. Brachial plexus

See colour plate section.

What critical features in the history and examination of injury to this structure would help you decide the course of management?

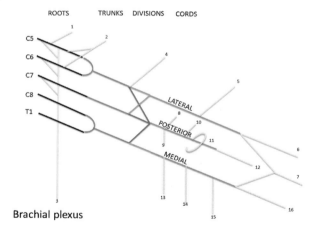

Brachial plexus

9. Shoulder spaces and intervals

What are the boundaries of 2? What structures exit at 3?

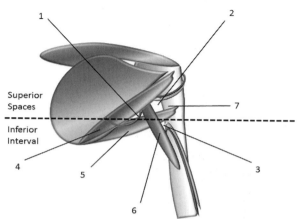

Shoulder spaces and intervals

10. Disc prolapse

What are the differences in the clinical manifestation of 1 and 2? What are the clinical features of 3 and how would you treat this pathology?

Disc prolapse

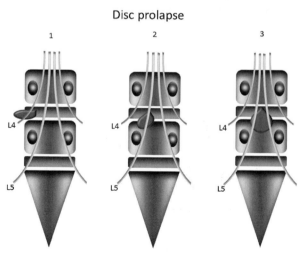

11. Spinal stenosis

What are the clinical features of this condition? Discuss the treatment options. How would you differentiate these symptoms from vascular claudication?

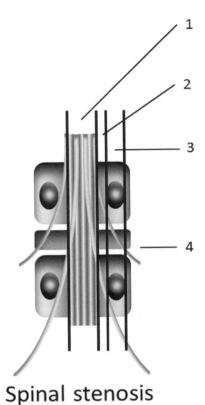

Spinal stenosis

12. Intervertebral disc

Describe the changes that happen to this structure with age. Tell me the composition of the disc.

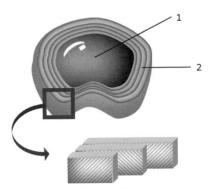

Intervertebral disc

13. Spinal cord anatomy

See colour plate section.

What are 4 and 6? How do the sensory nerve fibres arrange in the spinal cord?

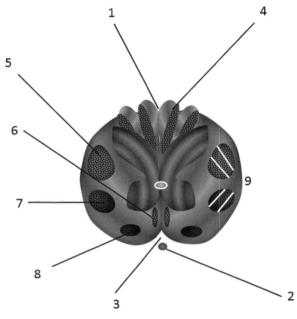

Spinal cord anatomy

14. Articular cartilage

What is 5 and what happens when you have a penetrating injury to 3?

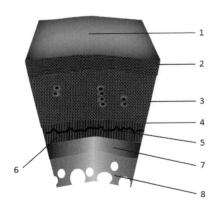

Articular cartilage

15. Growth plate

What is 2? Why is the orientation in this manner? What are Benninghoff arcades?

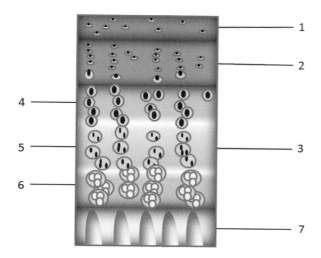

Growth plate

16. Menisci

Describe the structure of menisci. What happens if zone 2 is injured?

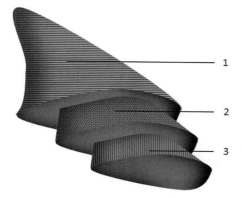

Menisci – Arrangement of collagen fibres

17. Tension band wire

Describe the principle of fracture fixation by this method.

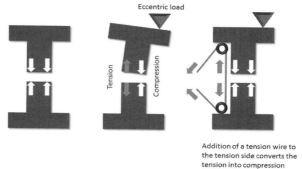

Addition of a tension wire to the tension side converts the tension into compression

Tension band wire - principle

18. Finger flexor pulley

Describe the anatomy of the flexor pulleys. What are the two important pulleys? What happens when they are injured? Tell me the sites the avulsed FDP tendon gets retracted to. What is the significance of the amount of retraction of avulsed FDP in terms of deciding the urgency of treatment?

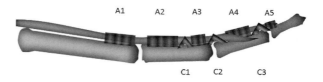

Finger flexor – pulley

19. Thumb pulley

Describe the pulley system of the thumb. Draw me the incision for Trigger thumb release.

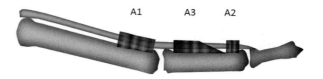

Thumb - pulley

20. Ligaments of PIP joint

Describe the ligaments around the PIPJ. Draw the structure of a volar plate.

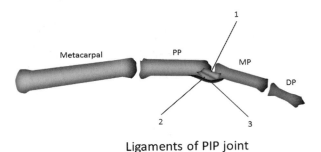

Ligaments of PIP joint

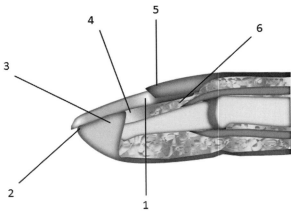

Nail anatomy

21. Finger extensor tendon

See colour plate section.

Describe the extensor tendons of the finger. What happens to the tendons in Boutonnière's deformity and swan neck deformity? How would you differentiate an acute Boutonnière from chronic? Tell me the causes for swan neck deformity. How would you treat a mallet finger?

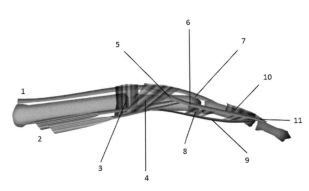

Finger – Extensor tendon

22. Nail anatomy

See colour plate section.

What is the function of nails? Draw me the incision to drain a finger pulp abscess. Tell me about the Seymour fracture. How will you differentiate subungual malignant melanoma from haematoma?

23. DeLee and Charnley and Gruen zones

Describe these zones of loosening. What is their significance in revision surgery?

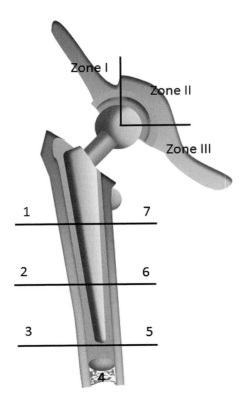

24. Glenohumeral joint arthroscopic view

See colour plate section.

What is the importance of structures 4 and 11? Describe the stabilizers of the glenohumeral joint. What is the Buford complex?

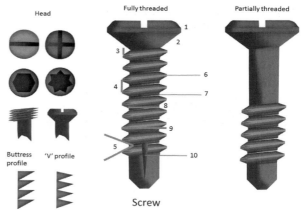

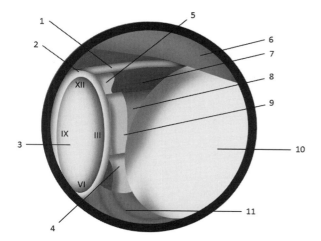

Glenohumeral joint arthroscopy view

25. Scratch profile

Draw the scratch profiles of a metal and ceramic. How does a scratch in a metal THR head coupled with polyethylene affect the life of the implant? What is the difference between these two materials?

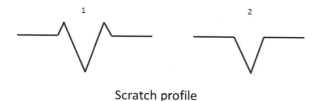

Scratch profile

26. Screw

What are the characteristics of these two screws? What are 4 and 7 and how do they differ in cortical and cancellous screws?

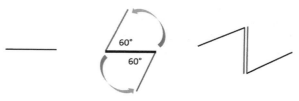

Screw

27. Z plasty

See colour plate section.

Draw a Z plasty and explain how it works. What are its uses?

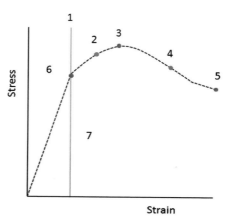

Z Plasty

28. Stress–strain curve

See colour plate section.

What is 1? What is 7? What happens at point 3?

Stress–strain curve

29. Stress–strain curve

See colour plate section.

Define yield point and ultimate tensile strength.

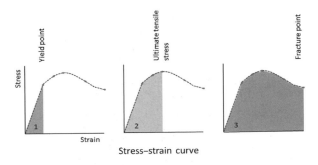

Stress–strain curve

30. Fatigue–failure curve

Where should an ideal material be in this curve? What is the endurance limit of a material?

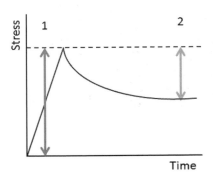

Fatigue–failure curve

31. Viscoelasticity

What is this and define creep?

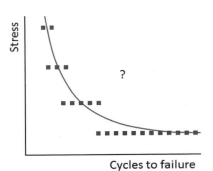

Viscoelasticity

32. Viscoelastic behaviour

What properties are described here? Give me an example of such a structure.

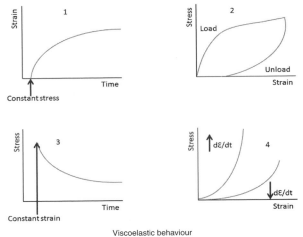

Viscoelastic behaviour

33. Mid thigh cross-section

See colour plate section.

What is structure 8? Where would you insert the pins of an external fixator?

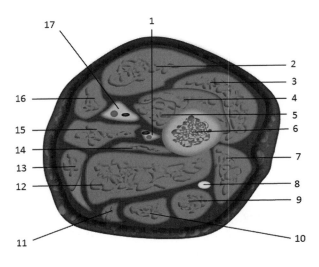

Mid thigh – cross-section

34. Mid leg cross-section

See colour plate section.

What are the different compartments? How would you do a fasciotomy?

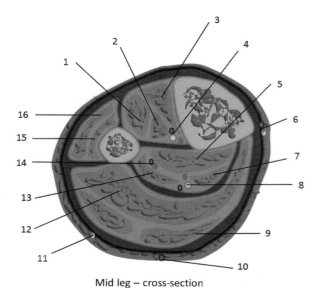

Mid leg – cross-section

35. Mid arm cross-section

See colour plate section.

Where would you place the pins of an external fixator in an open fracture of this bone? Take me through the anterolateral approach to the humerus.

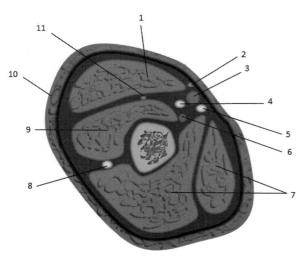

Mid arm – cross-section

36. Mid forearm cross-section

See colour plate section.

Describe how you would decompress the various compartments. Take me through the tendon transfers for a chronic wrist drop.

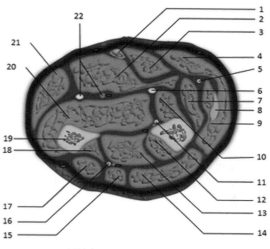

Mid forearm – cross-section

37. Distal forearm – cross-section

See colour plate section.

Where would you place your incision to perform synovectomy? What are the different extensor compartments of the wrist? Take me through the flexor carpi radialis (FCR) approach to the distal radius fracture.

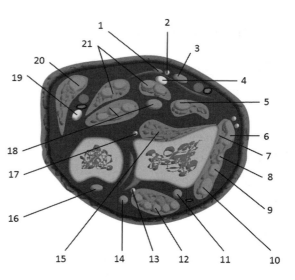

Distal forearm – cross-section

275

38. Carpal tunnel cross-section

See colour plate section.

What is 11? How are the flexor tendons of the fingers arranged inside this tunnel? What is pillar pain and how would you prevent its occurrence? Draw me the landmarks of carpal tunnel decompression incision. Which nerve supplies the cutaneous sensation of thenar eminence? Which thenar muscle has dual nerve supply?

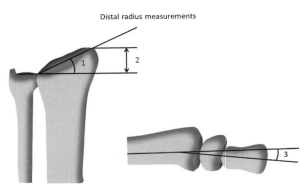

Distal radius measurements

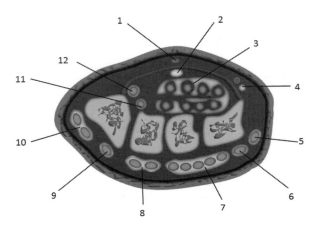

Carpal tunnel – cross-section

39. Distal radius measurements

What are these angles and how are they important? What is the carpal alignment index?

40. Femoral head vascular supply

See colour plate section.

Describe the blood supply of the proximal femur.

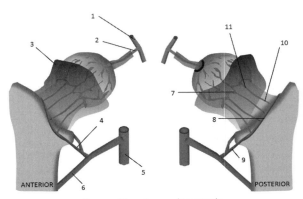

Femoral head vascular supply

Illustrations for Viva

Asir Aster and Muthu Jeyam

Parts for the illustrations

1. Nerve
   1. Nerve
   2. Epineurium
   3. Interfascicular epineurium
   4. Perineurium
   5. Endoneurium
   6. Schwann cell
   7. Axon

2. Nerve cell
   1. Dendrite
   2. Cell body
   3. Nucleus
   4. Axon
   5. Schwann cell
   6. Node of Ranvier
   7. Axon terminals

3. Bone architecture
   1. Haversian system or osteon
   2. Haversian canal
   3. Osteocyte
   4. Lamellae
   5. Canaliculi
   6. Lacunae

4. Proteoglycan
   1. Link protein
   2. Hyaluronic acid
   3. Protein core
   4. Link protein
   5. Chondroitin sulphate
   6. Keratin sulphate

5. Skeletal muscle
   1. Muscle
   2. Perimysium
   3. Fasciculus
   4. Endomysium
   5. Nuclei
   6. Muscle fibre
   7. Myofibril
   8. Myofilaments

   Sarcomere
   9. Z
   10. M
   11. H
   12. A

6. Tendon – vasculature
   1. Tendon
   2. Blood vessel: Segmental blood supply
   3. Blood vessel: Continuous blood supply
   4. Visceral layer
   5. Parietal layer
   6. Mesotenon
   7. Paratenon

7. Immunoglobulin
   1. Sulphur bridge
   2. Light chain
   3. Heavy chain
   4. Hinge region
   5. Antigen binding site
   6. Variable region
   7. Constant region
   8. Carbohydrate
   9. CH3 domain

8. Brachial plexus
   1. Nerve to subclavius
   2. Dorsal scapular N
   3. Long thoracic N
   4. Suprascapular N
   5. Lateral pectoral N
   6. Musculocutaneous N
   7. Median N
   8. Upper subscapular N
   9. Lower subscapular N

10. Thoracodorsal N
11. Axillary N
12. Radial N
13. Medial pectoral N
14. Medial cutaneous N of arm
15. Medial cutaneous N of forearm
16. Ulnar N

9. Shoulder spaces and intervals

1. Triangular space – Circumflex scapular A
2. Quadrilateral space – Axillary N, Post circumflex humeral A
3. Triangular interval – Radial N, Profunda brachii A
4. Teres minor
5. Teres major
6. Long head of triceps
7. Medial border of humerus

10. Disc prolapse

1. Far-lateral – Unilateral L4
2. Postero-lateral – Unilateral L5
3. Central – Bilateral L5

11. Spinal stenosis

1. Central
2. Lateral recess
3. Foraminal
4. Extraforaminal

12. Intervertebral disc

1. Nucleus pulposus
2. Annulus fibrosus

13. Spinal cord anatomy

1. Sulcus
2. Anterior spinal A
3. Fissure
4. Dorsal column – deep touch, proprioception and vibration
5. Lateral corticospinal tract – motor
6. Ventral corticospinal tract – motor
7. Lateral spinothalamic tract – pain and temperature
8. Ventral spinothalamic tract – light touch
9. Arm: Trunk: Leg

14. Articular cartilage

1. Articular surface
2. Superficial tangential zone – 10–20%
3. Middle zone 40–60%

4. Deep zone 30%
5. Tide mark
6. Calcified cartilage
7. Subchondral bone
8. Cancellous bone

15. Growth plate

1. Reserve zone
2. Proliferative zone
3. Hypertrophic zone
4. Maturation zone
5. Degenerative zone
6. Provisional calcification
7. Primary spongiosa

16. Menisci – arrangement of collagen fibres

1. Superficial – radial
2. Surface – irregular
3. Middle – circumferential

17. Tension band wire – principle

1. Explain the principle of the tension band wire.

18. Finger flexor – pulley
19. Thumb – pulley
20. Ligaments of PIP joint

1. Collateral ligament proper
2. Accessory collateral ligament
3. Volar plate

21. Finger extensor tendon

1. EDC
2. Intrinsics
3. Sagittal bands
4. Oblique fibres
5. Lateral slip
6. Lateral band
7. Central slip
8. Transverse retinacular ligament
9. Oblique retinacular ligament
10. Triangular ligament
11. Terminal extensor tendon

22. Nail anatomy

1. Lunula
2. Hyponychium
3. Paranychium
4. Sterile matrix
5. Eponychium
6. Germinal matrix

23. DeLee and Charnley acetabular zones and Gruen femoral zones
24. Glenohumeral joint arthroscopy view
    1. LHB
    2. Labrum
    3. Glenoid
    4. Anterior IGHL
    5. SGHL
    6. Supraspinatus
    7. Rotator interval
    8. Subscapularis
    9. MGHL
    10. Humeral head
    11. Inferior recess
25. Scratch profile
    1. Metal
    2. Ceramic
26. Screw
    1. Head
    2. Countersink
    3. Run out
    4. Pitch
    5. Thread angle
    6. Crest
    7. Root
    8. Root (core) diameter
    9. Thread diameter
    10. Tip with self-tapping groove
27. Z plasty
28. Stress–strain curve
    1. Yield point
    2. Work hardening
    3. Ultimate tensile stress
    4. Necking
    5. Fracture point
    6. Elastic
    7. Plastic
29. Stress–strain curve
    1. Elastic
    2. Toughness
    3. Energy to failure
30. Fatigue–failure curve

    When the stress decreases the number of cycles to failure (fatigue life) increases
31. Viscoelasticity

    1. Elastic
    2. Viscous
32. Viscoelastic behaviour
    1. Creep – deformation of a material over time to a constant load
    2. Hysteresis – under cyclical loading there is loss of energy in the material during each cycle (the stress–strain relationship during the loading process is different from that in the unloading process)
    3. Stress relaxation – with a constantly applied strain the stress in the material decreases
    4. Time rate dependent stress–strain behaviour – increasing the strain rate increases the stress
33. Mid thigh – cross-section
    1. Deep femoral A & V
    2. Rectus femoris
    3. Vastus lateralis
    4. Vastus intermedialis
    5. Vastus medialis
    6. Femur
    7. Short head of biceps femoris
    8. Sciatic N
    9. Long head of biceps femoris
    10. Semitendinosus
    11. Semimembranosus
    12. Adductor magnus
    13. Gracilis
    14. Adductor brevis
    15. Adductor longus
    16. Sartorius
    17. Femoral A & V
34. Mid leg – cross-section
    1. EDL
    2. EHL
    3. Tibialis anterior
    4. Anterior tibial A & V/Deep peroneal N
    5. Tibialis posterior
    6. Long saphenous V/Saphenous N
    7. FHL
    8. Posterior tibial A & V/Tibial N
    9. Gastrocnemius medial head
    10. Short saphenous V
    11. Sural N
    12. Soleus
    13. FDL

14. Peroneal A & V
15. Peroneous brevis
16. Peroneous longus

35. Mid arm – cross-section

1. Biceps brachii
2. Medial cutaneous nerve of forearm
3. Basilic vein
4. Median N
5. Ulnar N
6. Brachial A
7. Triceps
8. Radial nerve
9. Brachialis
10. Cephalic vein
11. Lateral cutaneous nerve of forearm

36. Mid forearm – cross-section

1. Palmaris longus
2. FDS
3. FCR
4. Brachioradialis
5. Superficial branch of radial N
6. Median N
7. Pronator teres
8. ECRL
9. ECRB
10. FPL
11. AIN
12. APL
13. EPB
14. EDC
15. EDM
16. PIN
17. ECU
18. EPL
19. Ulna
20. FDP
21. FCU
22. Ulnar N & A

37. Distal forearm – cross-section

1. Palmaris longus
2. Palmar cutaneous branch of Median N
3. FCR
4. Median N
5. EPL
6. APL

7. Brachioradialis
8. EPB
9. ECRL
10. ECRB
11. EPL
12. EDC
13. PIN
14. EDM
15. Pronator quadratus
16. ECU
17. AIN
18. FDP
19. Ulnar N
20. FCU
21. FDS

38. Carpal tunnel – cross-section

1. Palmaris longus
2. Median N
3. FDS & FDP in common flexor tendon sheath
4. Ulnar N
5. EDM
6. ECU
7. EDC & EIP
8. ECRL & ECRB
9. EPL
10. APL & EPB
11. FCR
12. FPL

39. Distal radius measurements

1. Radial inclination – 23°
2. Radial length – 12 mm
3. Volar tilt – 11°

40. Femoral head vascular supply

1. Obturator artery
2. Foveal artery
3. Capsule
4. Lateral femoral circumflex artery
5. Femoral artery
6. Profunda femoris artery
7. Subsynovial intracapsular arterial ring
8. Extracapsular arterial ring
9. Medial femoral circumflex artery
10. Ascending cervical artery
11. Retinacular artery

Index

AAOS. *See* American Academy
   of Orthopaedic Surgeons
   (AAOS)
abdominal injuries, 147–148
abrasive wear, 33
abscess
   epidural, 71–72
   finger, 272
absolute SpPins and SnNouts, 245
acetabular component/cup (THA)
   cemented, removal, 24
   in DDH, 40–41
   optimal positioning, 18
   survival rates, 214
acetabulum
   bone loss, 22
   defects, 22–23, 178–181, 183–185
   fracture, 113–120, 135–139, 141
   in DDH, 39–42
   revision THA, 202, 215
adhesive wear, 33
adipose tissue tumours, 108–109
adolescents
   malignant tumours, 104–107
   scoliosis, 76–77
adverse reaction to metal debris
   (ARMD), 214
AGC (Biomet) knee prosthesis,
   216
age. *See* elderly patients; paediatrics
Agility total ankle replacement, 57
Aitken's classification, 184–185
alkaline phosphatase (AlkPhos), 37
all or none studies, 244
allografts, 16, 24, 225, 239
American Academy of Orthopaedic
   Surgeons (AAOS)
   classifications
      acetabular defects, 22
      bone loss, 22
      femoral defects, 22
   guidelines, periprosthetic
      infection, 46
anatomical axis, knee joint, 225
Anderson and D'Alonzo classification,
   83, 145
Anderson and Montesano
   classification, 83

Anderson Orthopaedic Research
   Institute (AORI) classification,
   51–52
aneurysmal bone cysts, 71, 107
ankle
   arthritis, 56–58
   fractures, 117, 205–206
   fusion surgery, 57–58
   in pes planus, 63
   instability, 55–56
   osteomyelitis, 218–219
   pronation external rotation injury,
      205–206
   surgical approaches, 117, 205–206
   trauma, 116–118
ankylosing spondylitis, 85
annulus fibrosus, 238
anterior capsular release, shoulder, 89
anterior cord syndrome, 83, 144
anterior cruciate ligament (ACL),
   44, 49–51
anterior drawer test, 55
anterior talofibular ligament (ATFL),
   55–56
anterior tibiofibular ligament, 205
antibiotic-loaded spacer, 16, 46
antidromic potentials, 264
anti-TNF alpha medication, 158
AO classification, 82
arm
   mid arm anatomy, 275, 280,
      See also forearm
arm pain, nerve roots, 206–207
arthritis
   ankle, 56–58
   knee, 43, 53
   pes planus, 62
   thumb base, 153–154
   wrist, 153, *See also* osteoarthritis
      (OA); rheumatoid arthritis
      (RA)
arthrodesis
   ankle, 63
   foot
      MTP joint, 59–60, 65–67
      triple, 63–64
arthrograms, 177, 260
arthrogryposis, 60, 192

arthroplasty
   hip, 263–264
   knee, 46–48
   toe, 67, *See also* hemiarthroplasty;
      total hip arthroplasty (THA);
      total knee arthroplasty (TKA)
arthroscopic portals, elbow, 96–97
arthroscopic procedures
   Bankart's repair, 218
   capsular release, 89
   cruciate reconstruction, 49–50
   debridement, 57
   knee assessment, 112
arthroscopic view, glenohumeral,
   273, 279
arthrotomy, 30
articular cartilage, 234, 270, 278
articular surface replacement
   (ASR), 230
AS IT GRIPS 3Cs, 27
aseptic lymphocyte-dominated
   vasculitis-associated lesion
   (ALVAL), 18, 230
assessment, principles, 10–12
astrocytoma, 71
atlanto-axial joint, 95–96
atlanto-occipital joint subluxation,
   83
atlas (C1) fractures, 83
atypical lipoma, 109
autografts, 40, 85, 225, 239
avascular necrosis (AVN), 27–36
   dislocated hip risk, 178
   foot, navicular bone, 125
   hip, bilateral, 27
   lunate, 153–155
   SUFE and, 160
   THA, 209
axis (C2) fractures, 83

Babinski's sign, 79–80
back pain, 72, 104
Bado classification, 130
Bankart's repair, 218
Barlow's test, 172
basic science, buzz topics, 238–240
benign tumours, 71, 100, 108–109
   femur, 101–102

benign tumours (*cont.*)
    foot/feet, 102–103
    spine, 71, *See also* haemangiomas;
        lipomas
beta tricalcium phosphate, 226–227
bias, clinical trials, 243
biological agents, 59–60
biomechanical properties, 225–227
biopsy, 100
    giant cell tumour, 210
    osteomyelitis or malignancy, 219
    soft tissue swellings, 258
    spinal tumours, 69
    ultrasound-guided, 258
bisphosphonates, 37, 197, 208
blood supply
    bone, 238
    femoral head, 164
    menisci, 44
Bloom's taxonomy of assessment,
        10–11
Blount's disease (idiopathic tibia vara),
        187–189
bone
    architecture, 268, 277
    basic science, 233–236
    biomechanical properties,
        225–227
    blood supply, 238
    brittle, 196
    Hounsfield units, 258
    loss
        classification, 22
        in DDH, 42
        THA loosening, 21–29
        TKA loosening, 51–53
    metabolism, disordered, 36, 84
    necrosis, 166
bone cement. *See* cement (bone
        cement)
bone densitometry, 261–262
bone graft substitutes, 226–227
bone grafts/grafting, 225, 239
    ACL repair, 50–51
    AVN hip, 29–30
    DDH revision, 42
    spine, 80, 85
    TKA revision, 52–53
    tumour cavity, 210,
        See also allografts; autografts;
        vascularized fibular graft
        (VFG)
bone marrow fat cell hypertrophy,
        28
bone mineral density (BMD),
        236–237
bone morphogenetic proteins
        (BMPs), 236
bone pain, Paget's disease, 37

bone patella tendon bone (BPTB)
        graft, 50–51
bone scanning, 262–264
boundary lubrication, 225
Boutonnière deformity, 157, 272
bowed legs (genu varum), 186
brace/bracing
    elbow, 95–96
    humerus, 133
    hyperextension, 148
    spine, 76
brachial plexus, 269, 277–278
British Orthopaedic Association/
        standards of Trauma
        (BOAST), 135–136
Brostrom ligament repair, 56
Brown–Sequard (hemi-cord)
        syndrome, 83, 144
bucket handle tear, meniscus, 44
buttress plate, 112

calcaneal fracture, 115–116
calcaneocuboid joint, 60
calcaneofibular ligament (ATFL),
        55–56
calcium deposits, 90–91
candidates, appearance and affect, 7
carpal alignment index, 276
carpal tunnel, 276, 280
carpometacarpal (CMC) joint,
        153–154
cartilage
    articular, 234, 270, 278
    changes in OA, 26
    types, 233–234
cartilage-producing matrix, 104
cartilaginous structures, menisci, 44
case–control study, 245
categorical data, 248
Catterall classification, 167
cauda equina syndrome, 73–74,
        210–212
CAVE mnemonic, 190
cavus foot, 60–62
cells of bone, 233–236
cement (bone cement)
    biomechanics, 229
    cementing techniques, 20–21
    filling/augmentation, 71, 210
    removal, 21, 24, 202
cement mantle scale, 21
central cord syndrome, 83,
        143–144
central slip rupture, 157
cephalomedullary nail, 120
ceramic implants
    scratch profile, 273, 279
    THA, 31
    wear particles, 34

cerebral palsy (CP)
    feet, cavus, 60
    hips, 181, 183
    spine, scoliosis, 75, 77
cervical discs
    discectomy, 80, 143
    prolapse, 73–74, 206–207
    replacement, 80
cervical myelopathy, 79–80
cervical spine
    anterior approach, 80, 206–207
    distraction injuries, 84
    facet dislocation, 148
    flexion injuries, 84
    fractures
        C1 (atlas), 83
        C2 (axis), 83
        C3–C7 (subaxial), 83–84
        hangman's fracture, 83, 146
        odontoid peg, 145–146
        trauma, 81
Chance fractures, 147–148
Charcot arthropathy, 62
Charcot–Marie–Tooth (CMT) disease,
        60–61
Charnley THA, 229, 251
cheilectomy, 67
chemotherapy, 106–107
chondroitin sulphate, 26
chondrosarcoma, 71, 104–105
chordoma, 71
Chrisman–Snook procedure, 56
chromium ions, 18, 32, 214, 230
claustrophobia, MRI and, 261
clinical trials
    cohort *vs* case–control study, 245
    design aspects, 242–243
    hypothesis testing, 244–245
    sampling, 242–244
    study power, 245
    types, 244
club foot (talipes equinovarus).
        See talipes equinovarus
        (club foot)
cobalt ions, 18, 32, 214, 230
Cobb angle, 75
Codman's triangle, 106
cohort study, 245
Coleman block test, 62
collagen, 231–232
collagenase injections, 156
common peroneal nerve, 205
compartment syndrome, 115
compression injuries, 83–84
computed tomography (CT),
        258–259, 261
conduction velocity, nerves, 264
conduit graft, 237
confidence interval (CI), 244

congenital scoliosis, 75, 78
congenital vertical talus, 192–194
consent, 125, 156
constrained implants, TKA, 52
corticosteroids, AVN induced by, 28
cotyoplasty, 17
courses, oral exam practice, 3, 9
Craig splint, 175
crescent sign/line, 27–29
crosslinked UHMWPE, 35
Crowe classification, 39–40
cruciate ligaments, 44, 49–52
cruciate retaining (CR) implants, 52
Curling's ulcer, 145
cysts, aneurysmal bone, 71, 107
cytokines, 26, 34–35

data
    analysis, 246, 248–249
    interpretation, 246–251
    types, 248
decompression surgery, spinal
        tumours, 70–71
DeLee and Charnley zones, 272, 279
deltoid ligament, 205
Denis classification, 84, 140
Denise–Browne (DB) boots, 190, 192
developmental dysplasia of the hip
        (DDH), 39–42, 171–176
    guidelines, 175
    leg length discrepancy, 40–42
    risk factors (mnemonic), 171–172
    screening, 252
    sonographic grading, 175
diagnosis, absolute SpPins and
        SnNouts, 245
diffuse idiopathic skeletal hyperostosis
        (DISH), 85
digital radiography, 257
Dimeglio scoring system, 192
discitis, 72, 238
discs. See intervertebral discs
disease-modifying anti-rheumatic
        drugs (DMARDs), 60
distal interphalangeal (DIP) joint, 157
distal metatarsal articular angulation, 65
divot sign, 18
Drennan and Levine
        metaphyseal–diaphyseal angle,
        187–188
dual energy X-ray absorptiometry
        (DEXA), 261
Duchenne muscular dystrophy,
        75, 77
Dunn osteotomy, 162
Dupuytren's diathesis, 155
Dupuytren's disease (DD), 89,
        155–156
dysplasia, discussed, 33–40

Eaton classification, 153
effective joint space, 34
elasticity, 226
elastohydrodynamic lubrication, 225
elbow, 92
    dislocated, 98–99
    flail elbow, 95–96, 98
    fractures, 128–130
        fracture dislocation, 130
    ligaments, 98
    loose body in, 93–95
    osteoarthritis, 96–98
    painful, 92–95
    painless lump, 108–109
    rheumatoid arthritis, 95–96, 98
elderly patients
    degenerative changes, 87–88,
        90–91
        spine, 84
    fractures
        femur, 113–114, 120–123
        hip, 137–139
        tibia, 121–123
    malignant tumours, 104
electromyography (EMG), 265–266
Elmslie–Trillat procedure, 53
Elson's test, 157
enchondromas, 102–103, 149–150
end plate activity, on EMG, 265
Enneking's classification, 101
ependymoma, 71
epidemiology, incidence and
        prevalence, 251–252
epidural abscess, 71–72
equivalence trials, 244
evidence
    from literature, 4, 9–10
    grades of recommendation, 245
    levels of, 241–242, 248–249
evidence-based practice,
        introduction, 241
Ewing's sarcoma, 107–108, 219
examiners
    conduct, 7–9
    roles, 3
Exeter THA, 25, 208–209, 229
explanatory trial, 244
extended trochanteric osteotomy
        (ETO), 21, 29–24, 202
extensor carpi radialis brevis
        (ECRB), 93
extensor digitorum communis
        (EDC), 93
extensor indicis (EI) tendon, 149
extensor pollicis longus (EPL)
        tendon, 149
extensor tendons
    illustrations, 278
    rupture, 95–96

external fixators, 128, 229
external iliac artery, 141
extracellular matrix (ECM),
        231–232

F waves, 264
fasciculation potentials, 265
fasciotomy (fasciectomy), 156, 275
fat cell hypertrophy, 28
fat embolism, risk, 122
fatigue–failure curve, 274, 279
FATSAT, MRI sequence, 260
femoral component (THA), 214
    rupture. See also femoral stem
        (THA component)
femoral component (TKR), 54, 216
femoral condyle, deficient, 43
femoral head
    AVN, 31–32
    blood supply, 164
    core decompression, 29–30
    Legg–Calvé–Perthes disease,
        164–174
    PFFD classification, 185
    vascular supply, 276, 280
femoral neck, 18
femoral nerve, risks to, 201–203
femoral replacement, 213
femoral stem (THA component)
    cemented, removal, 24
    in DDH, 41
    loosening, 20–24
femur
    bone loss, 21
    defects, 22, 39–42
    fractures
        intertrochanteric, 120–121
        intracapsular neck, 113–114
        paediatrics, 176
        pathological, 105, 212–213
        periprosthetic, 220–222
        with tibia, 121–123
    in DDH, 40–42
    osteoporosis index, 261–262
    physeal injury, 196
    short dysplastic (paediatrics),
        183–185
    tumours
        benign, 101–102
        malignant, 105–107, 219–220
fibrillations, on EMG, 265
fibroblast growth factor (FGF), 236
fibroma, non-ossifying, 103–104
fibula hemimelia, 184
fibula, fractures, 116–118, 205–206
Ficat and Arlett classification,
        27–30
fingers
    abscess, 272

fingers (*cont.*)
Boutonniere deformity, 157, 272
extensor tendons, 272, 278
flexor pulleys, 271, 278
flexor tendons, 276
nail anatomy, 272
PIP joint ligaments, 278
rheumatoid, 157–158
tumours, 272
ulnar drift, 157,
See also Dupuytren's disease;
metacarpophalangeal (MCP)
joints
fish osteotomy, 162
fixation systems, 227–229, 275
Blount's disease, 188–189
bridging plate, 122–123
circular frame, 122, 123
external, 128, 229
intramedullary nail, 121
pathological femoral fracture, 213
pelvic vertical shear fracture, 137
periprosthetic femoral fracture,
220–221
tension band wire, 271, 278
fixed model effects, 248
flail elbow, 95–96, 98
flare phenomenon, 263
flat foot (pes planus), 62
fleck sign, 114
flexor digitorum longus (FDL), 63–64
flexor hallucis longus (FHL), 64
flexor pulleys, 271, 278
fluid-film lubrication, 225
^{18}F-fluorodeoxyglucose (FDG), 262
foot/feet
cavus foot, 60–62
club foot, 189–192
fracture dislocation, 114–115
fractures, 115–116, 123–121
hallux rigidus, 66–67
hallux valgus, 58–60, 64–66
hallux varus, 66
high arch, 60–61
pes planus, 62
rheumatoid arthritis, 58–60
surgical risks, 125
tumour, benign, 102–103
vertical talus, 189–194
footwear. *See* orthotic treatment
forearm
anatomy, 275, 280
fractures, 132–134
displaced, 203–204
non-accidental, 196–198
osteogenesis imperfecta (OI),
196–197
radius, 130–132
forefoot deformities, 58–60, 189–190

Forestier's disease, 85
Fracture Risk Assessment Tool
(FRAX), 261
fractures
bone scanning, 262
fixation
biomechanics, 227–229
healing, 238–239
open, 129
pathological, 105
Frankel grading system, 83
free radical stabilization, 35
fretting wear, 33
Friedrich's ataxia, 60
frozen shoulder, 88–89
Fs (6x) mnemonic, 171–172
Fulkerson procedure, 53
funnel plot, 246–251

gadolinium contrast, 260
Galleazzi test, 171
gallium, bone scan, 263–264
ganglion, wrist, 152
Gantz osteotomy, 162
Gelberman classification, 154
General Medical Council (GMC),
125
geniculate blood vessels, 44
genu valgus (knocked knees), 186
genu varum (bowed legs), 186
giant cell tumour, 209–210
Gillespie and Torode classification,
184
glenohumeral joint, 273, 279
Goldthwait–Roux procedure, 54
golfer's elbow, 92–93
Graf classification, 172–175
grafts/grafting
ACL, 49–51
hamstring, 50–51,
See also allografts; autografts;
bone grafts/grafting;
vascularized fibular graft
(VFG)
greater tuberosity fracture, humerus,
126–127
grind test, 153
Gross and associates classification, 22
growth plate. *See* physis (growth plate)
Gruen zones, 272, 279

H reflex, 264–265
haemangiomas, 71, 103
hallux rigidus, 66–67
hallux valgus, 58–60, 64–66
hallux varus, 66
halo vest/jacket, 83–84, 145–146, 148
hamartomatous lesions, 104
hamstring graft, 50–51

hands
enchondroma, 103, 149–150
paediatrics, 149–151
parts for illustrations, 278,
See also fingers; scaphoid;
thumbs
hangman's fracture, 83, 146
hard (Aspen) collar, 145
Hardinge surgical approach, 25,
201–202
Harris and Barrack scale, 21
Hartofilakidis classification, 39–40, 42
Hattrup and Johnson grading system,
66–67
Hauser procedure, 54
Hawkin's sign, 118
hemiarthroplasty
femoral neck fracture, 113
infected, 13–17
toe, 67
wear debris, 17
hemi-cord syndrome, 83, 144
Henry's approach, 203–204
hereditary motor–sensory neuropathy
(HMSN), 60–61
Herring classification, 167–168
heterogeneity, 241–242, 247–248
heterotopic ossification (HO), 37
Hibb's angle, 62
high tibial osteotomy (HTO), 43,
46–48
Hill–Sach's lesion, 217–218
hindfoot deformities, 60, 64, 189–190
hip, 13
avascular necrosis, 27
dislocation, 118–120, 141, 171–181,
183
fractures, 113, 120–121, 137–139
in trauma, 139–141
hemiarthroplasty, 13–17
infection
periprosthetic, 13–17, 15–16
sepsis drainage, 202–203
irritable, 181–183, 202
MR arthrograms, 260
osteoarthritis, 24–27, 213–215
osteonecrosis, 208–209
paediatrics, 159–186, 164–174,
171–181
Paget's disease, 36–39
painful
bilateral, 27, 39–42
differential diagnosis, 36, 38
paediatric, 181–183
post-hemiarthroplasty, 13–17
post-THA, 18, 20–24
pseudotumour, 18
resurfacing, 230
surgical approaches, 25–26, 136

ultrasound uses, 258,
   See also developmental
   dysplasia of the hip (DDH);
   Paget's disease; total hip
   arthroplasty (THA)
Hodgson's surgical approach, 75
Hoffman's sign, 79
homogeneity, 241–242
hormonal theory, in SUFE, 161
Hounsfield units, 258
humerus, fractures, 126–130, 132–134
Hungerford and Lennox classification,
   28
hydrodynamic lubrication, 225
hydroxyapatite, 226–227
hypothesis testing, 244–245

idiopathic tibia vara (Blount's disease),
   187–189
iliac wing, 104
iliosacral fixation, 141
illustrations, for viva, 277–280
immunoglobulin, 269, 277
implants. *See* prostheses
incidence, epidemiology, 251–252
infection
   control/prevention, 16
   gallium bone scan, 263,
      See also periprosthetic
      infection
inflammatory markers, sensitivity and
   specificity, 14, 46
insulin-like growth factor (IGF), 236
interleukin, 34
interleukin-1 (IL-1), 26
interleukin-1β (IL-1β), 34
interleukin-6 (IL-6), 14, 34
intermetatarsal angle, 65
interphalangeal joint (IPJ), 66
intervertebral discs
   age-related changes, 270
   anatomy, 238, 278
   congenital deformities, 78
   discitis, 72, 238
   hemivertebrae, 74–75, 78
   herniated, 74
   nerve supply, 238
   prolapse, 72–74, 206–207, 269, 278
      cauda equina syndrome,
         210–212
      facet dislocation and, 142–143
   structure, 84
   surgical approach, 74–75,
      See also cervical spine;
      lumbar spine
intradural tumours, 71
intraosseous blood supply, 154
irritable hip (transient synovitis),
   181–183, 202

Jefferson fractures, 83
Johnson and Strom classification, 63
joint aspiration, 14
joint lubrication, 224–225
joint space, effective, 34
juvenile rheumatoid arthritis, 95

K-wires, 132, 194
Keller's arthroplasty, 67
Kellgren and Lawrance Radiographic
   Criteria, 57
keratin sulphate, 26
Kerboull necrotic angle, 29
Kienbock's disease, 153–155
Klein's line, 160
knee
   anatomical and mechanical axes, 225
   aneurysmal bone cyst, 107
   arthroscopy, 112
   dislocation, 204–205
   genu valgus (knocked knees), 186
   genu varum (bowed legs), 186
   idiopathic tibia vara (Blount's
      disease), 187–189
   MR arthrograms, 260
   osteoarthritis, 46–48, 215–217
   paediatrics, 159–163, 186–189
   painful, post-arthroplasty, 44–46,
      48–49
   SUFE, 159–163
   surgical approaches, 204–205, 216
   tumour, 209–210, 219–220,
      See also patella
knocked knees (genu valgus), 186
knot of Henry, 64
Kocher–Langenbeck approach, 136
Kocher's criteria, 182–183
Kocher's manoeuvre, 217

labrum, 180–181
Langenskiold's classification, 188–189
lateral collateral ligaments (LCL), 98
lateral cutaneous nerve, risks to,
   203
lateral parapatellar approach, 216
lateral pillar classification, 167–168
lateral ulnar collateral ligament
   (LUCL), 98, 99
Lauge Hansen classification, 205
leg length discrepancy (LLD), 40–42,
   183–186
Legg–Calvé–Perthes disease (LCPD).
   See Perthes disease
levels of evidence, 241–242
Levine and Edwards classification, 83
Lichtman classification, 153
ligaments
   ankle, 55–56
   basic science, 231–233

insertion to bone, 239
PIP joint, 272
spine, 85, *See also* individual
   ligaments
limbus, 180–181
lipomas, 100, 108–109
Lisfranc tarsometatarsal fracture
   dislocation, 114–115
loose bodies
   hip, 113–120
   shoulder, 126–127, *See also* wear
      particulate debris
lower limb(s)
   anatomy, 274, 279–280
   congenital defects, 183–185
   leg pain, 72–73, 210–212
   trauma, intro, 111
   tumours, 105–107, 209–210,
      See also knee; leg length
      discrepancy (LLD)
lumbar spine
   disc prolapse, 74, 210–212
   fractures, 81, 139–141
   Paget's disease, 36, 37
   spinal stenosis, 78,
      See also thoracolumbar spine
lunate bone, 153–155
lunotriquetal (LTL) ligament, 151
lymphoma, 71

M wave, 265
macrophages, 35
Maffucci's syndrome, 103, 150
magnetic resonance imaging (MRI)
   arthrograms, 260
   lumbar spinal stenosis, 78
   metal artifarct reduction (MARS),
      18–19
   metal wear, 230
   quantitative MRI, 261
   scanners, 259–261
   T1 or T2 images, 259–260
malignant transformation,
   enchondromas, 103
malignant tumours, 100
   femur, 105–107, 219–220
   flare phenomenon, 263
   hip, 17
   pelvis, 104
   spine, 69–71
mallet finger, 272
Maquet procedure, 54
marking. *See* structured oral exam,
   marking
materials
   biomechanical properties, 225–227,
      279
   fatigue–failure curve, 274
   scratch profile, 273, 279

materials (*cont.*)
  stress–strain curve, 274
matrix metalloproteinases (MMPs), 26
Matsen's traction–countertraction
    reduction, 217
Mayfield classification, 150
Meary's angle, 62
mechanical axis, knee joint, 225
medial collateral ligaments (MCL), 98,
    216
medial patella–femoral ligament
    (MPFL), 53
medializing calcaneal osteotomy, 64
median nerve, 237
meniscus, 271, 278
  basic science, 44, 234
  bucket handle tear, 44
mesenchymal stem cells (MSCs), 233
meta-analysis, 241–242, 246–251, 246
metacarpophalangeal (MCP) joints
  rheumatoid, 95–96, 157–158
  silastic replacements, 157–158
  UCL injury, 156–157
metal artifact reduction sequence
    (MARS), 18–19, 230
metal implants, scratch profile, 279
metal particulate debris, 18, 34, 54, 214
metal-on-metal (MOM) hip
  biomechanics, 230
  complications, 18
  jumbo head, 32
  outcomes, 19–20
metal-on-plastic prostheses, wear
    debris, 17, 223–224
metaphyseal–diaphyseal angle, 187–188
metaphyseal–epiphyseal angle, 187–188
metastatic disease, 100
  femur, 105, 108, 212–213
  hip, 17
  knee, 106–107
  spine, 69–71
metatarsal heads, 58–60
metatarsophalangeal (MTP) joint
  arthrodesis, 59, 65–67
  movement range, 66
methotrexate, perioperative, 158
Meyerding's grading system, 80–81
micro-elastohydrodynamic
    lubrication, 225
Miller's pyramid of assessment,
    11–10
Mitchell osteotomy, 65
Moberg dorsal closing wedge
    osteotomy, 67
mobile bearing prosthesis, 224
Monteggia fracture dislocation, 130
Mose classification, 168, 169
motor unit action potential
    (MUAP), 265

multiple hereditary exostoses, 102
muramyl-tripeptide (MTP), 107
muscle
  contraction types, 239
  skeletal, 268, 277
muscles, electromyography, 265–266
muscular dystrophy, 60
musculoskeletal system tissues,
    intro, 231
Musculoskeletal Tumour Society
    staging system, 101
myeloma, 71
Myerson classification, 63
myokimic discharges, on EMG, 265
myopathy, EMG findings, 266
myositis ossification, 94

nail (finger), anatomy, 272, 278
nail fixation, 229
navicular bone, 121–123
neoplasm, definition, 100
nerve cells, 267, 277
nerve conduction studies, 264–265
nerve fibres, 237
nerve grafts, 237
nerves, 237, 267, 277
  injuries, classification, 237
  internervous plane, 206
  risks in surgery, 201–205
neurogenic claudication, 78–79
neurogenic shock, 81–82, 144
neurological injury, spinal trauma,
    82–83
neuromuscular foot deformity, 60
neuromuscular scoliosis, 75, 77
neurovascular system, knee
    dislocation, 204–205
non-accidental injury (NAI), 196–198
non-ossifying fibroma, 103–104
non-parametric tests, 248
nuclear imaging, 17, 46
nucleus pulposus, 238
null hypothesis, 244–245

obesity, TKA issues, 224
obturator nerve, risks to, 201–202
occipital condyle fractures, 83
odds, data analysis, 249–250
odontoid peg fractures, 83, 145–146
Ogden classification, 194
olecranon, 129–130
Ollier's disease, 103, 150
Omega approach, 201–202
oncology, 100, 105
  lesion characteristics, 104
  MDT team, 103–104,
    See also malignant tumours;
    metastatic disease
open fractures, 129

open reduction with internal fixation
    (ORIF), 139, 152
operating theatres, infection
    control/prevention, 16
orthodromic potentials, 264
orthotic treatment
  ankle arthritis, 57
  cavus foot, 62
  flat foot, 63
  hallux rigidus, 66
  pes planus, 63
  rheumatoid foot, 59
Ortolani's test, 172
osteoarthritis (OA), 26
  classification, 24
  elbow, 94–98
  hip, 24–27, 213–215
  knee, 46–48
osteoblastic regulators, 34
osteoblastoma, 71
osteoblasts, 36, 39, 233
osteochondritis dissicans (OCD),
    94–95
osteochondromas, 71, 101–102
osteoclasts, 36, 38–39, 233
osteocytes, 233
osteogenesis imperfecta (OI),
    196–197
osteolysis
  implant loosening, 34–36
  Paget's disease, 38
  wear debris, 223–224
osteomyelitis, 72, 218–219, 221–222
osteonecrosis, 208–209
osteopenia, 236, 261
  peri-articular, elbow, 95–96
  talus fracture, 118
osteoporosis, 137–139, 236–237,
    252
osteoprotegerin (OPG), 34–35
osteosarcoma, 71, 101, 105–107
osteosynthesis, 146
osteotomy
  chevron, 129–130
  extended trochanteric (ETO),
    21, 24–29, 202
  femoral, 162
  hallux rigidus, 67
  hallux valgus, 65
  hip, 30, 38
  knee, 47–48
  medializing calcaneal, 63–64
  Moberg dorsal closing wedge, 67
  olecranon, 129–130
  radius, distal, 154–155
  shortening, metatarsal, 59
  subtrochanteric, 42, 162
  tibial, 46–48
outcome measures, 253–256

paediatrics, 159
  ankle, 218–219
  elbow, 99
  feet, 189–194
  femoral head blood supply, 164
  femur, 176, 183–185
  forearm fractures, 196–198
  halo vest, 148
  hand, 149–150
  hip, 159–186
    dislocated, 171–181, 183
    irritable hip, 181–183
    septic, 202–203
    subluxation, 181
  intervertebral discs, 72–73, 238
  juvenile RA, 95
  knees, 159–163, 186–189
  lower limbs, bowed legs, 186
  osteogenesis imperfecta (OI),
    196–197
  Perthes disease, 164–174
  physeal injury, 196
  scoliosis, 75, 77–78
  septic arthritis, 182–183
  spondylolisthesis, 81
  tumours
    benign, 101–104
    spinal, 70, 71
  wrist, ganglion, 152
Paget's disease, 36–37, 84
  hip, 36–39
  long bones, 36–37
  lumbar spine, 36–37
  protrusio acetabuli, 37
  radiographic features, 36–37
  skull, 37
Paley classification, 184–185
Paprosky classification, 22–29
parametric tests, 248
paramyxoviral infection, 37
parosteal osteosarcoma, 219–220
pars interarticularis, 81, 83
patella, 43–44, 50, 53–54
patella baja, 47–48
patellofemoral maltracking, 54
pathological fractures, 105, 212–213
patient reported outcome measures
    (PROMs), 253–255
Pavlick harness, 175–176, 179
pelvis
  fractures
    classification, 139
    multiple trauma, 135–136,
      139–141
    vertical shear, 136–137
  malignant tumours, 104
periarticular fractures, 259
peripheral neuropathy, 58–59
periprosthetic fracture, 220–222

periprosthetic infection
  hip (THA), 13–17, 21, 221–222
  imaging, 17, 46, 263–264
  knee (TKA), 44–46
periprosthetic osteolysis, 34–36
periprosthetic regions, effective joint
    space, 34
peroneal nerves, 44
  at risk, 47, 205
peroneal tendon, 56
peroneus brevis tendon, 56
Perthes' disease
  classification, 165–169
  differential diagnosis, 165
  grading, 169
  paediatrics, 164–174
  prognostic signs, 169
pes planus (flat foot), 62
Peterson classification, 194
physis (growth plate)
  anatomy, 271, 278
  basic science, 234–236
  fractures, classification, 194, 234
  injury, 196
  layers, 194
  zones, 234–235
pillar pain, 276
pilon fracture, 116–118, 139–140
pinning in situ (PIS), 161–163
Pirani score, 190–191
pivot–shift test, 99
plasticity, 226
plate fixation
  buttress, 135
  calcaneal, 116
  dynamic compression, 203–204
  fixed angle, 120–122
  humerus, 133–134
  tibial plateau fracture, 228
platelet-derived growth factor
    (PDGF), 34, 236
polyethylene, 35
  wear debris, 17, 223–224
Ponseti's serial casting, 190, 192,
    194
popliteal fossa, 204–205, 219–220
positive sharp waves, on EMG,
    265
positron emission tomography
    (PET), 262
posterior cord syndrome, 83, 144
posterior cruciate ligament (PCL),
    44, 49–52
posterior distal tibiofibular
    ligament, 55
posterior interosseous nerve (PIN)
    palsy, 95–96
posterior longitudinal ligament
    (PLL), 143

posterior malleolus (PM), 206
posterior tibiofibular ligament, 205
post-traumatic arthritis, 56–58
Powers' ratio, 83
pragmatic trial, 244
prevalence, epidemiology, 251–252
pro-inflammatory cytokines, 26
pronation external rotation injury, 206
PROSTALAC spacer, 16
prostheses
  constrained, 52
  mobile bearing, 224
  surface biomechanics, 230
  wear in, 33–36, See also individual
    prostheses
proteoglycans, 26, 234, 268, 277
protrusio acetabuli, 37
proximal focal femoral deficiency
    (PFFD), 183–185
proximal interphalangeal (PIP) joint
  Boutonniere deformity, 157, 272
  ligaments, 272, 278
pseudotumour, 18, 32
pubic rami, fractures, 136–137,
    140–141
pulley system, thumb, 271, 278
pulses, peripheral, 79

quantitative CT, 261
quantitative MRI, 261

radial head, dislocation, 95–96, 98–99,
    130
radial nerve, risks to, 203
radial styloid, 127–128, 153
radial tunnel syndrome, 93
radiation, 257–258
radiocarpal joint, 127–128
radiographs, 257–258
radiological classification
  Blount's disease, 188
  Kellgren and Lawrence, 57
  Perthes' disease, 165–167
  SUFE, 160
radiology, introduction, 257
radiotherapy, 71
radioulnar joint, 130–132
radius
  fractures, 130–132, 139–140,
    203–204, 275
  measurements, 276, 280
  physeal injury, 196
  wrist levelling procedures, 154–155
Randall Loder grading system, 160
random model effects, 247–248
receptor activator of nuclear factor-κ
    B ligand (RANKL), 34–35
recommendation, grades of, 241,
    245–246

recurrent laryngeal nerve, 207
references, literature, 4, 9–10
Reimer's migration index (RIM), 181
respiratory disorders, 96, 122
reverse-polarity shoulder
    replacement, 92
revision courses. *See* structured oral
    exam, courses
rheumatoid arthritis (RA)
    elbow, 95–96, 98
    foot, 58–60
    hands, 157–158
    juvenile, 95
    knee, 43
risks, data analysis, 249–250
Risser's sign, 76
rod fixation, 141
rotator cuff, 87–88, 91–92

sacrum, fractures, 84, 140–141
Salter and Thompson classification,
    167
Salter–Harris classification, 194, 234
sampling, clinical trial, 242–244
saphenous nerve, 51
sarcoma, 100
sarcomere, 277
scaphoid, 150–153
scaphoid non-union advanced
    collapse (SNAC) wrist, 153
scapholunate angle, 150
scapholunate ligament (SL), 151–152
scarf osteotomy, 65
sciatic nerve
    in hip dislocation, 118
    in THA, 21, 25–26
    risks to, 40–41, 201–202
scoliosis, 74–78
    late-onset, 76–77
    paediatrics, 75, 77–78
scratch profile, 273, 279
screening, programme features,
    252–253
screws
    cannulated, 125, 162–163
    osteosynthesis, 146
    questions, 273, 279
    tibial fractures, 112–113, 227–228
seat belt injuries, 147–148
Seddon classification, 237
Selenius curve, 186
sensitivity and specificity, 14, 46, 253
septic arthritis, paediatrics, 182–183
septic hip, 202–203
Seymour fracture, 272
shoulder, 86
    dislocation, 87–88, 217
    fracture dislocation, 126–127
    frozen shoulder, 88–89

imaging, 258, 260
infection in, 86–87
instability, arthroscopy, 218
rotator cuff, 87–88, 91–92
spaces and intervals, 269, 278
subacromial impingement,
    90–92
Sillence classification, 196–197
Singh and Maini index, 261–262
single heel raise test, 63
single photon emission tomography
    (SPECT), 262
skeletal survey, 198
skeletal traction, 137–138
skull, Paget's disease, 37
slipped upper femoral epiphysis
    (SUFE), 159–163
small cell carcinoma, metastases,
    212–213
Smith Peterson approach, 202–203
soft tissue, 231
    damage, 115–117, 205
    release, 181, 194
    seat belt injuries, 147–148
    swellings, 258
    THA approaches, 201
solitary plasmacytoma, 71
sonographic grading, 175
Southwick radiological grading, 160
specificity. *See* sensitivity and
    specificity
spica cast, 175–177
'spilled tea-cup' sign, 150
spina bifida, 60
spinal cord
    anatomy, 270, 278
    injury, 143–145
spinal dysraphism, 60, 76
spinal fusion, 85
spinal ligaments, 85
spinal muscular atrophy, 75
spinal shock, 82, 144
spinal stenosis, 270, 278
    cervical, 79–80
    lumbar, 78–79
spinal tumours, 69–71
spine, 69
    anatomy, 278
    ankylosing spondylitis, 85
    basic science, 238
    epidural abscess, 71–72
    facet dislocation, 148–143
    hip pain from, 21, 25
    Paget's disease, 84
    trauma, 81–84, 148, *See also* cervical
        spine; lumbar spine; scoliosis
spino pelvic stabilization, 140
spiral cords, 155–156
splints, 175–180

spondylolisthesis, 79–81, 146
Staphylococcus aureus infection,
    46, 72
statistics, data interpretation,
    246–251
Steel's blanch sign, 160
Steinberg *et al.* staging system, 29
stem cell therapy, 30–31
Stener lesion, 157
steroids
    AVN induced by, 28
    intra-articular, 57
    joint infection and, 87
    perioperative, 158
    spinal trauma and, 82
    subacromial bursa, 90
Stimson dislocation reduction, 217
STIR, MRI sequence, 260
stress and strain, 226, 232–233, 274,
    279
stress ulceration, 145
structured oral exam
    answering questions, 3–9
    courses, 3, 9
    format, 3
    marking system, 3, 5–6, 9–10
    preparation, 2–3
    purpose and value, 1–2
    references from literature, 4, 9–10
    revision for, 2–3
    topics, 2, 9
study power, 245
Stulberg classification, 169
subacromial impingement, 90–91
subaxial (C3–C7) fractures, 83–84
subscapularis tendon, 88
subtalar joint, 60
subtrochanteric fracture, 212–213
subtrochanteric osteotomy, 42
Sunderland classification, 237
superficial peroneal nerve, 206
superior gluteal nerve, risks to,
    201–203
supination external rotation (SER)
    injury, 205–206
supracondylar fracture, femur,
    121–123
supra-maximal stimulation, 264
surgical approaches
    ankle fracture, 205–206
    cervical spine, 206–207
    forearm fracture, 203–204
    hip
        septic drainage, 202–203
        THA, 25–26, 201–202
    knee, 49, 204–205
survival analysis, 251
swan neck deformity, 272
synovial carcinoma, 94

synovial chondromatosis, 95
synovial fluid, 44, 183, 224
synovial joints, 224–225
synovitis, 26
systematic review, 241–242,
    246–251

T1 or T2 images, in MRI, 259–260
talar tilt test, 55
talipes equinovarus (club foot), 60,
    189–192
    correction (mnemonic), 190
    scoring system, 191–192
talonavicular joint, 60, 193–194
talus
    defects, 56, 192–194
    fractures, 116–118
tantalum rod decompression,
    31–32
tarsometatarsal fracture dislocation,
    114–115
technetium bone scan, 262–264
tendenosis, 93
tendonitis, calcific, 90–91
tendons, 231–233
    insertion to bone, 239
    ultrasound, 258
    vasculature, 268, 277
tennis elbow, 92–93
tension band wire, 271, 278
tests
    outcomes, 253
    parametric vs non-parametric,
        248–249
thenar muscle, 276
thigh skin fold sign, 171–172
thigh, anatomy, 274, 279
Thompson's hemiarthroplasty, 13–14,
    17
thoracic spine
    disc prolapse, 73,
        See also thoracolumbar spine
thoracolumbar injury classification
    and severity score (TLICS),
    83
thoracolumbar spine
    fractures, 82, 144–145, 147–148
    trauma, 81, 83
thrombophilic theory, Perthes
    disease, 164
thumbs
    arthritis, 153–154, 158
    EPL tendon rupture, 149
    pulley system, 271, 278
    ulnar collateral ligament injury,
        156–157
tibia
    aneurysmal bone cyst, 107
    Blount's disease, 187–189

fractures, 111–113, 116–118,
    121–123, 139–140
in knee replacement, 216
osteomyelitis, 218–219
physeal injury, 196
tumours, 103–104, 209–210
tibial component (TKR), 54
tibial nerve, 205–206
tibial plateau, 111–113, 227–229
tibial tubercle (TT), 53–54
tibialis anterior tendon, 194
tibialis posterior tendon, 62–63
tibiofemoral angle, 187–188
time/distance/shielding (TDS), 258
toes. See hallux rigidus; hallux varus
Tokuhashi grading system, 69–70
total ankle replacement, 57–58
total elbow replacement (TER), 95–98
total hip arthroplasty (THA)
    cemented, 208–209, 229
    cemented vs uncemented, 38
    ceramic, 31, 32
    dislocation risk, 113–114
    femoral neck fracture, 113
    jumbo head, 32
    loosening, 20–24, 272
    MOM hip resurfacing compared, 20
    ORIF and, 139
    osteoarthritis, 25–26
    Paget's disease, 37–38
    painful, bone scan, 263–264
    periprosthetic fracture, 220–222
    prostheses compared, 229–230
    revision surgery, 21, 202, 214–215,
        221–222
    surgical approaches, 25–26,
        201–202
    survival rates, 214
    uncemented, 38, 229–230
    wear in, 33–36
    younger patient, 213–215,
        See also wear particulate debris
total joint replacement, toe, 67
total knee arthroplasty (TKA)
    anatomical and mechanical
        axes, 225
    constrained implants, 52
    HTO revision, 47–48
    infected, 44–46
    loosening, 51–53
    malalignment, 54
    osteolysis, 223–224
    painful, bone scan, 263–264
    procedure, 216–217
    revision surgery, 46, 51–53
    UKA compared, 48–49
    valgus knee, 43–44
    wear in, 36
trabeculae of femur, 261–262

traction–countertraction method,
    217
tranexamic acid (TXA), 246–251
transcaphoid perilunate
    fracture–dislocation, 150–151
transforming growth factors
    (TGFs), 236
transient synovitis (irritable hip),
    181–183, 202
trapdoor procedure, 30
trapeziectomy, 153
trauma, multiple injuries, 139–140
Trethowan's sign, 160
trimalleolar fracture, 205–206
trochanteric osteotomy, 21, 24, 202
T-score BMD, 236
tumour necrosis factor (TNF),
    34, 236
tumours, 100
    differential diagnosis, 218–219
    margins, 101
    pathology, 209–210
    PET in diagnosis, 262
    reactive zones, 101
    staging, 101, See also benign
        tumours; malignant tumours

ulna
    fracture, 130, 139–140, 203–204
    ulnar minus variant, 154–155
ulnar collateral ligament (UCL),
    156–157
ultra-high molecular weight
    polyethylene (UHMWPE),
    33–36
ultrasound, 172–175, 258
unicondylar knee arthroplasty (UKA),
    46–49

Vaccaro et al. classification, 83
valgus deformity
    hindfoot, 64
    knee, 43–44, 215–216
Van der Vleuten utility index
    formula, 11
varus deformity
    hindfoot, 60
    knee, 46–47
vascular claudication, 79
vascular system
    bone, 238
    knee dislocation, 204–205
    menisci, 44
vascularized fibular graft (VFG),
    29–30
vastus lateralis muscle, 43–44
VATER syndrome, 78
Vaughn–Jackson syndrome, 95–96
vertebral body, 71, 83

viral infection, in Paget's disease, 37
viscoelasticity, 274, 279
viscosity, 226
vitamin E, 35
viva voce, old style, 4
volar capsule, 127–128
volar plate, 272

Waldenstrom radiographic
        classification, 165–167
water
    in cartilage, 26
    in collagen, 234
Watson–Jones approach, 201–202

wear, 33, 224
wear particulate debris
    ceramic implants, 34
    metal, 34, 54, 214
        pseudotumour, 18, 32
    metal-on-plastic prostheses,
        17, 223–224
Weber classification, 205
websites, oral exam questions, 2
Weil osteotomy, 59
Wilson radiological grading, 160
Wiltze classification, 81
wrist
    arthritis, 153

diagrams and questions, 275
dislocation, 130–132
fracture, displaced, 127–128
fusion, 158
ganglion, 152
joint levelling procedure, 154–155
MR arthrograms, 260
pain, Kienbock's disease, 153–155
SNAC, 153, See also carpal tunnel

Xiapex® injections, 156
X-rays, 76, 257–258

Z-plasty, 156, 273, 279